NEONATAL NURSING

NEONATAL NURSING

Edited by

Doreen Crawford

RGN, RSCN, ENB 405, ENB 870, ENB 998

Senior Clinical Nurse

and

Maryke Morris

BSc(Hons), RGN, ENB 405

Senior Clinical Nurse

Neonatal Unit

Leicester Royal Infirmary

Leicester, UK

CHAPMAN & HALL

London · Glasgow · Weinheim · New York · Tokyo · Melbourne · Madras

Published by Chapman & Hall, 2–6 Boundary Row, London SE1 8HN, UK

Chapman & Hall, 2–6 Boundary Row, London SE1 8HN, UK

Blackie Academic & Professional, Wester Cleddens Road, Bishopbriggs, Glasgow G64 2NZ, UK

Chapman & Hall GmbH, Pappelallee 3, 69469 Weinheim, Germany

Chapman & Hall USA, One Penn Plaza, 41st Floor, New York NY 10119, USA

Chapman & Hall Japan, ITP-Japan, Kyowa Building, 3F, 2-2-1 Hirakawacho, Chiyoda-ku, Tokyo 102, Japan

Chapman & Hall Australia, Thomas Nelson Australia, 102 Dodds Street, South Melbourne, Victoria 3205, Australia

Chapman & Hall India, R. Seshadri, 32 Second Main Road, CIT East, Madras 600 035, India

Distributed in the USA and Canada by Singular Publishing Group Inc., 4284 41st Street, San Diego, California 92105

First edition 1994

Typeset in 10/12pt Palatino by Mews Photosetting, Beckenham, Kent
Printed in Great Britain by St Edmundsbury Press, Bury St Edmunds

ISBN 0 412 48730 6 1 56593 290 0 (USA)

A catalogue record for this book is available from the British Library

Library of Congress Catalog Card Number:

Printed on permanent acid-free text paper, manufactured in accordance with ANSI/NISO Z39.48–1992 and ANSI/NISO Z39.48–1984 (Permanence of Paper).

Charles-Michel Billard (1800–1832) stated that:

> *During uterine life man can suffer from many afflictions ... the consequences of which are brought with him into this world ... children may be born healthy, sick, convalescent, or entirely recovered from former disease.*

This amazing perception from a neonatal pioneer still applies today.

Contents

Contributors

Ms Gosia Brykczńska
RCN Institute of Advanced Nursing Education
20 Cavendish Square
London, UK
W1M 0AB

Mr Ian Costello
Pharmacy Department
St George's Hospital
Blackshaw Road
Tooting
London, UK
SW17

Mrs Doreen Crawford
Neonatal Nursing Unit
Leicester Royal Infirmary
Leicester, UK
LE1 5WW

Mrs Ann Dooley and Mr Daniel Dooley
Paediatric High Dependency Unit
Leicester Public Health Laboratory
Leicester Royal Infirmary
Leicester, UK
LE1 5WW

Mrs Helen Gardiner
Freelance Nutritionist
Formerly Company Nutritionist
Scientific Department of Milupa Limited
Milupa House
Uxbridge Rd
Hillingdon
Middlesex, UK
UB10 0NE

Mrs Claire Thomson Greig
Dalgety Bay
Fife, UK

Ms Emily Logan
Ward 5C
Hospitals for Sick Children
Great Ormond Street
London, UK
WC1N 3JH

Ms Christine Midgley
Course Director of Pre-Registration Midwifery
Birmingham and Solihull College of Nursing and Midwifery
Midwifery Education Centre
Good Hope Hospital
Rectory Road
Sutton Coldfield
Birmingham, UK
B75 7RR

Miss Maryke Morris
Neonatal Unit
Leicester Royal Infirmary
Leicester, UK
LE1 5WW

Ms Kathy Sleath
Hammersmith Hospital
Du Cane Road
London, UK
W12

Miss Margaret Sparshott
Tamerton
Plymouth
Devon, UK

Mrs Marjorie Tew
Wollaton
Nottingham, UK

Mrs Marie-Claire Turrall
Therwil
Switzerland

About the authors

Gosia Brykczyńska BA, BSc, Cert Ed, RGN, RSCN, RNT ENB 273 is currently a lecturer in ethics and philosophy at the Institute of Advanced Nursing Education, Royal College of Nursing. She is a humanities graduate who has specialized in paediatric nursing. She has written numerous articles and chapters and edited several books, including a book on health care ethics. She is the nurse representative on the British Paediatric Association Ethics Advisory Committee, and is a member of the RCN Ethics Committee. She is currently enrolled as an MPhil/PhD candidate.

Ian Costello BPharm (Hons), MSc, MRPharmS is Senior Pharmacist (Neonatal and Paediatric Services) at St. George's Hospital in Tooting, London, a post he has held for the past year. His research interests include parenteral nutrition, pharmacokinetics and therapeutic drug monitoring in neonates.

Doreen Crawford RGN, RSCN, ENB 405, ENB 870 is currently a Senior Clinical Nurse on the Neonatal Unit at the Leicester Royal Infirmary, where she has worked for the last 5 years. She is also doing a BSc (Hons) degree at King's College, University of London. Doreen is a member of the Association of British Paediatric Nurses, Society of Paediatric Nurses and a member of the Neonatal Nurses Association. Her special interests include teaching neonatal nursing care, the enhancement and promotion of neonatal nursing by writing for various nursing publications, and undertaking speaking engagements. She is currently doing research into the benefits of teaching resuscitation skills to the parents of new babies.

Ann Dooley RGN, ENG 405 is currently undertaking postregistration RSCN training in Leicester. She has previously worked as a Staff Nurse in both the Neonatal Unit and the Paediatric High Dependency Unit at the Leicester Royal Infirmary. She has a special interest in the implementation of family-centred care.

Daniel Dooley, BSc (Hons), State Registered Medical Laboratory Scientific Officer is a microbiologist currently working for the Public Health Laboratory Service at the Leicester Royal Infirmary. He has a special interest in foodborne infection, particularly when caused by *Listeria monocytogenes*. He is undertaking postgraduate study leading to an MSc in biomedical sciences.

Helen Gardiner BSc(Hons) SRD is a freelance nutritionist. She was previously the Company Nutritionist in the Scientific Department of Milupa Limited.

Claire Thomson Greig RGN, SCM, Neonatal Certificate, ADM, BN, MSc (Nursing Education) has wide clinical experience of neonatal nursing in Scotland and Canada. She is currently a midwifery teacher in Lothian College of Health, where she coordinates Professional Studies II modules in Neonatal Care. Claire is a member of the Royal College of Midwives and the Neonatal Nurses Association. She is also the educational representative for the Scottish Neonatal Nurses Group.

Emily Logan RSCN, RGN, ENB 136 has been Sister on the Paediatric Nephrology Unit at Great Ormond Street Hospital for the past 3 years. She is presently undertaking an MSc in Health Psychology.

Christine Midgley, MEd, RGN, RM, MTD is the Course Director for Pre-Registration Midwifery education at the Birmingham and Solihull College of Nursing and Midwifery. Christine has occupied this post since its inception in August 1990. Previously she worked as a midwife teacher at the Leicester Royal Infirmary, where she was responsible for the ENB 405 Course. An interest in frameworks for nursing and midwifery stems from studying for her bachelor's degree.

Maryke Morris BSc(Hons), RGN, ENG 405 was a Senior Clinical Nurse on the Neonatal Unit at the Leicester Royal Infirmary, where she has worked for 4 years since graduating from the University of Surrey. Maryke is a member of the University of Surrey Nurses' Association and a member of the Neonatal Nurses Association. Her special interests include teaching and research into the extended role of the neonatal nurse.

Kathy Sleath RSCN, ENB 402 is currently Senior Nurse Specialist on the Neonatal Unit at Hammersmith Hospital, London. Kathy was an award winner in the *Nursing Times*/3M competition for innovative and pioneering work with oxygen-dependent infants. Kathy currently holds a joint post involving both her interests, in research and clinical practice.

Margaret Sparshott RGN, RM, ENB 405 is a Senior Staff Nurse on the Neonatal Intensive Care Unit at Derriford Hospital, Plymouth where she has worked since 1986. Her previous experience in Neonatal Nursing includes 6 years on the Premature Baby Unit at the Aghia Sophia Children's Hospital in Athens and 6 years on the Neonatal Unit at the Cantonal University Hospital in Geneva. She is a member of the Neonatal Nurses Association and is particularly interested in the environmental problems of the newborn, writing and lecturing on the subject.

Marjorie Tew MA is a Research Statistician at Nottingham Medical School. When Marjorie became a statistician to medical research she observed that the available statistics, when analysed, did not support the widely held theory that the great decrease in maternal and infant mortality after 1950 was caused by the great increase in hospitalization and obstetric management of childbirth. The findings of her wider and deeper researches confirmed her early conclusions and, despite strong opposition from the obstetric profession and its supporters, she succeeded in having these reported in many articles in medical journals or as chapters in books. In 1990 her book *Safer Childbirth? A Critical History of Maternity Care* was published. Its importance was acknowledged in the House of Commons Health Committee's report in 1992 of the findings of its

Inquiry into the Maternity Service. She is a member of the steering committee of the Royal Society of Medicine's Forum on Maternity and the Newborn.

Marie-Claire Turrall RGN, RSCN, ENB 405, Diploma Professional Studies in Nursing qualified in 1985 and has held a number of posts caring for children and infants in theatres, intensive care and cardiology wards. Most recently she worked as a Senior Clinical Nurse on the Neonatal Unit at Leicester Royal Infirmary. Marie-Claire currently resides in Switzerland and is actively involved in the local childbirth trust, counselling mothers with breastfeeding problems and helping those who have children in neonatal intensive care.

Preface

There are many books on the care of the sick infant and some are excellent. Most, however, are written with medicine in mind. This book is written mainly by experienced neonatal nurses, although some chapters have been written by the appropriate specialists. It is intended primarily for nurses who look after sick infants and is not intended to be an exhaustive reference but to address some of the issues and concepts of neonatal care in the 1990s. Nursing models are an important part of neonatal care in the 1990s but this book has not been written within this framework. There are several reasons for this: arguably no current model is ideally suited to neonates and the favouring of one particular model might restrict the book's applicability. Also, as contributors from other disciplines were invited to contribute we were anxious that these chapters did not stand out as oddities. Additionally, much neonatal care overlaps and were a framework to be used in its entirety for each nursing care chapter we felt that there could be some repetition; conversely, if a framework was fragmented in some chapters to cover specific areas of care, we were concerned that the overall effect would have been 'bitty'. We felt that such treatment of nursing models would have been unjustifiable.

In this book, the terms 'infant' and 'baby' are used interchangeably and where the term 'he' is used, the term 'she' is equally appropriate. The term 'neonatal nurse' applies to any person who is professionally involved in the nursing care of a sick baby, be he or she a nurse, midwife or student.

As long ago as 1907, Pierre Buddin, one of the founders of the art and science which we now call neonatology, wrote that 'the lives of the little ones have been saved but at the cost of the mother's'. Today nurses and doctors are partners, with the parents, in the care of the sick infant.

We have moved forward, away from the fairground exhibition of tiny and premature babies to the curious. It is not that the fascination for the small no longer exists, nor that we are reticent to display the hi-tech environment in which we work; nor even that these babies are so vulnerable that a passing stranger is a fearsome infection risk. The reason for our low profile is that these babies, like any other sick human beings, are entitled to privacy, peace and dignity in which to either recover or to die.

We wish to express our thanks and gratitude to family and friends who tolerated the stress and strain of writing this book and never gave up hope.

ACKNOWLEDGEMENTS

Maryke Morris and Doreen Crawford wish to acknowledge Karen Allyene, Play Specialist, for her advice on the developmental needs of a baby in a neonatal unit; Dennis Crawford for his computer skills, patience during indexing and for printing all the numerous drafts; Mr and Mrs Hayes for their personal account as parents of baby Joshua who was resident on the NNU; Margaret Sparshott for allowing us to use her drawing for the front cover.

1

Neonatal care today

Maryke Morris

There are many facets to the care of sick babies. This chapter provides a holistic overview of neonatal care today.

The care of sick or high-risk newborn babies takes place in a variety of settings. These range from the highly sophisticated and technologically advanced neonatal units for the acutely and critically ill to the special care baby unit, where the infant who requires additional care or monitoring to that available in the transitional care ward can be nursed alongside his mother. The criteria that differentiate each type of unit are defined by the British Paediatric Association but often, practically speaking, the differences lie only in the name, the sickness of the inhabitant and the number of staff on each shift.

With advances in life support and biochemical assessment, the lives of even smaller babies and those at the extremes of prematurity can be saved, but often not without cost in long-term hospitalization or follow-up care. Neonatal medicine is now advancing to the stage that some operations can be performed on the fetus, where the uterus can provide natural intensive care for the patient. The neonatal nurse's work, in these situations, begins before birth.

THE NEONATAL ENVIRONMENT

Anyone entering a neonatal unit (NNU) for the first time will be struck by the sight of a tiny baby in an incubator surrounded by all the machinery, wires, tubes and other paraphernalia. The NNU environment, like any critical care setting, has an emphasis on technical and continuous monitoring which may create barriers to humane care (Rushton, 1991). This involves some of the most technically advanced respiratory support systems, computerized and digital monitors, electrical pumps and incubators. Each has a fascinating display of figures, current status trends and audible/visible alarm signals. At times nurses act more like engineers (Catlett and Holditch-Davies, 1991) as they set up and operate the vast range of equipment.

The noise from such machinery, along with the lighting necessary for full visualization of the unstable baby, creates a very stressful environment to which the acutely ill newborn child is very vulnerable. This often creates adverse reactions in heart rate, oxygen saturations, blood pressure, sleep deprivation and increasing aggravation (Sparshott, 1989 and Chapter 14). The sick baby is unable to segregate the amount of environmental disturbance received. The nurse needs to remember to provide the restful and healing surroundings that are essential for recovery and development.

The neonatal nurse is caught at a 'crossroads of humanity and technology' (McHaiffe, 1987); she is caring for a baby in an environment that is far removed from the image that the parents had of their new baby sleeping contentedly in a crib.

A conducive environment

A bright, friendly-looking unit facilitates parent and child interaction (Rivers *et al.*, 1982) and the baby's level of responsiveness is increased when excessive and repetitive stimuli are reduced. A homely atmosphere, with appropriate pictures, mobiles and patterned drapes and linen gives a welcoming impression to parents and the absence of the 'goldfish bowl' of viewing corridors means that visitors must approach the baby, thus creating a more natural environment and helping to convince the family that they have a useful and constructive role to play (Thornes, 1985).

Many units are organized so that babies of similar dependency are nursed together, i.e. an intensive care area and special care nurseries. Slade (1988) found this layout to have a beneficial effect on parents as they translated the improvements into physical terms and were able to talk with other parents in similar situations. A low-dependency area, with a relaxed and supportive atmosphere, is conducive to learning essential parenting skills.

Provisions for parents

Facilities for parents in terms of sitting rooms, kitchen and bedrooms are important, as they allow the family to take a break from the stressful environment surrounding the baby. A bedroom can be a refuge for parents to have time alone and adjust to having a baby, reducing their reliance and dependence on the nursing staff. The privacy that a bedroom offers can help promote and maintain breastfeeding and the acquisition of parenting skills.

ADMISSION TO THE NEONATAL UNIT

If it is known in advance of the birth that a baby will need admitting to the unit, arrangements should be made for the parents to visit and familiarize themselves with some of the sights and sounds. By introducing them to the world of the sick baby, some of the myths and fears surrounding a neonatal unit may be alleviated.

Before the baby is taken to the unit, he should be given (or shown) to the mother and father. This first glimpse can be very rewarding and the father may want to accompany the baby, seeing for himself that the baby is settled in, so that he can then help to reassure the mother (Redshaw, Rivers and Rosenblatt, 1985). Involving the family from the start reinforces the understanding that the baby belongs to them and not to the hospital (Barnes, 1985).

A photograph, given to the mother (and one for the father if possible), will help to fill the void of a missing baby (Slade, 1988) and provide a focus for discussion (Redshaw, Rivers and Rosenblatt, 1985).

Transferring the baby to another hospital

If the baby has to be moved to another hospital, transferring the mother as well maintains the integrity of the mother–baby bond, benefitting them both and enabling the mother to participate in the baby's care (Warwick, 1983). Chapter 4 discusses the nursing care involved when a sick baby has to be transferred to another hospital.

RESPONSE TO HAVING A SPECIAL CARE BABY

Admitting the baby to the neonatal unit prevents the early contact of parent and child so that, instead of the parents providing warmth, food and love, the baby is removed into a strange environment. This leaves the parents feeling helpless and stripped of responsibility (Rivers *et al.*, 1982). These parents need care, not as patients but as individuals with parental responsibilities (Rivers *et al.*, 1982). Time must be given for parents to air their own views, opinions and feelings regarding having a baby admitted to a neonatal unit. This has been likened to the grieving process, described by Kübler-Ross (1969), which the family have to work through and resolve if they are to accept the reality of the baby and experience feelings of attachment. Parents also need to be kept informed about their baby's condition and any investigations performed, as well as the equipment used.

One family's experience

The following statements are the personal accounts of a mother and father whose baby was born preterm and had a prolonged stay on a neonatal unit.

The mother's reaction

'I knew at 25 weeks' gestation that my baby would have to be delivered at 30 weeks. While I waited, I decided to familiarize myself with the Neonatal Unit. There was so much machinery: endless bleeping monitors, wires, tubes and such tiny babies . . . ! Well, at least I knew what I was facing and I felt sure that, after a couple of months, all this technology would be behind me and life would get back to normal; how ill prepared I was!

My baby was born by caesarean section and I remember someone saying 'You have a lovely baby boy' but all I had were two photographs of him. Two days later, I first saw my baby; he had tubes coming out of his mouth, pads shielding his eyes from the ultraviolet light, so there was very little to see. As I stared into the plastic box, I felt cheated of my motherhood. I could not touch him, cuddle or feed him, there was a void between us with no mother love; just a terrible fear: a fear that he would not make it. The baby was so tiny and I did not want to get too close to him in case he died.

As the weeks went by, the baby seemed to get one infection after another, drips were sited in both hands, feet and even in his head; there appeared to be no end to it. He would really look well one day, then the next day he would be at death's door. During these harrowing months, my husband and I both lived on our nerves, jumping every time the phone rang, in case it was the hospital with bad news. We would ring the unit every day to enquire about the baby but I would make any excuse to avoid being the one to phone, because I did not want to be the one to hear any bad news.

During one appointment with the consultant, I remember him saying 'We are not out of the woods yet, a cold at this stage could kill him'. I felt shattered, I had heard nothing else all along and could not cope any more. But, when it is your baby, you have no choice, you go on from day to day.

When he started picking up, progress was slow but the frequency of setbacks diminished. One day, the phone rang to tell us he was in the nursery, out of intensive care! The family could not wait to see him that night and soon I could have my first cuddle without all the monitors on. His stay in the nursery was short, another infection meant a return to intensive care.

Our baby's yo-yo health was going nowhere and a negative-pressure box was brought on to the scene. This was his last chance at a kick-start, and it worked! He started putting on weight and before long he was back in the nursery. This time he was much bigger and looked a lot better, even his face had filled out. I learnt how to take him out of the box myself and I was able to change and feed him. I started to count the hours till I could be with him.

Even now, we still have our moments. For example, when he was due to have his vaccinations, I felt he was not well enough and it took a talk with the consultant to postpone them for a week. The support I have had from the nursing staff, especially in the difficult days, has earned my deepest gratitude and praise.

I have cried more tears over this baby than I have in the rest of my life but one thing is for sure, I love my son desperately and when they tell me he can come home, what a celebration we will have!'

The father's reaction

'Minutes after my son was born, the nurses called me into the small room next to the theatre to have my first look at him; wonderful!! I was then able to concentrate on what was happening to my wife. A little later, a nurse brought a photograph of the baby to be put at my wife's bedside.

During the afternoon I visited the neonatal unit and met the nurse who was looking after the baby. He was very straightforward and a good communicator who conveyed a feeling of optimism. Most things were explained to me, the ventilator, incubator and all the monitoring systems; the only thing that really bothered me was the fact that the baby had to be paralysed. At this stage, I do not think that we realized just how ill our baby was; perhaps just as well considering that my wife was also very ill.

The things that disturbed us most were the changes in treatment which had not been explained to us. For instance, during a phone call to the unit, my wife was told 'he's fine, he's just had a blood transfusion'!! No explanation for the transfusion was given. My wife never rang again. Another time, when he was on low-flow oxygen by nasal prongs, we arrived to find him back in a headbox and receiving more oxygen; nobody seemed able to tell us why except that it had happened during the night. X-rays were done without explanation and the results were not forthcoming.

The positive side was that the staff were very friendly, informative and admirably dedicated. As his condition improved, some nurses even took the trouble to phone us at home when he came off the ventilator, when he moved into the nursery and when he started to breathe air. When we had to refer to the doctors or consultants, our wishes were always followed.

The only criticism I have concern the different personalities, a cheerful person and a more sober person will supply the same information in different ways. It sounds better to be told 'He'll only be in the box for six or seven weeks' rather than 'He'll be in the box for at least six or seven weeks'. There is no way to overcome this except for the nurse to remember to phrase sentences as optimistically as possible.

As parents we needed to be given as much information as possible and like to know the reasons behind the investigations and care given. Unknown actions and the ignorance it causes create fear and apprehension.'

Visiting

Open unrestricted visiting allows the family to decide who can visit and when, maintaining the family unit (McGovern, 1984). Liberal visiting increases contact with the baby at the same time as keeping some sort of order to the family's life.

CARING AS A NEONATAL NURSE

Neonatal nursing encompasses all the skills and abilities that are acquired during training and practice. Additional emphasis on the psychosocial aspects of caring are necessary when nursing the sick baby and his family.

To be able to care, one must know the baby's and the family's needs and, by understanding them, respond appropriately, thus helping the family to 'grow' (Mayeroff, 1971). Patience and trust are necessary in this relationship for the family to develop and learn (sometimes through their mistakes) (Mayeroff, 1971). The nurse must be honest with the family (Mayeroff, 1971; Goodley, 1986). Presenting all the facts in an open and as positive a manner as possible can give hope and courage. Courage is essential with the very sick baby as a 'trip into the unknown' (Mayeroff, 1971) is taken with no guarantee of the outcome.

Parents and nurses use their past experiences and knowledge in caring for a sick baby. They have to be ready and willing to learn from each other, without feeling embarrassed by what is unknown. The neonatal nurse can have no pretentious claim in her care: McGovern (1984) noted that mums and dads give the best special care.

Caring gives meaning to life and enables someone to find their place in the world (Mayeroff, 1971). By this, it is understood that caring becomes the centre of activities, values and experiences, harmonizing one with another. This is visible in the parent, caring for a baby who canot be independent and responsible for his own needs and interests, which must be understood by those in charge (Sparshott, 1990). To do this, the parents have to understand the baby and interpret the world as if seen through the baby's eyes (Mayeroff, 1971).

FAMILY-CENTRED CARE

The origins

The original special care baby units excluded the family and other visitors because of the risk of cross-infection. With the acceptance of the work of Klaus and Kennel, who studied the effects of mother–child separation in the newborn period, visiting was then encouraged and from this evolved parental participation, which gradually developed into family-centred care as the benefits shown outgrew the perceived risks (McGovern, 1984). The involvement of the family has become part of the philosophy of many units.

Who is the family?

There are many views and opinions as to who and what constitutes a family, and all have to be respected in a heterogenous society (Cox, 1983), especially as many units cover a wide cross-section of society.

The family can be defined physically as being either a nuclear family consisting of parent(s) and children, as is common in modern western society, or an extended family unit, including grandparents and other relatives (Moore and Hendry, 1982). In today's society the family can be any mixture of these: there does not always have to be a relationship through marriage or birth. Wilson (cited by Moore and Hendry, 1982) considered the family to be no more than a 'specialist agency of affection', which can and does benefit its members to meet their physical and emotional needs. Anderson (1971) looked at the extended family as a surrogate welfare and mutual aid network, with support being gained from everyone, so to some extent everyone is involved in the care of the baby. Any of these relatives may need to be included in the care of a baby in an NNU.

Assessing the needs of the family

The nurse must get to know the family members and social circumstances, accepting all and every variation, so that personal and familial needs can be understood (Goodley, 1986). The nurse can then direct her care appropriately, enabling the parents to gain skills and become competent and thus evolves the partnership between the parents and the nurse (Stewart, 1990). This exemplifies family-centred care and is highlighted by Sparshott (1990): since the long term well-being of the infant is also dependent on the relationship with the parents, their role as care givers is fundamental from the beginning, even in the case of the ill or preterm baby'.

First-time parents have to redefine their roles so as to be able to identify themselves as parents, caring for and bonding with the newborn (Baker, Kuhlman and Magliaro, 1989).

Parental participation

The best care for the infant is provided when parents and nurses become partners. The extent of family intervention in either giving or receiving care, depends on the skills and knowledge of the individual family members (Barnes, 1985).

Involving the parents and family as much as possible can easily be achieved on the NNU. The parents then begin to take care of their infant, facilitating interaction and, ultimately, bonding. The family can perform many of the care activities (Goodley, 1986), provided that they are taught how to perform the task correctly.

SOME ASPECTS OF NURSING THAT ENHANCE FAMILY-CENTRED CARE

Communication

Goodley (1986) realized that in discussions with the family, the nurse must be honest about the baby's condition. This information may need to be reiterated many times, with leaflets and handbooks given to reinforce verbal explanations (Goodley, 1986). The nurse, parents and family should represent the baby's best interests.

A communication chart can be used to record the type and amount of contact that the family is having with the baby (or it can be written in the nursing process). Thornes (1985) noted that parental participation did not develop as quickly as it should because of the inconsistencies in staff attitudes to parental involvement and the nurses' adeptness in carrying out procedures.

Nurse allocation

Reducing the number of staff who have contact with the baby, as occurs with team, primary or key nursing, enhances the establishment of a trusting relationship between the parents and the nurse. Whichever method of organizing nursing care is employed, the baby should have an identified named nurse available to answer any questions, worries or problems that might arise when the parents begin caring for their child (McGovern, 1984), and to provide ongoing and realistic communication (Baker, Kuhlman and Magliaro, 1989).

Feeding the baby

Feeding the baby is seen as the ultimate expression of care and love (Stewart, 1990). Teaching parents to tube feed, as well as helping to establish breast or bottle feeding, helps the parents to relate to their baby.

Touching and handling the baby

Encouraging the family to touch and handle the tiny baby, and even cuddling a ventilated baby, helps to break down some of the physical and psychological barriers (Rivers *et al.*, 1982). If the baby is too sick to tolerate a cuddle then the parents can touch him through the incubator portholes. They can master nappy changes around the various tubes and wires and the baby soon becomes more responsive and rewarding, thus promoting bonding and strengthening the relationship between the baby and the family (Goodley, 1986). The less sick or growing preterm baby can be dressed, which is of considerable importance to the parents as their infant looks much more normal (Holt, 1987).

Reducing pain and discomfort

The family have a special part to play in reducing the trauma surrounding some procedures by distracting the baby and soothing him afterwards (Redshaw, Rivers and Rosenblatt, 1985), as well as identifying their baby's likes and dislikes. Including the family in planning and giving care helps them to assume their normal responsibilities and eliminates their feelings that the nurse is in charge of their infant's welfare (McHaiffe, 1987).

Play and stimulation

All members of the family can be involved in stimulating and playing with the baby, using toys, mobiles or pictures. Cuddling and talking to the baby is important. The sick or preterm baby requires stimulation, just like a well full-term baby, to maximize development and reactions to the environment, thus promoting normal baby behaviours.

CARING FOR THE DYING BABY

In the sad instance where all the technology and the best care available are unable to save the baby, then he has the right to die peacefully and naturally, in the presence of those who love him (Sparshott, 1990). The full range of intensive care should be continued until the parental consent to discontinue therapy has been given. This can be a frustrating time as the infant, in his hopeless condition, still needs intensive nursing. If other cases are transferred or refused admission owing to shortage of beds, then there is guilt and pressure added to grief. Even so, no pressure should be put on parents to agree to the withdrawal of support. This short time is all that they will have with their child and they need to make the most of it.

The family of a dying baby should be able to share the last few moments of their baby's life in privacy and comfort (preferably in a family room or quiet room). Removing the child from intensive care and letting the family cuddle and get to know him provides a tangible memory (Baker, Kuhlman and Magliaro, 1989). This can be supported by photographs and baby items. Some parents may like to have a verse placed in a Book of Remembrance. The parents' wishes are paramount and should be respected along with any ceremonies and protocols that a family with a different culture or religion from one's own may wish to follow. The family can then begin to grieve the baby they have lost.

STRESS AND THE NEONATAL UNIT

All the care in the world cannot mitigate the stress that is encountered when a baby is admitted to a neonatal unit. Nursing and medical staff are not immune to these stresses, and neither are grandparents, siblings and other people close to the family.

Stress and the neonatal nurse

A neonatal nurse has many commitments which demand her involvement, time and energy. These are not only physical, but also mentally and emotionally draining. The nurse supports and interacts with the family and other members of the multidisciplinary team. She also has to address her own feelings regarding the decisions that are made in the care of a very ill or dying baby, and employ defence mechanisms to enable her to cope (Vas Dias, 1987). The unit as a whole has to be supportive of the individual members, as decisions concerning life, death and morbidity are regular occurrences (Wittenberg, 1990; Proctor, 1990). Burn-out is a well recognized phenomenon.

Reducing staff stress

To reduce the likelihood of burnout, time should be allowed for group discussions about the dilemmas and strains of the unit. Being appreciated as a valuble member of the nursing team increases self-esteem and confidence. It is not incompatible with good nursing care to admit to feelings of stress (stress may also be identified by others), so that the causes can be identified and help offered. The remedy may involve taking time out from the tense situation to regain composure, or talking with another member of staff or a clinical psychologist.

Causes of parental stress

The early birth of a baby or an unplanned admission to a neonatal unit presents a crisis for the parents (Gorski, 1984) for which they were psychologically and socially unprepared. These parents have their total responsiblity for physically caring for the baby removed, and may have a poor perception of being parents. Negative feelings of aggression, anxiety, guilt, shock, fear and confusion surround the situation (McGovern, 1984).

Nursing away parental stress

The neonatal nurse needs to be aware of how the family are coping with their sick baby and respond appropriately. This may mean letting the parents talk about their worries. Problems unrelated to the baby are just as important and can play a role in preventing the parents from adapting to the situation. By identifying and resolving any anxiety or distress in the parents, the nurse and multidisciplinary team can help to remove any inhibitions to the parents' ability to visit and form a relationship with their baby (Bass, 1991).

Actively involving the parents in the care and decision making reinstates the parental responsibilities. Communicating in a positive and empathetic manner (even when the news may not be good), using easily understandable sentences, is more useful to the parents (Bass, 1991) than confusing statements full of jargon.

Support for the parents

Parents may gain support from each other, members of the family, friends, other parents on the unit, religious ministers and health care professionals, notably the nurse who has most contact with their child (McHaiffe, 1989). This nurse represents a familiar face, who is kind to the baby and provides a non-judgmental listening ear. This helps the parents to feel more relaxed and trusting of the caregiver (McHaiffe, 1989).

A family psychotherapist, working in conjunction with the neonatal staff, can explore problem areas in individual, family or group meetings, allowing parents to voice feelings and fears. Identifying anxieties is the first step towards understanding and resolution.

Parent support groups, organized either by nursing staff or the parents themselves, encourages mutual support, reassurance and understanding from people who know what it is like to have a baby on the NNU.

REFERENCES

Anderson, M. (1971) *Sociology for the Family*, Penguin, England.

Baker, K., Kuhlman, T. and Magliaro, B.L. (1989) Homeward bound. *Nursing Clinics of North America* **24**(3), 655–64.

Barnes, A. (1985) The continuity of care in the family. *Nursing* **2**(36), 1051–4.

Bass, L.S. (1991) What do parents need when their infant is a patient in the NICU? *Neonatal Network* **10**(4), 2–33.

Catlett, A.T. and Holditch-Davies, D. (1991) Environmental stimulation of the acutely ill preterm infant: physiological effects and nursing implications. *Neonatal Network* **8**(6), 19–26.

Cox, C. (1983) *Sociology: An Introduction for Nurses, Midwives and Health Visitors*, Butterworths, London.

Goodley, S. (1986) Family care and the preterm baby. *Midwives' Chronicle* **99**(1176), 8–10.

Gorski, P.A. (1984) Experience following premature birth: stresses and opportunities for infants, parents and professionals, in *Frontiers of Infant Psychiatry*, Vol 2, (eds J.D. Call, E. Galenson and R.L. Tyson), Basic Books, New York.

Holt, M. (1987) A special care baby. *Nursing Times* **83**(36), 56–8.
Kübler-Ross, E. (1969) *On Death and Dying*, MacMillan, New York.
McGovern, M. (1984) Caring for special babies 2: Separation of the baby from the family. *Nursing Times* **80**(4), 28–30.
McHaiffe, H.E. (1987) Isolated but not alone. *Nursing Times* **83**(28), 73–4.
McHaiffe, H.E. (1989) Mothers of very low birthweight babies: who supports them? *Midwifery* **5**(3), 113–21.
Mayeroff, M. (1971) *On Caring*, Harper and Row, New York.
Moore, S. and Hendry, B. (1982) *Teach Yourself Sociology*, Hodder and Stoughton, England.
Proctor, J. (1990) Experience of 'burnout' in the special care baby unit. *Midwives' Chronicle* **103**(1232), 266–8.
Redshaw, M.E., Rivers, R.P.A. and Rosenblatt, D.B. (1985) *Born Too Early*, Oxford University Press, Oxford.
Rivers, R.P.A. *et al.* (1982) Problems of parents with a baby in SCBU. *Midwife, Health Visitor and Community Nurse* **18**(5), 170–5.
Rushton, C.H. (1991) Humanism in critical care: a blueprint for change. *Pediatric Nursing* **17**(4), 399–402.
Slade, P. (1988) A psychologist's view of a special care baby unit. *Maternal and Child Health* **13**(8), 208–12.
Sparshott, M.M. (1989) Minimising discomfort of sick newborns. *Nursing Times* **85**(42), 39–42.
Sparshott, M.M. (1990) The human touch. *Paediatric Nursing* **2**(5), 8–10.
Stewart, A.J. (1990) Mums and dads need care too. *Professional Nurse* **5**(12), 660–5.
Thornes, R. (1985) Research–Parent Participation. *Nursing Mirror* **160**(13), 20–1.
Vas Dias, S. (1987) Psychotherapy in special care baby units. *Nursing Times* **83**(23), 50–2.
Warwick, G. (1983) Mother–baby separation – one of the dangers. *Nursing Times* **79**(39), 64–7.
Wittenberg, J-V.P. (1990) Psychiatric considerations in premature birth. *Canadian Journal of Psychiatry* **35**, 734–9.

2

Nursing models: suitable frameworks for care?

Christine Midgley

In the 1970s nursing saw the introduction of the nursing process, based on the assessment, planning, implementation and evaluation of care. The frameworks for nursing care, or models for nursing, followed the introduction of the nursing process. This sequence was unfortunate as it resulted in a process being implemented without reference to a basis for assessment. This made assessment of the patients difficult to achieve, because there was no frame of reference against which to assess patients.

For the skilled neonatal nurse the care of a baby with respiratory distress syndrome will present challenges which the nurse is able to meet. The psychological and sociological aspects of care, for both the parents and the baby, may present very different challenges. The parents may adhere to different values and beliefs from those of the nurse. Other members of the care team may have different views again. Whose views are upheld, and why?

Nurses are not the only caregivers on a neonatal unit: many other health care professionals are involved. The role of nurses needs to be identified and their responsibilities defined, distinct from those of others working in neonatal care. Role status and responsibility is not simply an academic exercise but a professional responsibility, particularly where financial accountability is concerned. Identification of the nurse's role and responsibilities is particularly important if claims are made about the professional status of nursing. Other health care workers may be waiting in the wings to take on nursing responsibilities, and to do so at less cost in salaries. A further reason for identifying the nurse's role is related to the extending role of nursing. Nurses need to ensure that this does not detract from their primary responsibilities of nursing. When nurses take over a task from doctors this does not necessarily elevate the status of nursing: rather, it may reduce nursing to a series of tasks.

The education of nurses has moved from an apprenticeship model to a theoretical model. Concepts such as health now form the basis of nursing education. The health concept includes all aspects of the individual: physical, psychological, social and mental wellbeing. Therefore, it becomes even more important that these concepts are reflected in nursing care. With nursing education being based in higher education, and less time being spent in the clinical areas, nurses need to identify quickly the concepts and theories surrounding neonatal nursing.

Models for nursing would address some of these issues, but is a satisfactory model available for neonatal nursing?

MODELS FOR NURSING

A model is a systematic approach to care based on philosophical beliefs about nursing. In neonatal care the baby will be at the centre of these beliefs. Are the beliefs about the care of the babies clearly identified in the neonatal unit philosophy? When developing a unit philosophy, should parents be involved? Are their beliefs about nursing relevant? Possibly they are: after all, neonatal nurses are caring for their baby, and secondly, indirectly, we are responsible to the public for funding of the health service.

Discussion should take place on the nursing staff's sociological views. An example of this may be the potential boundaries which may exist between 'acceptable' views and 'unacceptable' choices exercised by nurses and, possibly, parents. This could be attitudes towards a baby with major congenital abnormalities. Nursing staff may vary in their views regarding the care of the baby and this may present a conflict in the caring team. Such situations should be discussed openly. A framework could then be agreed. The frame of reference for the care would be the model for nursing. If a self-care model was chosen, then the discussion would centre around the choices for care, and the type of care the parents could give to their baby. This will mean that nurses need to justify their interventions on the basis of whether nurses must be responsible for the procedure, or whether parents can be taught to 'self care'. Although this may be considered accepted practice in most units, parents may not be free to do all they could for the baby.

STRUCTURE OF A MODEL

Pearson and Vaughan (1986) identify the structure of a model as 'Containing the theories and concepts of the practice and the theories and concepts reflect the philosophies, values and beliefs about both human nature and what it is that nursing is trying to achieve'. They continue by identifying three basic components of any practice model as:

- the beliefs and values on which the model is based;
- the goals of practice, or what the practitioner aims to achieve;
- the knowledge and skills the practitioner needs in order to gain these goals.

THE OREM SYSTEMS-ORIENTATED MODEL

Dorothea Orem based her model on health and the ability of individuals to care for themselves, which she terms self care. It is obvious that neonates cannot care for themselves, but this does not preclude the application of the Orem model. The aim of neonatal care is to maintain the life of the baby, and transfer that baby from hospital into the community. In order to achieve this aim, the contribution the parents make cannot be undervalued. If the parents and baby are considered as one, for the purposes of the model, then the Orem model could be used for neonatal care. Using the model in this way gives an example of the adaptation of models to meet a variety of nursing situations.

The beliefs and values of the model

Orem identifies nursing systems based on three types of care Orem (1980). These are wholly compensatory care, partly compensatory care and supportive–educative (developmental) care. With wholly compensatory care, the nurse and parents take full responsibility for the baby's requirements; ventilatory care, temperature regulation and nutritional needs being just some of the examples. Partly compensatory care is self explanatory, and supportive–educative care would apply to the nurse's role in assisting the parents to meet the needs of their baby. The latter would be likely to function alongside either of the two other roles.

The goals of practice

Orem (1980) states that 'Self care and care of dependents may be well intentioned but not therapeutic. It is necessary to determine the therapeutic value of practices prescribed by the general culture and even by health professionals.'

A single self-care practice or a whole system of self care is therapeutic to the degree that it actually contributes to the achievement of the following results: support of life processes and promotion of normal functioning. The nurse's role is to provide:

- maintenance of normal growth, development, and maturation;
- prevention, control or cure of disease processes and injuries;
- prevention of or compensation for disability.

Some of these results are required by all persons on a continuing basis during all stages of the lifecycle, but others are required only in the event of disease or injury. The nurse's role is to identify what level of care is to be given, and what results are to be achieved. These are the assessment and planning stages of the nursing process.

Knowledge and skills of the practitioner

Orem (1980) identifies these by writing, 'Nurses are not only major providers and managers of patients' self care, they are also the makers of judgments and decisions about the self care requisites of their patients and the designers of nursing care. Nurses have the responsibility to meet all three types of self care requisites'. She continues by stating, 'The social, interpersonal, and technological dimensions of thse nursing situations require that nurses be the major and, in some instances, the sole contributors to action systems produced to meet the self care requisites of patients and protect patients' powers of self care agency and their personal integrity'.

Some of the wording underlying the concepts of care will need adaptation to fit the work of neonatal nursing. The basis for a framework for care has been identified and, as with all models for nursing, it will require adaptation to meet the requirements of both the patients and the beliefs of the unit.

ROPER, LOGAN AND TIERNEY MODEL

This is a British model developed by members of the Department of Nursing at the University of Edinburgh.

The beliefs and values of the model

Roper, Logan and Tierney (1983) write, 'The model of living is made up of five components and these are labelled as follows:

- Activities of Living (ALs)
- Lifespan
- Dependence/independence continuum
- Factors influencing the ALs
- Individuality in living.'

Roper, Logan and Tierney (1983) discuss factors influencing the ALs and summarize these by writing, 'Factors influencing the ALs are described in five main groups as physical, psychological, sociocultural, environmental, politicoeconomic'.

The goals of practice

These are identified using the activities of living as well as the other components of the model and making a nursing care assessment. The assessment process includes identifying where the person can complete their own activities of living, and to ensure that these are continued to the individual requirements of the person concerned. In neonatal care the individual requirements would need to be identified by the parents: for example how the baby is dressed.

The baby may be independent in some of the activities of living, such as maintaining his own temperature.

Knowledge and skills of the practitioner

The nurse will need to have knowledge of the activities of living and the other components which make up the model of living. The practitioner will require the skills to implement these activities as well as knowledge of the standard to which care should be given.

The Roper, Logan and Tierney model has been implemented in some neonatal units in Britain. It is a straightforward model to use, although not a simplistic framework. There is the potential for the activities of living being used as a checklist, with little reference to the factors that influence the model for living. This reduces the meaning of the model and can result in a rote learning kind of approach.

Where the model has been used in neonatal units, some nurses have felt that expressing sexuality is not relevant to babies. If this activity is interpreted at a simplistic level then it may not be, but if it is considered in the wider context of the sociocultural and spiritual values of the individual, then it may well be relevant.

The Orem self-care model, and the Roper, Logan and Tierney activities of living model are similar, particularly in respect to the health care basis of both these frameworks.

OTHER FRAMEWORKS

The Neuman systems model

The author of the model, Betty Neuman, is an American nursing theorist. She has moved away from the traditional 'illness' model to one which encompasses a total approach to patient problems. Neuman (1980) writes, 'Nursing can use this model to assist individuals, families, and groups to attain and maintain a maximum level of total wellness by purposeful interventions'. The model emphasizes prevention, health education and wellness besides the management of ill health.

Neuman identifies some of the assumptions made in developing the model as, 'Though each individual is viewed as unique, he is also a composite of common "knowns" or characteristics within a normal, given range of response.' She continues, 'There are many known stressors. Each stressor is different in its potential to disturb an individual's equilibrium or normal line of defence. Moreover, particular relationship of the variables: physiological, psychological, sociocultural and developmental at any point, can affect the degree to which an individual is able to use his flexible line of defence against possible reaction to a single stress or combination of stresses'. The flexible line of defence can be affected by the amount of sleep a person has had. The Neuman model, with its emphasis on health prevention and stresses, is more suited to health visiting, psychiatric nursing or social work. The model does have relevance to the neonatal unit but this is more applicable to the family (and the staff on the unit) than to the baby. If neonatal nurses saw their role more in relation to health promotion, then Neuman could be a useful model. Health promotion in neonatal care could extend to areas such as reducing the incidence of premature onset of labour, for example. Possibly the health care professionals are too rigid in their spheres of work and nurses, midwives, health visitors and social workers need to work together for the benefit of the family. The individual profession approach may not be the most effective method for care. If a multiprofessional approach was initiated, then a framework for care and identified criteria for practice would be even more important.

A MODEL FOR NEONATAL CARE

The three models have been chosen from a range of models. These particular ones were selected on the basis of having some potential to lend themselves to neonatal care, but from a brief analysis it would appear that none exactly fits neonatal nursing. This is not a criticism or a shortfall in the models. What is required is for nurses to develop these models to meet neonatal nursing requirements. Readers are strongly advised to read each of these models in the original text before reaching any definite conclusions regarding their suitability for neonatal nursing. Models are not intended to fit perfectly into the diverse situations of nursing care; rather, they are intended to act as a basic framework identifying what nurses are doing. Models can also assist nurses in the evaluation of their care and in identifying any nursing research which may be relevant to care. They are also valuable in identifying 'nursing' and helping communicate this to others, in particular learners.

One criticism most often levelled at models is that they involve a lot of paperwork, but when a model is used correctly this criticism should not be valid. It may not be necessary to use every aspect of the model. Difficulties can arise in this respect when printed care plans are used. Aspects of the model should be used and discarded as the need arises, on a daily or even an hourly basis, as necessary.

Models for nursing should act as a catalyst for nurses' thought processes and, as such, enhance the opportunities for identifying research subjects. Research should not be an optional extra in nursing; rather, it should form part of the role and responsibility of each nurse. This will help to develop nursing on a professional basis.

A framework for nursing care is not a new method of nursing; rather, the models are a means of identifying what nurses do. A framework should produce uniformity of care but not conformity. Nurses continue to take the responsibility for decision making in regard to nursing. If a model is to be used in neonatal nursing, then either an existing model should be used or nurses will need to write their own model. It is unwise for nurses to look to higher education for drawing up a model, primarily because there are likely to be few nurses with sufficient experience in neonatal work in higher education.

Few models have been developed in Britain, and very few in relation to neonatal nursing. Is this because of a lack of analytical thinking? Witness for example, the limited amount of nursing research in the rapidly developing field of neonatal work, compared to the amount of medical research in the field.

Models for nursing may be one way forward in relation to the analysis and identification of the work of neonatal nurses. No professional can afford to remain static. Neonatal nurses need to ensure that their profession is moving in a direction which is led by them, and not by others.

REFERENCES

Neuman, B. (1980) The Betty Neuman health-care systems model, in *Conceptual Models for Nursing Practice*, 2nd edn, (eds J.P. Riehl and C. Roy), Appleton Century Crofts, New York.

Orem, D. (1980) *Nursing: Concepts for Practice*, 2nd edn, Appleton Century Crofts, New York.

Pearson, A. and Vaughan, B. (1986) *Nursing Models for Practice*, Heinemann, London.

Roper, N., Logan, W.W.Q. and Tierney, A.J. (1983) *Using a Model for Nursing*, Churchill Livingstone, Edinburgh.

3

Prenatal and intranatal care of the fetus, mother and father

Claire Thomson Greig

Care of the sick newborn infant involves consideration of his history and immediate family. It is therefore relevant to include, within this text, information that focuses on these aspects. Within the limits of this chapter, an overview of prenatal care will be described, specific aspects of intranatal care will be addressed and the care of the father will conclude the chapter.

PRENATAL CARE

Prenatal care is now a recommended part of every pregnancy (Field, 1990). The original aim of prenatal care was to try to reduce mortality rates, but today broader aims are sought. These can be summarized as follows (Sweet, 1988, p. 126):

- Maintenance and improvement of health in pregnancy.
- Early detection of any deviation from the normal.
- Preparation for labour and a safe, normal delivery that may be a pleasurable, fulfilling experience.
- Good recovery from childbirth and the successful establishment of breastfeeding.
- A live, healthy mature baby happily integrated into the family.
- Education of prospective parents.

Prenatal care is provided by the National Health Service (NHS) via midwives, general practitioners (GP) and obstetricians. Depending on local practice, her needs and/or choice, the woman may use a combination of the skills of all three professionals during her pregnancy. Prepregnancy care may have improved the health of both partners prior to conception (Shorney, 1990).

During the initial appointment, the woman undergoes assessment of health status, including weight and blood pressure (BP), urinalysis and general examination of her abdomen and genital tract. Interviews can reveal information relating to the woman's past history as well as her feelings, hopes, anxieties and plans for the pregnancy and childbirth. Blood is drawn for grouping, full cell count, infections and antibodies. Clinical examination can confirm the pregnancy and this can also be established by an abdominal ultrasound scan, which can give an estimate of gestation from standardized crown-to-rump length measurements in the first trimester (Robinson and Fleming, 1975).

Based on the findings of the assessment, prenatal care can be planned with the woman, and subsequent care usually includes reassessments of BP, urinalysis, general health and the progress of the pregnancy. If deviations from normal are detected, such as the development of pregnancy-induced hypertension (PIH), anaemia or poor fetal growth, the care plan can be revised to try to meet the changed needs of the woman and fetus. Hospitalization as part of the management of complications of pregnancy is less common; community midwives provide additional surveillance when required (Middlemiss *et al.*, 1989).

The woman may undergo specialized tests of fetal wellbeing. Biochemical tests such as serum oestrogen, human placental lactogen or human chorionic gonadotrophin levels are no longer considered helpful as a guide in the care of the woman or fetus (Alexander *et al.*, 1989). However, if there is a potential for genetic or chromosomal abnormality, chorionic villus sampling (CVS) performed between 8 and 12 weeks of gestation (Stringer, 1988) may assist in diagnosis. Maternal serum alphafetoprotein measurements taken between 16 and 18 weeks' gestation can indicate open neural tube defects or Down's syndrome if maternal age is a consideration

(Merkatz *et al.*, 1984). Amniotic fluid sampling after 18 weeks can also give chromosomal information, as can blood from the fetal umbilical cord. The development of specialized real-time ultrasound equipment is helpful in the prenatal diagnosis of structural congenital abnormalities such as cardiac defects, neural tube defects and renal abnormalities, as well as guiding CVS, fetal blood and amniotic fluid sampling. These invasive techniques can result in spontaneous abortion, and this risk must be taken into consideration when deciding whether to undertake these tests (Daker and Bobrow, 1989; Neilson and Grant, 1989).

Fetal breathing patterns, liquor volume, fetal movements and muscle tone can be assessed using ultrasound techniques. Standards against which to judge fetal health have been developed and a low score can indicate a compromised fetus. Doppler flow studies can reflect the flow of blood through the placental bed or the umbilical artery: reduced flow may give an early indication of fetal compromise. These biophysical assessments may be helpful in judging optimum delivery time, but their predictive value has yet to be fully evaluated (Neilson, 1987; Mohide and Keirse, 1989).

Women who are unlikely to develop problems during pregnancy are deemed to be 'low risk', but at any time the woman may be assigned 'high-risk' status based on identification of factors related to poor pregnancy outcome. This is intended to result in increased beneficial care, positively altering the outcome. However, most of the systems have limitations and may lead to unnecessary interventions, cause increased anxiety for the woman and ultimately result in a less positive outcome (Alexander and Keirse, 1989; Marshall, 1989).

Following the recommendations of the Short Report (House of Commons Social Services Committee, 1980), and the continuing dissatisfaction expressed by women (MacIntyre, 1984), revisions in the provision of prenatal care were undertaken. A reduced schedule of reassessments for the 'low-risk' woman results in shorter waiting times and longer, more thorough consultations (Hall, MacIntyre and Porter, 1985). Community or GP-based clinics can be more convenient for the woman to attend (McKee, 1984). Local schemes which offer 'low-risk' women continuity of midwifery care have proved satisfying for women and for the midwives (Flint, Poulengeris and Grant, 1989). To help them to meet their specific needs prenatally, some women choose an independent midwife and have reported positively on the care given (Isherwood, 1989; Leap, 1991).

Other initiatives include systems of planned prenatal clinic assessments enhanced by additional community-based midwifery care and support, some of which have been specifically organized to serve women who are particularly at 'high risk' due to their social circumstances (Davies, 1990). The most significant aspect of enhanced prenatal care is the social support offered by midwives, which has improved outcomes in respect of birth weight as well as other maternal and neonatal parameters (Oakley, Rajan and Grant, 1990).

Despite such changes, the most recent evaluation of the maternity services showed that significant improvements in the location and schedule of prenatal assessments, the continuity of care, information giving by professionals and individualized care led by midwives are still needed (House of Commons Health Committee, 1992).

Prenatal care also includes preparation for parenthood classes. Topics usually include preparation for labour, pain relief, relaxation/psychoprophylaxis and baby care. Women have expressed concern about the apparent poor organization of NHS run classes, conflicting advice, lack of realism and the wrong impression of parenthood being given by the midwife running the class (Oakley, 1981; Rees, 1982).

Classes are now more informal and held in a variety of locations suited to the women's needs (Evans and Parker, 1985; Smoke and Grace, 1988; Simkin and Enkin, 1989). Women may attend smaller group-specific classes, for example, for couples or unsupported women or for teenagers. Non-NHS preparation for parenthood classes, such as those run by the National Childbirth Trust, have been found to be more individualized and pertinent (Skevington and Wilkes, 1992).

One debatable topic for inclusion in these classes is information about preterm and sick babies. These topics have been thought frightening and unnecessary, but this information can reduce the fear and anxiety experienced by parents when such an infant is born. For the information to be relevant, it is necessary to run the programme from 20 weeks' gestation (Lynam and Miller, 1992).

INTRANATAL CARE

The achievement of an optimal delivery encompasses many aspects but the physical and emotional health of the woman and fetus are paramount.

MIDWIFERY CARE OF THE MOTHER

Prenatally the woman may have thought about how she would like to labour and deliver and have written these thoughts in the form of a birth plan. During labour the woman is assessed, taking into account her general physical and emotional condition as well as her vital signs and urinalysis. Assessment of labour involves abdominal and vaginal examinations to determine the length, strength and frequency of contractions, the descent of the fetus, the cervical effacement and dilatation and, if the membranes have ruptured, the nature of the liquor (Drayton, 1990).

Together, the woman and the midwife can plan interventions and care fulfilling her comfort, hygiene, hydration and elimination needs (Drayton, 1990). Continued reassessments may detect deviations from normal which necessitate revision of the plan to meet the changing needs of the woman and the fetus. Most women report satisfaction with their physical care, but efforts to meet emotional needs have been a source of dissatisfaction (Jacoby, 1988; McIntosh, 1988). Women are anxious about labour and delivery, and these anxieties are increased when deviations from normal occur (Jacoby, 1988). For some, the situation of a preterm birth is a crisis and the midwife's crisis intervention skills may have to be utilized to effect a resolution (Caplan, 1960; Wright, 1986).

One strategy to help women deal with their anxiety is to give information. They will then understand better what is happening to them, the nature of the deviation, what choices there are to deal with the problems or needs, what the consequences of these choices would be, thus helping them make decisions and feel more in control of their labour. When asked, midwives stress that information giving is important, yet in practice they are seen to avoid giving information, or give it inconsistently (Kirkham, 1989). It is also evident that the women who have most difficulty getting information are from the lower social classes (Jacoby, 1988; McIntosh 1988). Further improvements are necessary in midwives' abilities to listen, to identify non-verbal clues, to avoid making assumptions, to respond to questions and to give information in a way in which the woman can understand (Jacoby, 1988; Kirkham, 1989).

Another strategy which enhances the woman's experience of labour and delivery is the presence of a constant female companion who provides emotional support. Although the father may be present and provide support, it is the female supporter who appears to influence a more positive experience for the woman. She may be a midwife or a lay female, such as a member of the family or the community, who in some cultures is known as a 'doula'. Traditionally, a doula is the usual and only companion of labouring women in developing countries, but the concept is increasingly being successfully incorporated into other cultures (Kennell *et al.*, 1991; Rosen, 1991).

The onset of labour

Most pregnant women expect the spontaneous onset of labour, leading to delivery 'at term', i.e. around 40 weeks' gestation, but this may not occur. Preterm delivery is a major cause of morbidity and mortality and the association between preterm delivery and lower social class is well established. There are specific causes of preterm labour, such as fetal abnormality, polyhydramnios, multiple pregnancy and maternal infections but, in many instances, no cause can be determined (Chamberlain, 1991). Preterm labour can be difficult to diagnose accurately, which can delay relevant management (King, 1987).

Prelabour rupture of the membranes complicates 50% of all preterm labours, and further decision making depends on the presence of infection. If infection is present, labour will usually be induced. If absent and labour has not begun and the woman and fetus are well, treatment with antibiotics can allow prolongation of the pregnancy and fetal maturation (Keirse *et al.*, 1989b).

One factor which has significantly reduced the perinatal and neonatal mortality and morbidity associated with preterm delivery is the administration of corticosteroids to encourage maturation of fetal alveolar surfactant production. Reductions in the incidence and severity of respiratory distress syndrome and associated necrotizing enterocolitis and periventricular haemorrhage are significant if the delivery occurs more than 24 hours and less than 7 days after treatment starts. However, corticosteroids have side effects, which include maternal pulmonary oedema and infection. Also when PIH, poor fetal growth, diabetes mellitus or rhesus isoimmunization are diagnosed, the optimal administration of corticosteroids may not be possible (Ho, 1988; Crowley, 1989).

In order for corticosteroids to be administered, preterm labour usually has to be delayed using, for example, betamimetics such as ritodrine, which can be effective but has not proved to be as efficient as was originally hoped (Keirse *et al.*, 1989a). Side effects such as tachycardia, palpitations, sweating, headache and oedema are distressing for the woman, so the use of ritodrine is contraindicated in women who are hyperthyroid, diabetic, or who have cardiac disease (Chamberlain, 1991).

Indomethacin, a prostaglandin synthesase inhibitor, has proved more efficient in reducing uterine contractions but its use can only be short term due to the side effects of gastrointestinal bleeding and thrombocytopenia. It has also been linked to the development of postnatal pulmonary hypertension in the neonate, due to prenatal ductus arteriosus constriction (Keirse *et al.*, 1989a).

Prolonging pregnancy using betamimetics or prostaglandin synthesase inhibitors can also allow time for *in utero* fetal transfer to a regional centre for delivery, or to allow for further fetal maturation (Keirse and van Oppen, 1989).

To try to avoid significant mortality and morbidity, induction of labour may be warranted at any gestation when fetal or maternal health deteriorates and labour does not occur spontaneously. In order to improve the success of induction, the cervix should be 'ripe'. Assessment of the cervix using a modified Bishop scoring system can guide management and, if ripening is required, prostaglandins can be used effectively. Artificial rupture of the membranes, followed by oxytocin therapy if necessary, usually successfully induces labour (Keirse and Chalmers, 1989). Augmentation using artificial rupture of the membranes and/or oxytocin therapy at any stage of labour may also be beneficial when inefficient or ineffective uterine action interferes with progress or compromises the woman or the fetus (Keirse, 1989).

Route of delivery

Normally the infant will be delivered spontaneously, vaginally and from a cephalic presentation. Alternative routes and methods of delivery have to be chosen when either the maternal or the fetal status does not allow for a normal delivery. This status must be assessed between the delivery of each fetus in the case of multiple pregnancy. Presentation of the fetus by the brow or shoulder usually necessitates an elective caesarean section, as does severe cephalopelvic disproportion. Severe types of placenta praevia and placental abruption, and cord prolapse in the first stage of labour, are also usually managed by caesarean section. Other previously accepted indications for caesarean section, such as prolonged labour, fetal distress, breech presentation and previous caesarean section, are more controversial, as successful outcomes have been reported using other forms of management. The maternal and perinatal morbidity associated with caesarean section is high, and efforts to reduce the necessity for this common surgical operation, yet achieve a favourable outcome, continue (Hillan, 1990).

With a cephalic presentation and a fully dilated cervix, forceps may be used to assist delivery if there is fetal distress or significant delay in fetal descent through the birth canal, for example, due to deep transverse arrest on the ischial spines or ineffective maternal effort (Vacca and Keirse, 1989). A vacuum extractor can be a valid alternative to forceps in the above circumstances, but tends not to be used in English-speaking countries (Barclay, 1988). In vaginal breech births forceps can be used to assist delivery of the head (Vacca and Keirse, 1989).

Both forceps and vacuum extraction deliveries have been associated with lower APGAR scores and hypoxia, and can result in complications such as cephalhaematoma and scalp and facial injuries for the baby, and trauma to the structures of the birth canal (Vacca and Keirse, 1989), but no increase in the long-term risk of physical and cognitive disability (Seidman *et al.*, 1991).

Position for labour and delivery

Despite the prevalence of labour and delivery in bed, lying semirecumbent, many women can choose to be ambulant and mainly upright (Garcia and Garforth, 1989), using alternative postures such as squatting, kneeling, standing, all-fours and sitting, increasing the woman's control and satisfaction. There are advantages to not lying in bed, with a reported increase in the efficiency of contractions and reductions in the length of labour, the use of oxytocics for augmentation, the experience of backache, the use of narcotics and epidural analgesia, abnormal fetal heart rate patterns and fetal acidosis. However, some positions result in discomfort for the woman and the midwife, poor midwife visualization of the perineum and an increase in maternal blood loss. Even when there are physical restrictions such as epidural analgesia, intravenous infusions or electronic fetal monitoring, some alternatives can be implemented successfully (Hillan, 1985; Roberts, 1989).

Pain control

The pain of labour can be severe and women vary in their ability to cope, depending on their culture, previous experience and the influence of family and friends. The stress-related effects of uncontrolled pain may increase cardiac output, respiratory alkalosis and acidaemia and reduce placental flow, all of which can lead to fetal compromise. Nausea, fatigue, dizziness and confusion are unpleasant symptoms which may also result, and compromise the woman's experience (Dick-Read, 1969; Brownridge, 1991).

For an optimum labour and delivery experience, pain relief and the ability to cope with pain are discussed before labour. Some women choose to experience the pain, others choose non-pharmacological pain relief measures, and yet others want as pain-free a labour as possible. Non-pharmacological methods include psychoprophylaxis, massage, acupuncture, transcutaneous electrical nerve stimulation and hypnosis. These methods have few side effects (Simkin, 1989).

Opioid drugs, given intramuscularly or by intravenous or patient-controlled infusion, can effectively reduce pain. The side effects of these drugs can cause nausea, dizziness and sedation in the woman, and postnatal respiratory depression and some reduction in feeding ability in the baby (Matthews, 1989; Buchan and Sharwood-Smith, 1991). However, opioids may help decrease resuscitation-related hypertension and so reduce the incidence of neonatal intracranial bleeding (Dickerson, 1989).

Inhalational analgesia of 50% oxygen and 50% nitrous oxide mixtures can be administered via the Entonox apparatus using a face mask or mouthpiece. Used efficiently, so that the maximum influence is at the height of the contraction, this is still a valuable form of analgesia and major side effects have not been documented (Brownridge, 1991).

Epidural analgesia involves the administration of local anaesthetic (by bolus or continuous infusion) via an indwelling catheter in the epidural space, giving sensory loss from the uterus and upper vagina. It can be additionally 'topped up' if operative or instrumental delivery is necessary, so avoiding the risks of general anaesthesia. Unfortunately there can be significant side effects, including lack of spontaneous leg movement and micturition, hypotension, allergic drug reactions, dural tap and the loss of the reflex to bear down in the second stage of labour, with possibly a higher incidence of instrumental deliveries. The effects on the fetus are usually related to maternal hypotension, such as bradycardia and fetal distress (Sweet, 1988; Brownridge, 1991; Buchan and Sharwood-Smith, 1991).

Despite the plans made for her labour, the actual experience of pain can be more or less than expected and, when greater, '... emotional distress and loss of self esteem ...' can result (Brownridge, 1991, p. 70). Therefore it is the midwife's responsibility to continue to respond to the woman's individual needs for pain control during labour and delivery to try to optimize her experience without adversely affecting the fetus.

Fetal monitoring

Monitoring the fetus during labour usually involves intermittent auscultation (IA) with a fetal stethoscope and/or continuous electronic fetal monitoring (EFM) using an external transducer or internal electrode.

IA involves listening to the fetal heart at approximately 15 minute intervals during the first stage of labour and between each contraction during the second stage. This gives intermittent information about the heart rate but little about its relationship to uterine contractions or its variability. Continuous

EFM gives this additional information but the interpretation of abnormal patterns is very unreliable and can lead to unnecessary interventions. The unreliability of EFM needs to be overcome if the valuable information it can provide is to be used to advantage. Developments in computerized interpretation of the specifics of the electrocardiograph trace produced by the EFM internal electrode may prove useful in clinical management (Westgate *et al.*, 1992). EFM complemented by fetal scalp blood sampling (FBS) measuring fetal pH can give a more accurate assessment of fetal wellbeing, but FBS needs an experienced operator and time, and gives only intermittent information (Grant, 1989).

The effects on the woman and the baby of IA and EFM have been evaluated and the only significant difference was a reduction in the incidence of neonatal seizures. However, there was no difference noted in the long-term neurological outcome between the two groups. For the mothers using EFM there was an increase in operative deliveries, an increase in forceps deliveries when EFM was combined with FBS, and an increase in postnatal infections. Although most 'high-risk' women did not object to EFM, others reported that it made them more anxious, it was uncomfortable and distracting, and found that the midwife left them alone more than they would have liked (McDonald *et al.*, 1985; Grant, 1989).

IA appears to be an efficient method of assessing fetal wellbeing in the majority of labours. EFM combined with FBS should be used only during the labours of selected 'high-risk' women (Grant, 1989; Evans, 1992).

CARE OF THE FATHER

It has been suggested that the transition to parenthood can be as vulnerable a period for men as it can be for women (Brown *et al.*, 1991).

Preparation for fatherhood

Dodendorf (1981) categorized the changes in the expectant father according to the stage of pregnancy. In the first trimester, the father-to-be has mixed emotions and worries about the financial costs of the baby, and a resentment in the form of jealousy of the developing fetus. During the second trimester, the father may begin to imagine what his baby may look like, the responsibilities of actual fatherhood can become more clear and he may begin to make practical preparations for the baby. The final weeks of pregnancy see the father directing his feelings towards the reality of the baby and the impending labour and birth.

Some expectant fathers have been noted to exhibit the signs and symptoms of couvade during their partner's pregnancy. Ritual couvade in some preindustrialized countries involves changes in dress, sexual restraint and mock labour. Modern couvade has been noted to exist within industrialized societies, with variable incidence (Clinton, 1987). Symptoms experienced include weight gain, insomnia, restlessness and irritability. Expectant fathers who are most likely to experience couvade are black, working class, anxious and fathering an unplanned pregnancy (Connor and Denson, 1990).

May (1980) reported that fathers exhibited one of three levels of involvement during pregnancy, from being withdrawn and disinterested to being in complete partnership with the mother. The degree of involvement was thought to reflect the amount of sharing which normally existed within the relationship. Cultural influences can also determine the level of involvement.

It is suggested that fathers may have increased anxiety levels because of lack of knowledge about fatherhood. As the role of the midwife is towards the family, the needs of the father could be assessed and incorporated into the midwifery care plan. Fathers could also be included in the prenatal clinic visits and preparation for parenthood classes, although this would have implications for the timing, frequency, content and conduct of the classes (Bedford and Johnson, 1988; Brown, Rustia and Schappert, 1991).

Birth and the father

Generally, fathers who were prepared for and attended the birth, and those who simply attended, responded more positively and rated their experiences more highly than those who did not attend (Cronewett and Newmark, 1974).

Initially, the father's role was one of supporting his partner psychologically. The move from simply being with the woman to actually participating in her care was gradual. Fathers became involved in providing comfort measures and verbally encouraging breathing rhythms and relaxation. The term 'labour coach' developed. Many preparation for parenthood classes are designed with this aim central. Most women feel that the presence of their partner during labour and delivery is helpful (Niven, 1985). However, Berry (1988) found that fathers felt anxious during labour and delivery, and were more concerned about their usefulness and hiding their emotions than with coaching their partner.

More recently, Chapman (1992) identified three roles fathers assumed during labour and delivery, indicating varying degrees of involvement in the physical and emotional support of the woman. The most involved was that of coach; less directive was that of team mate, and the least involved was that of witness, which most men adopted. The partners appeared satisfied with the role the fathers assumed and Chapman proposed that the roles simply reflected the pattern of the couple's normal relationship with respect to sharing and working together, which can be influenced by the cultural expectations of what the father should do. These roles are similar to those which fathers were seen to adopt during pregnancy, indicating three levels of involvement there also (May, 1980).

Duvall's (1977) theory that a father has three tasks to achieve: to accept the reality of the pregnancy and child, to be recognized as a parent by his significant others, and to try to become an involved father, is still relevant today. However, the extent to and the ways in which individual fathers achieve these tasks vary, as there are some individuals and some cultures where childbirth and child rearing remain the sole prerogative of the woman. Therefore, rather than forcing a stereotypical role on fathers, their needs should be assessed. The options available to fathers can be explored prenatally and they can choose which suit their needs and those of their partners. Preparations for the role can then be individualized rather than generalized (Bedford and Johnson, 1988).

CONCLUSION

Neonatal nurses will not usually provide for the physical care of the mother during the prenatal and intranatal period.

However, there may be opportunities to cooperate with midwives and obstetricians to help meet the social, emotional and educational needs of the family, especially those deemed to be high risk. It is necessary to evaluate such involvement to determine its influence on the provision of optimum care.

REFERENCES

Alexander, S. and Keirse, M.J.N.C. (1989) Formal risk scoring during pregnancy, in *Effective Care in Pregnancy and Childbirth*, Vol. I (eds I. Chalmers, M. Enkin and M.J.N.C. Keirse), Oxford University Press, London, pp. 345–65.

Alexander, S., Stanwell-Smith, R., Buekens, P. and Keirse, M.J.N.C. (1989) Biochemical assessment of fetal well-being. *Effective Care in Pregnancy and Childbirth*, Vol. 1. (eds I. Chalmers, M. Enkin and M.J.N.C. Keirse), Oxford University Press, London, pp. 455–76.

Barclay, C. (1988) History and the use of vacuum extraction. *Midwife, Health Visitor and Community Nurse* **24**(8), 328–31.

Bedford, V.A. and Johnson, N. (1988) The role of the father. *Midwifery* **4**(4), 190–5.

Berry, L.M. (1988) Realistic expectations of the labor coach. *Journal of Obstetric, Gynaecologic and Neonatal Nursing* **17**(5), 354–5.

Brown, P., Rustia, J. and Schappert, P. (1991) A comparison of fathers of high risk newborns and fathers of healthy newborns. *Journal of Pediatric Nursing* **6**(4), 269–73.

Brownridge, P. (1991) Treatment options for the relief of pain during childbirth. *Drugs* **41**(1), 69–80.

Buchan, A.S. and Sharwood-Smith, G.H. (1991) *Handbook of Obstetric Anaesthesia*, W.B. Saunders, London.

Caplan, B. (1960) Patterns of parental response to the crisis of premature birth. *Psychiatry* **23**, 365–74.

Chamberlain, G. (1991) The A B C of antenatal care. Preterm labour. *British Medical Journal* **303**(6793) 44–8.

Chapman, L.L. (1992) Expectant fathers' roles during labor. *Journal of Obstetric, Gynaecologic and Neonatal Nursing* **21**(2), 114–20.

Clinton, J.F. (1987) Physical and emotional responses of expectant fathers throughout pregnancy and the early post partum period. *International Journal of Nursing Studies* **24**(1), 59–68.

Conner, G.K. and Denson, K. (1990) Expectant fathers' response to pregnancy: a review of literature and implications for research in high risk pregnancy. *Journal of Perinatal and Neonatal Nursing* **4**(2), 33–42.

Cronewett, L.R. and Newmark, L.L. (1974) Fathers' responses to childbirth. *Nursing Research* **23**(3), 210–7.

Cowley, P. (1989) Promoting pulmonary maturity, in *Effective Care in Pregnancy and Childbirth*, Vol I, (eds I. Chalmers, M. Enkin and M.J.N.C. Keirse), Oxford University Press, London, pp. 746–64.

Daker, M. and Bobrow, M. (1989) Screening for genetic disease and foetal anomaly during pregnancy, in *Effective Care in Pregnancy and Childbirth*, Vol I, (eds I. Chalmers, M. Enkin and M.J.N.C. Keirse), Oxford University Press, London, pp. 366–81.

Davies, J. (1990) Against the odds. *Nursing Times*. **86**(44), 29–31.

Dick-Read, G. (1969) *Childbirth Without Fear*, Pan, London.

Dickerson, K. (1989) Pharmacological control of pain during labour, in *Effective Care in Pregnancy and Childbirth*, Vol II, (eds I. Chalmers, M. Enkin and M.J.N.C. Keirse), Oxford University Press, London, pp. 913–50.

Dodendorf D. (1981) Expectant fatherhood and first pregnancy. *Journal of Family Practice* **13**(5), 744–51.

Drayton, S. (1990) Midwifery care in the first stage of labour, in *Intrapartum Care. A Research-Based Approach* (eds J. Alexander, V. Levy and S. Roch), Macmillan Press Ltd, London, pp. 24–41.

Duvall, E.M. (1977) *Marriage and Family Development*, 5th edn, J.B. Lippincott Company, Philadelphia.

Evans, S. (1992) The value of cardiotocograph monitoring in midwifery. *Midwives Chronicle* **105**(1248), 4–10.

Evans, G. and Parker, P. (1985) Preparing teenagers for parenthood. *Midwives Chronicle* **98**(1172), 239–40.

Field, P.A. (1990) Effectiveness and efficacy of antenatal care. *Midwifery*, **6**(4), 215–23.

Flint, C., Poulengeris, P. and Grant, A. (1989) The Know Your Midwife Scheme: a randomised trial of continuity of care by a team of midwives. *Midwifery* **5**(1), 11–16.

Garcia, J. and Garforth, S. (1989) Labour and delivery routines in English consultant maternity units. *Midwifery*, **5**, 155–62.

Grant, A. (1989) Monitoring the foetus during labour, in *Effective Care in Pregnancy and Childbirth*, Vol II, (eds I. Chalmers, M. Enkin and M.J.N.C. Keirse), Oxford University Press, London, pp. 846–82.

Hall, M., Macintyre, S. and Porter, M. (1985) *Antenatal Care Assessed*, University Press, Aberdeen.

Hillan, E. (1985) Posture for labour and delivery. *Midwifery* **1**(1), 19–23.

Hillan, E. (1990) Recent trends in Caesarean section. *Nursing Standard*, **4**(35), 24–7.

Ho, E. (1988) Prenatal corticosteroid in preventing respiratory distress syndrome. *Midwifery* **4**(1), 24–8.

House of Commons Health Committee (1992) *Second Report. Maternity Services*, Vol. I, (Chairman N. Winterton), HMSO, London.

House of Commons Social Services Committee (1980) *Second Report. Perinatal and Neonatal Mortality*, (Chairman R. Short), HMSO, London.

Isherwood, K. (1989) Independent midwifery in the UK. *Midwife, Health Visitor and Community Nurse* **25**(7), 307–9.

Jacoby, A. (1988) Mothers' views about information and advice in pregnancy and childbirth: findings from a national study. *Midwifery* **4**(3), 103–10.

Keirse, M.J.N.C. (1989) Augmentation of labour, in *Effective Care in*

Pregnancy and Childbirth, Vol. II, (eds I. Chalmers, M. Enkin and M.J.N.C. Keirse), Oxford University Press, London, pp. 951–66.
Keirse, M.J.N.C. and Chalmers, I. (1989) Methods for inducing labour, in *Effective Care in Pregnancy and Childbirth*, Vol. II, (eds I. Chalmers, M. Enkin and M.J.N.C. Keirse), Oxford University Press, London, pp. 1057–79.
Keirse, M.J.N.C. and van Oppen, A.C.C. (1989) Preparing the cervix for induction of labour, in *Effective Care in Pregnancy and Childbirth*, Vol. II, (eds I. Chalmers, M. Enkin and M.J.N.C. Keirse), Oxford University Press, London, pp. 988–1056.
Keirse, M.J.N.C., Grant, A. and King, J.F. (1989a) Preterm labour, in *Effective Care in Pregnancy and Childbirth*, Vol. I, (eds I. Chalmers, M. Enkin and M.J.N.C. Keirse), Oxford University Press, London, pp. 694–45.
Keirse, M.J.N.C., Ohlsson, A., Treffers, P.E. and Kanhai, H.H.H. (1989b) Prelabour rupture of the membranes preterm, in *Effective Care in Pregnancy and Childbirth*, Vol. I (eds I. Chalmers, M. Enkin and M.J.N.C. Keirse), Oxford University Press, London, pp. 666–93.
Kennell, J., Klaus, M., McGrath, S., Robertson, S. and Hincley, C. (1991) Continuous emotional support in labour in a US hospital. A randomised controlled trial. *Journal of the American Medical Association* **265**(17), 2197–201.
King, J.F. (1987) Dilemmas in the treatment of preterm labour and delivery, in *Recent Advances in Obstetrics and Gynaecology*, (ed J. Bonnar), Churchill Livingstone, Edinburgh, pp. 65–82.
Kirkham, M. (1989) Midwives and information-giving during labour, in *Midwives, Research and Childbirth*, Vol. I, (eds S. Robinson and A. Thomson), Chapman and Hall, London, pp. 117–38.
Leap, N. (1991) Independent midwifery. *Midwives Chronicle* **104**(1237), 34–8.
Lynam, L.E. and Miller, M.A. (1992) Mothers' perceptions of the needs of women experiencing preterm labour. *Journal of Obstetric, Gynaecologic and Neonatal Nursing* **21**(2), 126–36.
McDonald, D., Grant, A., Sheridan-Pereira, M., Boylan, P. and Chalmers, I. (1985) The Dublin Randomised Trial of Intrapartum Foetal Heart Monitoring. *American Journal of Obstetrics and Gynaecology* **52**, 524–39.
McIntosh, J. (1988) Womens' views of communication during labour and delivery. *Midwifery* **4**(4), 166–70.
Macintyre, S. (1984) Consumer reaction to present-day antenatal services, in *Pregnancy Care for the 1980s*, (eds L. Zander and G. Chamberlain), The Royal Society of Medicine and The Macmillan Press Ltd, London, pp. 9–17.
McKee, H. (1984) Community antenatal care: the Sighthill community antenatal scheme, in *Pregnancy Care for the 1980s*, (eds L. Zander and G. Chamberlain), The Royal Society of Medicine and The Macmillan Press Ltd, London, pp. 32–48.
Marshall, V.A. (1989) A comparison of two obstetric risk assessment tools. *Journal of Nurse-Midwifery* **34**(1), 3–7.

Matthews, M.K. (1989) The relationship between maternal labour analgesia and delay in the initiation of breast feeding in healthy neonates in the early neonatal period. *Midwivery* **5**(1), 3–10.

May, K. (1980) A typology of detachment/involvement styles adopted during pregnancy by first time expectant fathers. *Western Journal of Nursing Research* **2**, 443–53.

Merkatz, I.R., Nitowski, H.M., Macri, J.N. and Johnson, W.E. (1984) An association between low maternal serum alpha fetoprotein and foetal chromosomal abnormalities. *American Journal of Obstetrics and Gynecology*, **148**, 886–91.

Middlemiss, C., Dawson, A.J., Gough, N., Jones, M.E. and Coles, E.C. (1989) A randomised controlled study of a domiciliary antenatal care scheme: maternal psychological effects. *Midwifery* **5**(2), 69–83.

Mohide, P. and Keirse, M.J.N.C. (1989) Biophysical assessment of foetal wellbeing, in *Effective Care in Pregnancy and Childbirth*, Vol. I, (eds I. Chalmers, M. Enkin and M.J.N.C. Keirse), Oxford University Press, London, pp. 477–92.

Neilson, J.P. (1987) Doppler ultrasound. *British Journal of Obstetrics and Gynaecology* **94**, 929–34.

Neilson, J.P. and Grant, A. (1989) Ultrasound in pregnancy, in *Effective Care in Pregnancy and Childbirth*, Vol. I (eds I. Chalmers, M. Enkin and M.J.N.C. Keirse), Oxford University Press, London, pp. 419–39.

Niven, C. (1985) How helpful is the husband at childbirth? *Journal of Reproductive and Infant Psychology* **3**(2), 45–53.

Oakley, A. (1981) Adjustment to motherhood. *Nursing* **1**, 889–901.

Oakley, A., Rajan, L. and Grant, A. (1990) Social support and pregnancy outcome. *British Journal of Obstetrics and Gynaecology* **97**(2), 155–62.

Rees, C. (1982) Antenatal classes: time for a new approach. *Nursing Times* **78**(34), 1446–8.

Roberts, J. (1989) Maternal position during the first stage of labour, in *Effective Care in Pregnancy and Childbirth*, Vol. II, (eds I. Chalmers, M. Enkin and M.J.N.C. Keirse), Oxford University Press, London, pp. 883–92.

Robinson, H.P. and Fleming, J.E.E. (1975) A critical evaluation of crown rump length measurements. *British Journal of Obstetrics and Gynaecology* **82**, 702–10.

Rosen, M.G. (1991) Doula at the bedside of the patient in labour. Comment. *Journal of the American Medical Association* **265**(17), 2236–7.

Seidman, D., Laor, A., Gale, R., Stevenson, D.K., Mashiach, S. and Danon, Y.L. (1991) Long-term effects of vacuum and forceps deliveries. *Lancet* **337**(8757), 1583–5.

Shorney, J. (1990) Preconception care – the embryo of health promotion, in *Antenatal Care. A Research-Based Approach*, (eds, J. Alexander, V. Levy and S. Roch), Macmillan Press Ltd, London, pp. 1–19.

Simkin, P. (1989) Non-pharmacological methods of pain relief during labour, in *Effective Care in Pregnancy and Childbirth*, Vol. II, (eds I. Chalmers, M. Enkin and M.J.N.C. Keirse), Oxford University Press, London, pp. 893–912.

Simkin, P. and Enkin, M. (1989) Antenatal classes, in *Effective Care in Pregnancy and Childbirth*, Vol. I, (eds I. Chalmers, M. Enkin and M.J.N.C. Keirse), Oxford University Press, London, pp. 281–334.

Skevington, S.M. and Wilkes, P. (1992) Choice and control: a comparative study of childbirth preparation classes. *Journal of Reproductive and Infant Psychology* **10**(1), 19–28.

Smoke, J. and Grace, M.C. (1988) Effectiveness of prenatal care and education for pregnant adolescents: nurse midwifery intervention and team approach. *Journal of Nurse-Midwifery* **33**(4), 178-84.

Stringer, J.R. (1988) Chorionic villus sampling. A nursing perspective. *Journal of Obstetric, Gynecology and Neonatal Nursing* **17**(1), 19–22.

Sweet, B. (1988) *Mayes' Midwifery*, 11th edn, Baillière Tindall, London.

Vacca, A. and Keirse, M.J.N.C. (1989) Instrumental vaginal delivery, in *Effective Care in Pregnancy and Childbirth*, Vol. II, (eds I. Chalmers, M. Enkin and M.J.N.C. Keirse), Oxford University Press, London, pp. 1216–33.

Westgate, J., Harris, M., Curnow, J.S.H. and Greene, K.R. (1992) Randomised trial of cardiotocography alone or with ST waveform analysis for intrapartum monitoring. *Lancet* **340**(8813), 194–8.

Wright, B.(1986) *Caring in Crisis*, Churchill Livingstone, Edinburgh.

4

Resuscitation – flying squad transfer

Doreen Crawford

The majority of infants are in excellent condition at birth; observe them closely but leave them alone and the majority will stay that way. There is a direct correlation between the amount of intervention given and the amount of intervention subsequently required. If an infant does genuinely need your help, the chances are that he is going to need medical help as well. Do not delay calling for urgent help.

With good midwifery and obstetric care, there is only a small percentage of newborn infants who require intervention and resuscitation to support or establish cardiopulmonary function. For this small minority a clean, fully equipped and warm resuscitation area should be available (Milner, 1986). This should be checked daily and rechecked after each use. Staff should be drilled and assessed as competent in resuscitation skills, which should be revised and updated at least every 6 months.

The majority of infants who need initial support, and possibly subsequent neonatal care, can be anticipated. Effective communication between the departments of midwifery/obstetrics and neonatology ensures that a paediatrician is present at the birth and that the neonatal unit is on standby. Success is greatest when care is initiated from the start by competent and well equipped personnel.

INFANTS MOST LIKELY TO NEED SUPPORT

- Infants of mothers who have suffered a major incident, e.g. massive haemorrhage or sudden eclamptic fits.

- Infants of mothers who suffer from a severe or chronic condition which has a known effect on the fetus.
- Prolonged rupture of membranes.
- Those with gestations of less than 35–36 weeks.
- Malpresentations and cord prolapse.
- Those needing major obstetric interventions, e.g. high forceps, caesarean section etc.
- Severe intrauterine growth retardation.
- Those who have displayed fetal distress and/or have been compromised by delivery and may have inhaled meconium.
- A prenatal diagnosis which suggests that the infant will need expert care.
- Twins and multiple births.
- Rhesus incompatibility.
- Infants of drug-dependent mothers.

The list is not exhaustive. Many emergencies are sudden and unexpected, occurring at any time of the day or night, Christmas and Bank Holidays especially!!

TRANSITION FROM INTRA- TO EXTRAUTERINE EXISTENCE

The lungs are unnecessary to sustain existence until the moment of birth. Because of the high pulmonary vascular resistance, there is restriction to blood flow from the heart to the lungs. Only about 7% of the right ventricle output flows through the lungs in fetal life. The right-sided cardiac output is redirected through the foramen ovale and the ductus arteriosus. During the last moments of the second stage of labour, the umbilical cord is compressed and fetal circulation to the placenta is inhibited. This results in hypoxia sufficient to initiate gasping. For the majority of infants, this gasping coincides with birth; they then take their first breath and all is well.

With the first few breaths, marked cardiovascular changes begin. The lung fluid is cleared and the alveoli expand and become able to exchange gas. With the exchange of gas, the oxygen tension rises and the carbon dioxide tension falls. The pulmonary arterioles dilate and pulmonary vascular resistance falls. This results in increased pulmonary blood flow. Decreased pulmonary pressure means that there is a reduction in blood flow through the ductus. Increased pulmonary blood flow raises the pressure in the left atria, which closes the foramen and reduces the flow between right and left sides of the heart (see Chapter 9).

Neonatal asphyxia

The pathophysiology of neonatal asphyxia is well documented; however, an overview is given briefly here.

The vicious cycle of neonatal asphyxia occurs when impaired gas exchange results in a rising fetal $Pa\text{CO}_2$ and a decreasing $Pa\text{O}_2$. This initiates gasping respiration. Unless this gasping results in satisfactory gas exchange and blood gas adjustment, the respiratory effort is temporarily suspended. This is known as primary apnoea and may last about 10 minutes. After this period, respiratory activity again commences, with rhythmic gasps of ever-increasing frequency and desperation. If gas exchange occurs at this point, spontaneous recovery is still possible. However, if satisfactory oxygenation exchange still does not take place the respiratory activity will decrease and once again cease. This is called terminal apnoea, and animal studies suggest that respiration will not spontaneously recommence (Dawes *et al.*, 1963).

The above are the respiratory patterns of the two stages, although both primary and terminal apnoea have associated effects on the cardiovascular system and profound implications for body tissues.

The debate as to whether the infant is in primary or secondary apnoea is not one that is likely to concern the midwife/neonatal nurse faced with initial resuscitation: it is largely of academic interest only. At the time, one does whatever is necessary to try and bring the infant round. The question becomes more important later, as the infant, once fully resuscitated and supported, starts to display behaviour associated with prolonged hypoxia/anoxia.

How long to continue resuscitation is a question which is often asked and there is no easy answer. Successful recovery has taken place in primates after 20 minutes of complete oxygen deprivation, but anecdotal evidence is all that is available for many cases of prolonged resuscitation of human babies. Abandonment of resuscitation is a decision which should be made by the most senior member of the team present at the time, after all reasonable methods have been tried. Often, the thought of having to tell or support the parents keeps people going far longer than is really justifiable.

BASIC EMERGENCY RESUSCITATION OF THE NEWBORN

There are several ways to identify the infant who needs resuscitation and to remember the priorities. This type of situation can overwhelm many people, who are not necessarily inferior nurses. Some people need longer to adjust to a situation but can then be more rational than those who adjust rapidly. Staff need to support each other during and after resuscitation calls.

The elderly but effective APGAR scoring system remains as useful in today's delivery rooms as it was when it was first developed in 1953. For convenience it is reproduced here as Table 4.1. Another aid is the alphabet prompt 'ABCDE', as described by Henderson (1988). An example of practice based on this logical sequence is given below.

Table 4.1 APGAR score

	Score		
Clinical feature	*0*	*1*	*2*
Heart rate	0	<100	>100
Respiration	Absent	Gasping or irregular	Regular or crying lustily
Muscle tone	Limp	Diminished or normal with no movements	Normal with active movements
Response to pharyngeal catheter	Nil	Grimace	Cough
Colour of trunk	White	Blue	Pink

A: Action

Start the clock, if you have one, or verbally announce the time. Someone will (hopefully!!) remember what time the resuscitation commenced. The clock is useful as a stopwatch to time heart and respiratory rate as well as being a time check on the length of resuscitation. Switch on oxygen and overhead heater, if available. Remove any wet towels from around the infant. Dry him and keep him warm.

A: Assessment of the infant

For the midwife/neonatal nurse there is little practical difference between the actions used to resuscitate term or preterm infants. From the nursing perspective, all potentially viable infants should be resuscitated, even if this means working on questionably viable infants of less than 24 weeks' gestation or those weighing less than 500 g. Resuscitation may fail or may be called off, but there is a difference between what a senior medical clinician will decide and what midwifery/nursing staff feel able to do. Midwives and neonatal nurses are not covered professionally or legally to diagnose death, however obvious, and have no legal duty to complete death certificates. In many cases the actual cause of death has to await a postmortem and certificates have to be completed by doctors. In view of the recent increase in litigation, the advice to continue with resuscitation until the arrival and support of medical colleagues is probably sound.

If you, as an experienced midwife/neonatal nurse, feel anxious then so will the senior house officer, so call someone senior. For the purpose of this book we assume that medical help is delayed.

A: Airway

A common reason for failing to establish a good respiratory pattern at birth is the presence of copious secretions in the upper airway. Once these are cleared, by suctioning, often no further intervention is needed and the infant can go, with his mother, to the postnatal areas. Such infants are usually vigorous and rate a high APGAR score in all other respects. They have been known to fight off would-be resuscitators. Time and experience with newborns in transitional status between womb life and independent existence allows one to distinguish between the genuine and the fraudulent.

B: Breathing and bagging

Infants who are making no respiratory effort at all, who are pale or blue, inactive and floppy need more vigorous attention. Typically these infants have low APGAR scores. After clearing the airway, tilt the head to the 'sniff position' and commence bag and mask ventilation with warm, humidified oxygen at a rate of approximately 60 breaths/min. It is vital that the appropriate size of bag and mask is used. A bag with a 250 ml reservoir may be insufficient to ventilate the very large infant, and 500 ml would probably be better. There is some debate as to which face mask is the most effective. Palme, Nystorm and Tunell (1985) suggested that a one-piece bag and mask was best as it did not come apart during resuscitation. When you next review the types of bag and mask in use, you may like to consider factors such as simplicity of use and ease of cleaning, as there have been reported cross-infections from bag use (Mehtar *et al.*, 1986).

Currently, a blow-off valve set at 30 cmH_2O is used but there is evidence that normal term infants use pressures in excess of 40–60 cmH_2O with their initial breaths, to open up their alveoli (Klause and Fanaroff, 1986), so that current practice may not be physiologically sound and may change with further research. In any case, maintain ventilation until the infant picks up and pinks up.

If bagging is prolonged a secure airway and continued ventilation is best achieved by assisting the doctor with endotracheal intubation. This is most often achieved using direct laryngoscopic vision, although finger intubation has been described (Hancock and Peterson, 1992). Severely compromised or small premature infants do not usually require sedation for intubation. Unless your paediatrician is very confident, muscle relaxants, given to aid intubation, are usually only used by anaesthetists.

Beware the big, term infant with sudden collapse and an empty-looking abdomen with a large hyperinflated-looking chest. Diaphragmatic herniation is rare, but manual bagging compromises this infant and intubation is preferable (Whitten, 1989).

C: Circulation and infant's colour

While bagging, get someone to check the apex heart rate

and react accordingly. If the heart rate is over 80 beats/min and improving, leave well alone but recheck in a few moments. If less than 80 and not improving, the infant's circulation needs supporting and so do you. If help is not already on the way, call for it now. Cardiac massage should be commenced at a ratio of five sternal compressions to one inflation, and this is sufficient to support the infant until senior medical help arrives. At any point during the resuscitation the infant may decide to self support: if this happens leave him to it but watch carefully.

Once the infant has picked up, pinked up and is self-supporting, keep the oxygen mask close to his face. Gradually reduce the amount of oxygen flowing but ensure that his colour remains pink.

D: Doctors, drugs and dextrose sticks

Once help arrives, the infant will be assessed and further medical intervention prescribed. He may be intubated to secure the airway and manual ventilation and cardiac massage may be continued if necessary. Pharmacological stimulation, manipulation and support of the heart may be prescribed and initiated. Venous access is crucial and should be obtained.

Get someone to record all medication that is given to support the infant. From experience, it is easy to lose track of what is given during an extended resuscitation – much more seems to be opened than is ever used (Table 4.2).

D: Decision

Does one transfer an apparently well infant to the NNU for observation or allow him to stay with his mother on the postnatal ward? There is no easy answer to this. Some postnatal wards are better equipped than others and some regions have excellent facilities, such as intermediate or transitional care units. Where the infant is nursed is irrelevant, as long as adequate observation is given to ensure a safe environment (Crawford, 1990).

E: Environment and evaluation

Keep the infant warm and get someone to check that the parents are aware of what is happening. Every resuscitation

Table 4.2 Drugs used in resuscitation

Naloxone	Occasionally, the type and amount of analgesic, e.g. pethidine, given to the mother during labour, can depress the infant's respiratory drive. Naloxone is an opiate antagonist and is best given intravenously; intramuscular administration is slower to act but allows for longer action.
Sodium bicarbonate	This is used to correct acidosis. It should be given well diluted, slowly, and with great care, as it is highly corrosive to tissue. Sudden infusions of base have been implicated in the development of intraventricular haemorrhage.
Adrenalin and calcium	These are occasionally used to increase the heart rate in persistent asystole or bradycardia. A major vein such as the umbilical vein should be used as calcium burns tissue. They should be diluted and given slowly. The dose should be flushed through with saline, prior to administration of subsequent medication. Calcium precipitates readily out of solution, so caution and care are required. Rarely, and in desperation, in the total absence of access lines to the circulation, adrenalin may be given down the endotracheal tube, but how much of it is usefully absorbed, when given this way, is debatable.
Dextrose	The badly asphyxiated infant is often hypoglycaemic. Instant reaction to the result of the dextrose stick is required. If possible, aim to avoid large bolus injections of strong dextrose solutions. Sudden swings to hyperglycaemia can cause the infant to release large amounts of insulin in response, and rebound hypoglycaemia can occur. Small amounts, given with care, and a maintenance infusion of 10% dextrose will be sufficient for many infants. Repeated checking of blood dextrose levels, until stable for 4–8 h is recommended.
Plasma protein fraction	This is useful as a volume expander in the hypotensive and shocked infant. It is also a 'buffer' and can help correct a mild acidosis. During resuscitation it requires time to deliver via an infusion pump and its action is not instant. It is mostly used during follow-on care.

is different; if they all seem to be the same, check that you are reacting to the individual needs of the infant and not in an automated policy-constrained manner. As soon as possible, after every resuscitation and regardless of outcome, evaluate the actions and performance of everyone involved, honestly. Much can be learned from the experience.

In many hospitals, ABCDE is insufficient to meet the needs of the infant, and then F: Flying squad transfer, is required.

FLYING SQUAD TRANSFER

The decision to part a newborn infant from his mother is not one which is taken easily. In addition, the plight of the father is not an easy one. Does he travel with his new infant or stay and comfort his wife? What about the infant's siblings who are marooned at home? There are no easy answers. Each case is different, but there should be clear benefits to the infant from transfer. Many transfers need not be the middle-of-the-night dramatic dash to a distant receiving centre. Many cases, e.g. those with Hirchsprung's disease, anal atresia etc., could be maintained for a few hours at the referring centre to allow the family to get to know their child.

Transfer is possible by road, helicopter or fixed-wing aircraft. All have advantages and disadvantages. The advantage of flying is only fully realized over long distances which, in the UK, is unusual; helicopter transfer could be used more in congested cities but depends on suitable landing facilities. The majority of transports in the UK are done by road. Let the ambulance personnel make the travel arrangements for you; it will save time and headaches. Occasionally the RAF and local flying clubs get involved and, if one is not careful, the entire transfer can degenerate into a media circus. The help of the police is useful; they know the quickest and most direct routes in strange cities, can miraculously clear a road of traffic and find somewhere to park the ambulance even at the most traffic-congested hospitals.

Emergency flying squads are not without risk. According to Clarke (1985), one of the major risks of neonatal transfer is exposure to inadequately trained personnel. This indictment was echoed by Macnab (1991), who analysed the mortality from paediatric transfers and recommended that all transport coordinators should review the qualifications and experience of their transport teams. There are few specialist neonatal transport teams in the UK, most probably for reasons of cost.

Ideally all transfers should be carried out by experienced people trained and equipped to deal with the situation. Working together as a team is one of the most important aspects of a successful transfer. Emergency situations tend to bring out the best in some people but the worst in others, and people whose personalities clash should not be sent together. Mutual respect and maximum cooperation between the respective team members can be assured by the sharing of training and study days. The composition of team members and equipment will vary between units and according to the different needs of the infant being transferred. Usually it includes:

- some form of transfer incubator. The ideal transport system is yet to be built. The latest, although expensive, are an improvement. They are lighter in weight and contain a lot of built-in supportive equipment, such as a suction unit with compartments for gloves and catheters etc. Supportive equipment and accessories for the older models needed to be fastened on 'somehow', and inevitably accessories got scattered, lost or damaged. Preset the suction strength to the optimum for the infant in transit; the back of an ambulance is not the place to have to fiddle with dials.
- ventilator and method of hand bagging;
- oxygen and spare cylinders, air compressor or cylinders;
- oxygen analyser and oxygen saturation monitor;
- cardiac monitor and spare leads;
- temperature monitor with probes
- apnoea monitor;
- means of measuring blood pressure. Runcie *et al.* (1990) were critical of the accuracy of oscillotonometric methods of measurement, and recommended direct measurement.
- infusion pumps, fluids and lines;
- crash case containing equipment for chest drains etc. and drugs;
- infant's notes, X-rays, details of identity, family etc.

Everything should be checked and rechecked to ensure that it is working properly and all batteries are fully charged. The ritual of checking is tedious and sometimes neglected when the unit is busy or when there has been a long period between squad calls; some units ensure regular and efficient checking by having a nurse or technician designated as responsible.

Also, when equipment is scarce, poaching from the transport system is liable to occur. This should be strictly prohibited.

The back of an ambulance is a hostile place in which to perform mobile intensive care. There is a big difference between what is ideal and what is actually possible. No infant who is critically unstable should be transferred, but there is a very real need to get him to expert help as soon as possible. This desire for infant stability often means spending time at the referring centre, working with the staff there, to stabilize his condition. Experienced assessment is needed to gauge the optimum time for travel.

Management of the squad call is an art: timing is vitally important. Once the request for a transfer comes through, the squad personnel should be contacted and assembled in time to meet the waiting ambulance. The emergency equipment should be checked (ideally by the people who are going to use it) and the referring unit telephoned to give estimated time of arrival and last-minute instructions on maintenance of the infant. Have some loose change for public telephones (or a mobile phone) and coffee machines handy; it could be a long haul.

On arrival at the referring centre

On arrival at the referring unit, do not go straight in and trespass on the infant, as this is liable to alienate people. Perhaps their methods are not the same as yours, but does it really matter? They have worked hard, often in poorly equipped and staffed situations. They have kept the baby alive, and in many cases have done much more. They deserve credit where due. If possible, take five minutes to read the baby's notes and record all the details you need. A proper handover is essential once the baby is stabilized.

Assess the baby's immediate needs. Use this as your baseline and measure all changes from this. Confer and plan (with your medical colleagues) any intervention needed. The main points are as follows:

- Evaluate the infant's respiratory status, with close attention to protecting the airway. If there is any question of his ability to self sustain, elective intubation is infinitely preferable to emergency intubation in the back of the ambulance. This also applies to a poorly secured endotracheal tube: if in doubt replace or retape the tube.

- Evaluate the infant's circulatory status, with assessment of the heart rate, pulse volumes, blood pressure and capillary refill time. Any deficit should be corrected by intravenous fluids. If this is insufficient and his circulation needs further support, inotropic vasopressors may be required. Large-volume fluid loss, during the trip, from open abdominal wall or spinal defects, can be minimized by the use of plastic wrap on the lesion (Paxton, 1990). Blood glucose can be maintained by appropriate infusion of dextrose.
- Evaluate the infant's thermal stability. Hypothermia causes an increase in metabolic rate and the increased use of glucose and oxygen may result in acidosis. If he is cold he should be slowly rewarmed, and careful attention to temperature during transit is vital.
- Evaluate the infant's gastrointestinal system. Disturbance of the middle ear, due to motion, can occur and may result in vomiting. Passage and aspiration of a nasogastric tube is recommended. Fitter infants should not be fed before or during transfer.
- Introduce yourselves to the parents as soon as possible.

Once the infant is stabilized, check all lines and secure all that could potentially fall out. Invariably the equipment will be of a different manufacture from your own transport equipment and time is spent applying probes and leads, in order to monitor the infant during transit. Synchronize the settings of the transport system (as closely as possible) to the system already supporting him. If he is intubated and ventilated, suck him out before transfer into the transport system, then recheck air entry. Give him a few moments to settle. Hopefully, he will remain pink, warm and well perfused.

Frischer and Gutterman (1992) considered the emotional impact on parents of transported infants: throughout this book we emphasize how vital the parents are to the infant, and their article is recommended reading. Try to spend a few last moments with the parents and check the infant's identity details. Give them detailed information regarding the receiving unit and back this up in writing. Take a last-minute photograph of the infant for the parents and find out when they will be able to visit. Then go.

In transit

Really accurate assessment of the infant during transit is difficult owing to lack of space, supportive equipment, noise, vibration and poor light. The squad team tends to rely on the readings of his vital signs as supplied by the monitors.

By air

Problems with transport are compounded if the transport is by air, due to noise, poor light and, usually, a cramped environment (Paxton, 1990). Altitude affects the management of the infant's physiology, especially if there are pneumothoraces or abdominal pathology, with trapped gas. With increasing altitude the barometric pressure will decrease and the volume of trapped gas will increase. Any air trapped in body cavities will expand proportional to the increase in altitude, and this may compromise the infant. Appreciation of this will enable the transport squad to anticipate and, to some extent, ameliorate difficulties in transporting an infant with a diaphragmatic hernia.

Another law of physics for the transport team to contend with is the fact that, with increasing altitude, the partial pressure of oxygen decreases. This results in a reduction in efficiency of oxygen diffusion across the alveolar membrane. To maintain a satisfactory level of oxygenation, there may need to be increasing adjustments made to the infant's inspired oxygen.

By road

This is slower, and going into a city at peak times can be frustrating, but many road users respect the blue light and will take evasive action. Looking over the shoulder of the driver to see what is happening on the road is usually more horrendous than anything that is happening in the back of the ambulance. The ambulance team know their vehicle and their job. They can be of immense help, especially during long hauls. Transport ventilators quickly use the oxygen in their small transport cylinders: ambulances carry large cylinders and the transport system can be reconnected to run on the ambulance supply. In addition, you can harness the ambulance's power supply and conserve the battery power of the transport system.

It is best not to recommend that the parents or relatives follow behind the ambulance. Motorists may tolerate assertive driving by an ambulance displaying a blue light, but will not be so forgiving for following vehicles. Fast driving puts people at risk, so it is best to let the relatives find the receiving hospital at their own pace. In some cases the parents may travel with the infant, but this is at the discretion of the transfer team and dependent on hospital policy.

In-transit documentation

The condition of the infant during transit must be documented. Light is often poor and time is at a premium. If time is spent writing copious notes, who is observing the infant? On the other hand, in an eventful action-packed journey details not noted at the time of occurrence risk being forgotten, owing to ever more urgent demands on the team's attention. The paperwork works best if it is simple in design and user friendly. Important details such as fluids administered in transit and changes to ventilator settings should be included. Figure 4.1 shows an example of 'in transit' documentation.

Measurement of quality in emergency neonatal transport

One of the major issues for neonatal nurses in the 1990s is the measurement of quality in the service we provide. Lesley (1993) has adapted a scoring system for use during transfers which takes into account five of the infant's physiological parameters: blood sugar, pH, Po_2, blood pressure and temperature, as a baseline on arrival at the referring centre, after stabilization prior to departure and on arrival at the receiving centre. Such a tool is doubly useful in that, as well as measuring the efficiency of a transfer team, it can add weight to any argument that transport by any means other than the optimum specialist paediatric team is false economy.

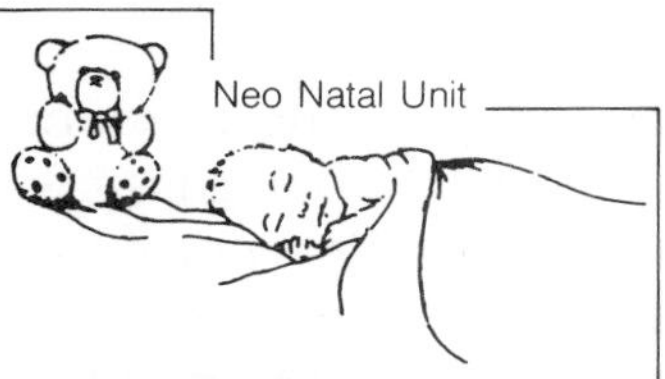

Neo Natal Unit

Leicester Royal Infirmary

Flying Squad / Transfer Record

Name of baby	Date of birth
Gestation	Age on transfer

Time of referral	Parent's names and emergency contact number
Referring Consultant	
Referring hospital	Names of ambulance crew
Accepting hospital	Nurse responsible for transfer
Accepting Consultant	Doctor responsible for transfer

Expected condition of baby / Information given to referring hospital.

Journey out	Date	Departure time	Arrival time
Journey back	Date	Departure time	Arrival time

Condition of baby on arrival / Action taken.

Fluid support	Drugs	Intravenous	UAC	Arterial	Long line	Other lines	

Time	Rate	Ratio	Pressures	FiO_2	S_aO_2	R.R.	H.R.	Probe temp	BM stix	Fluids	Fluids
		/	/								
		/	/								
		/	/								
		/	/								
		/	/								
		/	/								

Incidents during transfer / action taken

Figure 4.1 Flying squad transfer record.

Reverse transports

When considering transfers, many people only think of the dramatic dashes for survival. Of equal importance, is the 'routine' transfer of an infant from a specialist centre back to the local hospital. In theory this should go easily, as the infant is no longer so sick that he needs specialist intervention. It should be seen as promotion for the infant: a measure of his success and proof of his ability to survive. The benefits to the parents should be clear: it is closer to home and one step nearer discharge. From the specialist unit's point of view, it is a cost-effective means of ensuring continuing care which will free resources for more critical cases.

From the parents' point of view, the situation is less simple. Pleasure that the infant is well is tempered by anxiety that the hospital which, in their view, could not cope before is being asked to do so now and the staff who have become trusted and familiar will be replaced by strangers. To try and prevent potential problems arising from reverse transportation, the desirability of such a move should be introduced to the parents early on during the infant's stay. Staff from the referring hospital should be actively encouraged to keep in contact with the family and maintain links with the infant. The specialist hospital should consider sending regular written updates back to the hospital of referral.

Foundations for good interhospital relations can be maintained if staff at specialist hospitals are not dismissive of the referring hospital's actions and abilities. Parents should understand that there are several ways of applying care and approaching situations; one way is not necessarily superior to another.

Overdependence by parents on the staff of the specialist hospital can be overcome by including the family in all decisions concerning their infant. Their opinions should be respected and contributions valued. In this way, the staff act as facilitators in the relationship bond between the infant and the family by boosting the family's confidence and feelings of self worth. Once established, this will persist after transfer.

The largest boost to a successful transfer is planning and effective communication between the two hospitals and between the two sets of care staff. To best ensure this, Croop and Kenner (1990) suggested the formulation of protocols to meet the needs of these families. These will differ from unit to unit, but the idea is an excellent one.

Follow-up and continuing care

This should be arranged in advance of the transfer or discharge and should be the culmination of planned agreement with the families. There is often much stress and anxiety suffered by the parents on the discharge home of their infant, and doubts regarding their ability to cope. Often these are centred on fears of cot death, which the teaching of resuscitation skills to parents (Crawford and Marro, 1993) may help to alleviate.

ACKNOWLEDGEMENT

The author wishes to thank Andy Lesley RGN RSCN ENB 405, Neonatal Transport Co-ordinator, Nottingham Neonatal Service, for his generous help and advice in reviewing this chapter and for making helpful suggestions.

REFERENCES

Clarke, T. (1985) A review of neonatal transports. *Irish Medical Journal* **78**(2), 40–3.
Crawford, D.A. (1990) Transitional care – who cares? *Nursing* **4**(23), 9–12.
Crawford, D.A. and Marro, G. (1993) As easy as ABCD. *Paediatric Nursing* **5**(3) 12–13.
Croop, L. and Kenner, C. (1990) Protocol for reverse neonatal transports. *Neonatal Network* **9**(1), 49–53.
Dawes, G., Jacobson, H. *et al.* (1963) Treatment of asphyxia in newborn lambs and monkeys. *Journal of Physiology* **169**, 167–84.
Frischer, L. and Gutterman, D. (1992) Emotional impact on parents of transported babies. Consideration for meeting parents' needs. *Critical Care Clinics* **8**(3) 649–60.
Hancock, P. and Peterson, G. (1992) Finger intubation of the trachea in newborns. *Pediatrics* **89**(2), 325–7.
Henderson, C. (1988) Overwhelmed by infant resuscitation? Remember your ABCDE's. *Neonatal Network* **7**(3), 35–9.
Klaus, M. and Fanaroff, A. (1986) *Care of the High Risk Neonate*, W B Saunders, Philadelphia, pp. 31–5.
Lesley, A. (1993) Neonatal transport – quality issues. *Neonatal Nurses Yearbook*, CMA Medical Data Ltd., Cambridge.

Macnab, A. (1991) Optimal escort for interhospital transport of pediatric emergencies. *Journal of Trauma* **31**(2) 205–9.

Mehtar, S., Drabu, Y. *et al*. (1986) Cross infection with *Streptococcus pneumonia* through a resuscitare. *British Medical Journal* **292**(513), 25–6.

Milner, A. (1986) ABC of resuscitation; resuscitation at birth. *British Medical Journal* **292**, 1657–9.

Palme, C., Nystorm, B. and Tunell, R. (1985) An evaluation of the face masks used in resuscitation of the newborn. *Lancet* **1**, 207–10.

Paxton, J. (1990) Transport of the surgical neonate. *Journal of Perinatal and Neonatal Nursing* **3**(3), 43–9.

Runcie, C., Reeve, W., Reidy, J. and Dougall, J. (1990) Blood pressure measurement during transport. A comparison of direct and oscillotonometric readings in critically ill patients. *Anaesthesia* **45**, 659–65.

Whitten, C. (1989) *Anyone Can Intubate – a Practical Step by Step Guide for Health Professionals*, Medical Arts Press K-W Publications, San Diego, California.

5

Nursing care of babies who are born too soon or too small

Maryke Morris

The neonatal unit is renowned for having small babies in its care, but who are they and what are the special requirements of these patients?

TERMINOLOGY

The World Health Organization has set guidelines for the terminology of babies, depending on the length of gestation or birth weight. Gestation can be assessed from the mother's menstrual cycle, with gestation being measured from the first day of the last normal period, counting completed days or weeks only (Figure 5.1). Ultrasound scans of the fetus can also be performed to assess gestational age. Birth weight is taken as the first weight of the naked newborn, measured as soon after birth as possible (WHO, 1977).

Gestational classification

- Term: pregnancy lasting from 37 up to 42 completed weeks (259–293 days)
- Preterm: birth occurring before the 37th completed week (259 days)
- Post-term: birth occurring during or after 42 completed weeks (294 days)

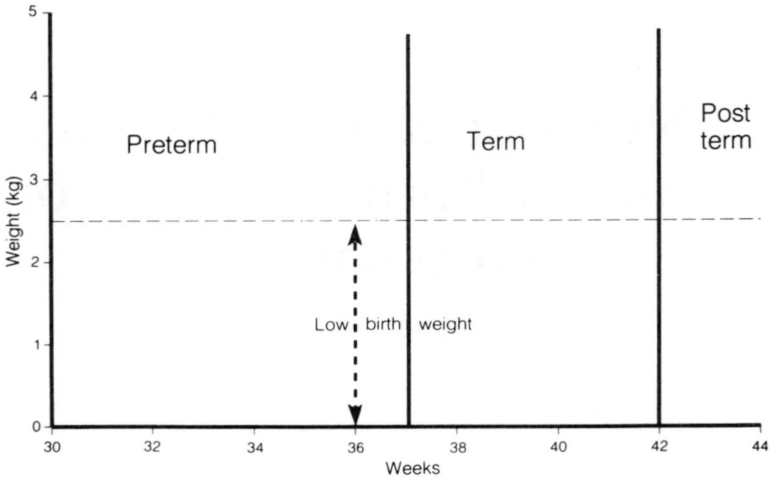

Figure 5.1 Classification by menstrual (gestational) age of fetus.

Assessment of maturity can be performed after birth by examination of external characteristics, combined with neurological signs. These include reflexes and posture exhibited by the newborn, for example, Dubowitz assessment (Appendix 2), which is carried out in the first 5 days of life (Dubowitz, Dubowitz and Goldberg, 1970).

Birth weight classification

- Low birth weight (LBW): birth weight less than 2.5 kg
- Very low birth weight (VLBW): birth weight less than 1.5 kg
- Extremely low birth weight (ELBW) or very very low birth weight (VVLBW): birth weight less than 1.0 kg

These classifications (gestation and birth weight) work independently of each other. To compare these two variables, a third classification system exists which draws its data from centile charts and is constructed appropriate for race and sociogeographic circumstances.

Weight for gestational age (Figure 5.2)

- Light for dates (LFD): babies below the 10th centile
- Heavy for dates (HFD): babies above the 90th centile

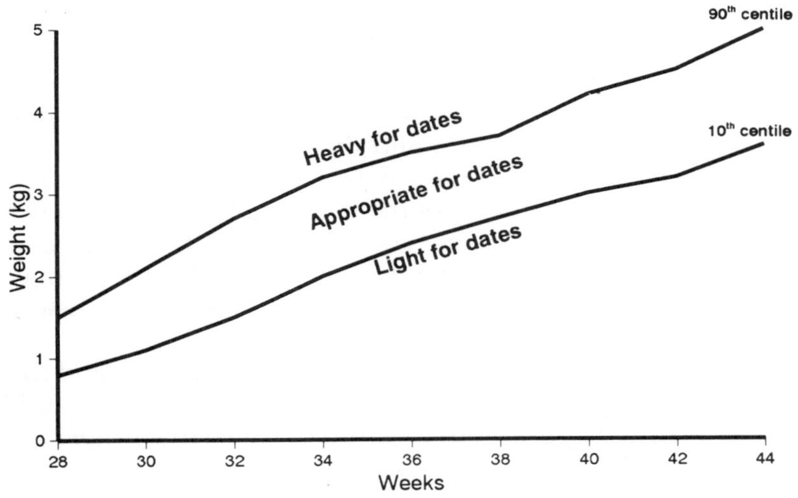

Figure 5.2 Weight for menstrual (gestational) age of fetus.

If other measurements are taken into account, for example length, chest and head circumference, and plotted on centile charts then an infant can be assessed as:

- small for dates (SFD) or small for gestational age (SGA): babies below the 10th centile;
- appropriate for dates (AFD) or appropriate for gestational age (AGA): babies between the 10th and 90th centiles;
- large for dates: babies above the 90th centile.

Intrauterine growth retardation (IUGR) is another term that is used synonymously with small for gestational age.

CHARACTERISTICS OF THE PRETERM BABY (BORN TOO SOON)

The preterm baby is a long-limbed tiny, skinny but fully formed infant, with a head and abdomen that appear out of proportion to the rest of his pink and hairy (lanugo) body. The finger- and toenails are perfectly formed, although the infant less than 24 weeks' gestation may have fused eyelids and very soft ears which can be easily bent due to the absence of cartilage. The bones of the skull are poorly mineralized and often overlapping, and can appear to move when the head is held. The preterm 'frog-like' posture is due to poorly developed muscle tone which cannot overcome the forces of gravity. Immature external genitalia are possible, the testes may not have descended into the scrotum and the female has a predominant labia minora due to the small labia majora. Respiration is controlled by movements of the diaphragm initiated via the abdomen, the ribs may be visible through the soft, thin transparent skin, and the baby will have a feeble cry. He may have a low birth weight and can be appropriate, light or heavy for dates.

Preterm birth can prevent the maturation of organs and the acquisition of passive immunity. Poor adaptation to extra-uterine life predisposes him to jaundice, digestive problems, metabolic and haematological disturbances.

CHARACTERISTICS OF THE LIGHT-FOR-DATES BABY (BORN TOO SMALL)

The light-for-dates baby does not always represent the term baby but smaller, although similarities may exist. The light-for-dates baby can be born at any stage of gestation, will have a weight below the 10th centile and may have a malnourished appearance, with folds of lax skin over the joints due to little subcutaneous fat and possible muscle wasting. The skin itself may be dry and rough and appear cracked over the hands, feet and abdomen. As growth retardation may take place at any time during pregnancy, the effects are variable depending when, and for how long, growth was suppressed. The baby, if born towards term, will have a mature cry and activity and muscle tone will be normal for gestation.

The absence of subcutaneous tissue and the relatively large surface area predisposes the light-for-dates infant to problems with thermoregulation. This, associated with small reserves of glycogen in the small liver, causes problems with hypoglycaemia. Feeding may not pose any problems, due to mature organ systems, but the baby is at risk of functional disturbances, and may have haematological problems. The light-for-dates infant may encounter difficulties around the time of birth, such as birth asphyxia and meconium aspiration because of hypoxia during the last part of pregnancy and fetal distress causing the passing of meconium *in utero*. Table 5.1 shows the contrasting features of appropriate-for-dates, preterm and light-for-dates malnourished infants.

Table 5.1 Contrasting features of appropriate-for-dates, preterm and light-for-dates malnourished infants. (From *Craig's Care of the Newly Born Infant* reproduced by kind permission of Churchill Livingstone)

Feature	*Preterm*	*Light for dates*
Definition	Born before 37 weeks' gestation	Birth weight below 10th centile for gestational age
Vernix	Present in variable amounts	Little or absent
Skin	Red and transparent	Dry, folds of lax skin
Subcutaneous tissue	Sparse	Sparse
Skull	Bones soft and pliable	Bones less pliable
Face	Doll-like	Mature
Abdomen	Prominent	Usually flat or scaphoid
Cord	Thick and fleshy	Thin, flabby and stained
Cry	Feeble	Mature
Muscle tone	Hypotonic, frog-like position	Variable, usually active
Complications	Hypothermia Respiratory distress syndrome Infection Cerebral haemorrhage Jaundice	Hypoglycaemia Hypocalcaemia Hypothermia

FACTORS CONTRIBUTING TO A PRETERM DELIVERY

Spontaneous premature labour can be caused by rupture of the membranes, placental abruption and intrauterine or urinary tract infection. Where there is an incompetent cervix, multiple pregnancy or less than 3 months between consecutive pregnancies, the risk of premature birth is increased. Maternal factors include poor nutritional status, small weight gain during pregnancy, very young age, history of a previous preterm delivery or midtrimester miscarriage, and some chronic disease states such as renal disease and hypertension. Preterm birth may be induced for the safety of the mother or baby in any of the following situations: severe pregnancy-induced hypertension, placental abruption, antepartum haemorrhage, severe IUGR, rhesus incompatibility affecting the fetus, or fetal distress.

FACTORS CONTRIBUTING TO A LIGHT-FOR-DATES BABY

Growth *in utero* can be reduced because of fetal, placental or maternal factors. Conditions in the fetus usually limit all aspects of growth, not just birth weight, and include dysmorphic syndromes and chromosomal abnormalities, along with congenital viral infection, exposure to X-rays and some drugs. Placental insufficiency, due to its small size, inappropriate siting on the wall of the uterus and reduced blood flow to one of twins can lead to a malnourished infant.

The health of the mother during pregnancy can influence the size of the fetus, with pregnancy-induced hypertension, and antepartum haemorrhage affecting growth. Preconceptual disease states, such as chronic hypertension, cyanotic heart disease, anaemia and malnutrition having the same effect. Maternal characteristics that predispose to a light-for-dates infant include having been a small baby herself or of small stature as an adult, extremes of age (less than 20 or older than 35 years), or being of Asian or West Indian origin. A firstborn child or a later-born infant of a mother who has previously had a light-for-dates infant, and the baby who is part of a multiple pregnancy, can all be small babies.

Socioeconomic factors exert an effect on birth weight. Smoking has a large influence on a baby being light for dates and has a synergistic effect when associated with social class. Lower social class and alcohol intake, unless in excess or associated with poor energy intake, may have little effect on birth weight (Brooke *et al.*, 1989).

NURSING CARE OF THE BABY BORN TOO SOON OR TOO SMALL

Nutrition

The preterm baby, born before 32–34 weeks' gestation, may

have a poor sucking and swallowing reflex. There can be difficulty in tolerating milk feeds, due to small gastric capacity and an immature digestive system, resulting in vomiting, reflux and regurgitation (Levene, Tudehope and Thearle, 1987), with the risk of aspiration, diarrhoea and poor weight gain (Kelnar and Harvey, 1987, p. 93).

Milk can be given via a nasogastric tube to overcome the absent suck reflex. This starts with small, frequent volumes (e.g. 1 ml/h), increasing this as it is tolerated (for example 1 ml every 4–12 h). If gastric feeds are not being tolerated, jejunal/transpyloric feeding or parenteral nutrition is required. Nasojejunal tube feeds involve a continuous infusion of milk, starting with low volumes.

The LFD infant may be able to suckle some of his feeds but the need for very frequent (1–3 hourly) feeding and the high energy expenditure associated with sucking may mean that some feeds are given by nasogastric tube to allow the infant to rest. If the baby is very sick, whether preterm or light-for-dates, gastric feeding may be poorly tolerated or contraindicated, especially if the baby has severe respiratory function, an umbilical catheter *in situ* or gastrointestinal disturbance. Chapter 7 discusses feeding the low birth weight infant in further detail.

Unstable blood sugars

Hypoglycaemia

These infants have reduced energy stores, a high rate of glucose utilization, and are at risk of hypoglycaemia (laboratory blood sugar less than 1.7 mmol/l or blood sugar stick reading less than 2.2 mmol/l (Fleming, Speidel and Dunn, 1986). Some form of feeding should be instituted as soon as possible and combined with keeping glucose utilization to a minimum by keeping the baby warm, well oxygenated and stress free.

Blood sugar estimates need to be performed at birth and repeated every 4 hours in the first 24 hours (or more) until stable. Unless the level is falling or the baby is hypoglycaemic, the interval between readings can then be increased. Coordinating all blood sampling together reduces the trauma to the infant.

Symptoms of hypoglycaemia include limpness, apathy, jittery limbs, slow feeding and apnoea attacks. Smaller, more frequent enteral feeds or a continuous intravenous dextrose infusion can be given to counteract falling blood sugar levels (Pildes and Pyati, 1986), and in severe hypoglycaemia a small bolus of dextrose may be necessary. In very low birth weight babies, blood glucose levels can fall very quickly and need careful monitoring during the infusion of drugs, plasma and blood, in which case a second i.v. access may be beneficial.

Hyperglycaemia

Hyperglycaemia (blood glucose levels greater than 8 mmol/l) (Fleming, Spiedel and Dunn, 1986) has been found to be a problem most usually in the preterm infant. This can be because of intolerance to the dextrose in an intravenous infusion, immaturity, stress, RDS, infection, dehydration, certain drugs and some surgical procedures (Pildes and Pyati, 1986). Nursing care involves monitoring blood glucose levels (as above) and testing urine for glycosuria using dipsticks or Clinitest tablets. Intravenous solutions may need adjusting to a lower concentration or insulin infusion commenced, as appropriate. Other causal factors have to be identified and treated appropriately.

Temperature regulation

Both the preterm and the light-for-dates baby have small deposits of brown adipose tissue and glycogen to act as an energy store. They have little subcutaneous fat to provide insulation from a cool environment and a source of energy. The extended posture of a preterm baby and the relatively large surface area increases the heat loss through the skin. This, coupled with the preterm baby's inability to shiver and immature hypothalmus, leads to poor thermoregulation, which is further impaired if a baby is infected, has low oxygen levels (less than 4 kPa), poor circulation, and/or if the energy intake is either inadequate or has to be used for tissue repair and/or maintaining respiration.

To help minimize the energy expenditure associated with thermoregulation and keeping the baby warm, thus preventing cold stress, the infant needs to be nursed in a thermally neutral environment (Appendix 3), which may mean that he is placed in an incubator or heated open cot, or is dressed and wrapped up in a cot in a warm room, depending on his size and ability to keep warm. The thermal neutral environment is the temperature of the surroundings which will maintain the baby's core temperature (36.5 °C–37 °C per axilla) with the minimum oxygen usage and energy expenditure (Kelnar and Harvey, 1987, p. 96). A baby who is too warm or too cold will try to regulate his temperature, often with detrimental effects in the preterm or light-for-dates baby.

An infant with a low core temperature (less than 36 °C) is at risk of cold stress, which increases oxygen requirements, energy expenditure, susceptibility to infection and cerebral haemorrhage. Enzyme activity and surfactant production is impaired. The cold baby with respiratory distress, cardiac or gastrointestinal problems can have his illness worsened, as he is unable to respond to the increased need for oxygen shown by apnoea and bradycardia, hypoxia and acidosis, whereas an unmet energy requirement and reduced efficiency of enzymes causes hypoglycaemia and an increased weight loss. The cold infant needs to be warmed up gradually at a rate of 1 °C/h. If the hypothermia remains untreated or is already severe, neonatal cold injury and death can occur.

Hyperthermia has similar effects on the body as the infant attempts to regulate his temperature by losing heat through increasing respiratory rate and fluid losses via evaporation, which can increase weight loss, dehydration and jaundice. Apnoea and restlessness can occur as the result of heat stress. Any of these cooling mechanisms can affect the infant's homeostasis and hold on life.

Heat exchange mechanism

Convection is the loss of heat from the baby to the cold air. A warmed incubator or heated cot with a lid, or a perspex heat shield, warms the air surrounding the baby, minimizing cooling. Opening the incubator porthole creates cool draughts and consideration of the baby's temperature stability is important every time access is required.

Conduction occurs when heat is transferred from the body to a surface in contact with the skin, and so a baby should never be laid on a cold surface. Dressing and wrapping the baby in blankets prevents heat loss to a cool mattress or unheated cot. In a baby too sick to dress, covering the mattress with sheepskin reduces heat loss. Cold hands and equipment, e.g. stethoscopes, or X-ray plates, touching the warm body can also cause the baby to lose heat.

Evaporation occurs when liquid condenses on the skin. Drying the baby at birth and keeping him as dry as possible, during washing and when nursed without a nappy, eliminates heat loss through evaporation. Similarly, warming any gases and infusions administered to ambient/body temperature prevents cooling. The very preterm baby may respond to the use of humidity and clingfilm coverings, especially in the first week of life when the skin is forming a waterproof keratin layer (Levene, Tudehope and Thearle, 1987, p. 109).

Radiation is the loss of heat from the baby to all surrounding areas. It can occur in the delivery room, in an incubator that has not been prewarmed, or when a baby is naked. The preterm baby and his splayed posture increases the surface area exposed to the environment and contributes to heat loss. A double-walled incubator and perspex shield over a naked baby can reduce radiant heat losss, as can dressing the baby and nursing him in a warm environment.

Temperature recording

Axillary temperature readings need to be taken with care: constant temperature recordings can be taken by skin probes attached to the abdomen (core) and shin (skin) temperature. A fall in the skin temperature occurs before changes to the core, and hence an early warning system exists. The preterm infant often experiences difficulties in maintaining warm peripheries (36–36.5°C) because of low blood pressure and vasoconstriction, detected by the shin probe, indicating the need for additional coverings and bootees, as his condition allows, and correction of the cause.

Breathing problems

Respiratory distress, caused by immaturity of the lungs, is a common problem in the preterm infant, necessitating the need for additional inspired oxygen or intubation and ventilation according to the severity.

The light-for-dates infant, although having mature lungs, may have experienced respiratory insults *in utero* or at birth. He may require careful and constant monitoring, headbox oxygen or total ventilatory support. The care of such a baby is discussed in Chapter 8. These infants are prone to apnoea and bradycardia, whch requires early detection. This is achieved by nursing the baby on an apnoea mattress with a cardiorater, with the alarms set. Periodic recordings of the vital signs of heart and respiratory rate, colour, respiratory difficulty and oxygenation levels are valuable in identifying trends and the current and previous status of the infant, thus enabling plans for care to be made and evaluated. Any bradycardic or apnoeic episodes (and the nursing intervention required) should be charted, along with any associated factors, e.g. during feeding. Chapter 9 gives further explanations as to the care of a baby with bradycardia.

Haematological and vascular disturbances

Intraventricular haemorrhage

Intraventricular haemorrhage (IVH) is common in the preterm baby. The baby's capillaries are fragile and can easily be ruptured as a consequence of hypoxia and variable cerebral blood pressure, causing bleeding into the germinal matrix. To reduce the risk of IVH, nursing care aims at preventing situations that can dramatically alter cerebral blood flow, such as turning the head sharply to one side and sudden handling (Kling, 1989), which is further discussed in Chapter 10. The term LFD infant has a more stable capillary network and IVH is a rarity *per se*, unless associated with other causative factors.

Anaemia

The sick preterm baby undergoes many investigations requiring blood samples, may suffer acute or chronic blood loss and has poor iron stores. Acute blood loss can occur intrapartum, for example due to placental abruption, or after a postpartum bleed, such as intracranial, pulmonary or gastro-intestinal haemorrhage, or from a leaking cannula or umbilical cord. Chronic anaemia may be the result of chronic blood loss (for example from the gastrointestinal tract or due to repeated blood sampling), haemolytic disease, prematurity, infection, drugs and vitamin deficiences (Fleming, Spiedel and Dunn, 1986). Twin to twin transfusion *in utero* can cause one infant to be anaemic during the first week of life and the other to be polycythaemic.

Treatment may be needed and involves the identification and resolution of the underlying cause as well as correction of the low haemoglobin status. A 'top-up transfusion' of packed paediatric cells may be prescribed if the baby has RDS, hypotension, a haemoglobin level of less than 8 g/dl or shows clinical signs of anaemia or heart failure (Roberton, 1987). Chronic anaemia occurring as a consequence of poor iron stores and vitamin deficiencies in the older preterm infant is treated with oral iron, folate or vitamin E preparations from 6 weeks of age, allowing the baby's own bone marrow to respond and produce red blood cells.

Polycythaemia

The LFD infant may also become anaemic if repeated blood specimens are taken, although the haemoglobin levels, to begin with, are often higher than normal for the newborn, because of placental insufficiency or transfusion, maternal smoking, twin to twin transfusion, cold stress or hypoxia, all of which can cause polycythaemia (Fleming, Spiedel and Dunn, 1986). A plethoric infant may exhibit neurological, cardiovascular and renal problems due to a diminished blood flow through the small capillaries, and is at increased risk of necrotizing enterocolitis. Observation and early detection of any of these problems, for example seizures, heart failure, cyanosis, oliguria, renal failure, transient tachypnoea, jaundice, poor feeding and hypoglycaemia, requires nursing vigilance and the appropriate care needs to be given. Polycythaemia is treated by a plasma infusion to dilute the blood (Leven, Tudehope and Thearle, 1987) and increasing the fluid input.

Hypotension

Low blood pressure is common in the sick preterm baby because of shock, low blood volume at birth, or as a consequence of haemorrhage, dehydration, drugs (e.g. pancuronium, tolazoline), sepsis and adapting to extrauterine life (Cabal, Larrazabal and Siassi, 1986; Roberton, 1987). It is further compounded by the reduction in venous return and cardiac function, as occurs in a ventilated baby (Roberton, 1987). Hypotension and poor perfusion require treatment with a continuous infusion of one or more vasolidators or a transfusion of plasma or blood, depending on the cause and packed cell volume (Roberton, 1987). Continuous arterial blood pressure monitoring with hourly recording or non-invasive manual readings are part of the nursing care of the sick preterm baby, and a gradual or sudden decrease in the mean blood pressure should be reported immediately to the medical staff. A table of the expected mean blood pressure according to age and weight appears in Chapter 9.

Ductus arteriosus

The ductus arteriosus often remains open or reopens in a sick preterm infant, giving rise to problems in maintaining oxygenation levels, increasing and prolonging the need for mechanical ventilation as well as the possibility of apnoea and cardiac failure. First-line therapy is restriction of the fluid intake, necessitating careful assessment of fluid balance as diuretic therapy may also be prescribed. The infant should be kept well oxygenated, with respiratory support increased as needed since hypoxia can keep the duct open (Fleming, Spiedel and Dunn, 1986). If the duct fails to close, then treatment is either with drugs (indomethacin), which have their own side effects, or ligation, in which case the baby has to be well enough to tolerate surgery. (See Chapter 9 for further details).

Jaundice

Jaundice is a problem that both types of infant may experience. In the preterm, it may be more pronounced and prolonged due to functionally immature organ systems. Jaundice results from haematological disturbances, e.g. polycythaemia and dehydration, in the light-for-dates infant. Serum bilirubin estimates need to be monitored and phototherapy instituted as necessary, with care given as in Chapter 13.

Renal function

The immature kidneys of a preterm baby are unable to conserve fluid and sodium, causing oliguria and metabolic acidosis, and are susceptible to damage by poor perfusion and certain drugs (Guignard and John, 1986). If the baby is very immature the kidneys may be unable to function, so that very little urine is passed. The LFD baby is prone to renal damage and failure as a consequence of hypoxia and polycythaemia.

Fluid balance requires the accurate charting of urinary output, and dipstick tests for specific gravity, pH, blood, glucose, bilirubin and protein have to be completed on each specimen in the first 24 hours and then daily unless there are abnormal results or urine output is still a cause for concern. If the infant is receiving parenteral or intravenous nutrition, then the nurse should obtain a urine specimen for electrolyte status and send this to the laboratory daily. Other measures of fluid balance, such as dehydration, oedema and urinary volume, need observation and appropriate action taken, as the preterm baby has a narrow tolerance range with respect to water and mineral load and is susceptible to damage from reduced perfusion and drugs (Richardson, 1991).

Insensible water losses need consideration in the preterm baby due to the thin unkeratinized skin and large surface area, and are increased with overhead radiant heaters, phototherapy and infant activity (Richardson, 1991). Care for susceptible infants is planned to reduce the loss of moisture from the skin. Newborn preterm babies may benefit from the addition of humidification to the incubator, and any infant receiving phototherapy should have his fluid requirements increased, depending on the unit policy.

Electrolyte imbalances can occur in both LFD and preterm infants, and these are corrected by additives to intravenous and milk feeds. Potassium supplements should not be given unless renal function is established (Richardson, 1991).

Prevention and control of infection

The preterm infant is susceptible to infection because little passive immunity was obtained *in utero* and the mechanisms for dealing with bacteria and viruses are immature. From the 20th week of gestation IgG is actively and passively transported across the placenta, and lymphocyte function is developed by 28 weeks. Antibodies can be synthesized by the B lymphocytes by the end of the second trimester, providing there is some IgG available. IgG assists in the synthesis of antigens and enables the baby to receive passive immunity from his mother. Immunoglobulin of the A and M types are not present in the newborn, and this reduces the phagocytic activity of leucocytes. Intravenous infusion of immunoglobulin can be given to the preterm very low birth weight baby (Roberton, 1993, p. 192).

Both types of infant are at risk of nosocomial infection, which the nurse can help to reduce by adhering to the infection control procedures of the unit, using clean equipment, strict and thorough handwashing between babies and procedures, and teaching parents the same. Chapter 12 deals specifically with infection.

The umbilical cord and its necrosis can be a focus of infection for bacteria that colonize the skin of the newborn. The risk of umbilical-related infection is increased when the infant is preterm, admitted to the neonatal unit, has an umbilical catheter inserted, or *in utero* had prolonged ruptured membranes (Korones, 1986; Roberton, 1993, p. 194). Care of the umbilical cord varies between units. Some advocate cleaning with an alcohol wipe, others suggest dusting with Sterzac powder, and elsewhere the cord stumps are left alone to heal. Bain (1993) found that cleaning the cord with an alcohol wipe and dusting with Sterzac powder resulted in less cord-related infection and a shorter time to cord separation, compared to any other cord care regime. The sick ventilated infant may have an umbilical catheter *in situ*, in which case no preparations are usually applied to the skin, but as the catheter can act as a mode of entry for pathogens (Roberton, 1986) the condition of the umbilical stump and surrounding skin is checked hourly for redness, inflammation, discharge and other signs of infection.

Care of the skin

Nappy changing is an important part of the infant's nursing care. The LFD baby may have no special care requirements and nappy changes can be performed 4–6 hourly, before feeds or as required. A sick or preterm baby, although needing to have a clean bottom, may also require minimal handling as even a simple nappy change could exhaust him. Eight to twelve-hourly nappy changes is not deficient nursing care with the sickest baby, provided that the perineum and buttocks are not reddened or sore and that the skin is intact. If the baby's buttocks are sore, then more frequent changes may be indicated, or nursing the baby with the buttocks exposed to promote healing and comfort and using a heat shield to maintain warmth.

The dry cracked skin of the LFD infant and friable skin of the preterm baby poses an infection hazard, which is minimized by keeping the skin clean and dry and preventing colonization. Any sore or broken areas require daily inspection and a swab for microbiology taken if the skin looks inflamed or weepy. Applying a dry, non-adherent dressing provides a barrier to ambient bacteria. Topical or systemic antibiotic therapy may be prescribed as a local infection can soon spread in the newborn.

Dry skin can be massaged with sunflower oil or baby lotion, provided the baby does not require phototherapy and the skin is not broken. A dressing may be applied for protection.

The amount, type and removal of tape requires forethought with the preterm infant, as the skin can easily tear and scar. Probes used against the skin, for example temperature and transcutaneous monitors, should be resited daily or 4 hourly, to prevent the skin from burning.

Pressure area care

Pressure sores can occur in the sick immobile or paralysed baby. Nursing on a sheepskin with covered intravenous fluid bags as a waterbed, with soft linen and blankets, combined with changing the baby's position with care procedures, are nursing activities which help maintain skin integrity. Position the baby so that any areas requiring constant observation are visible, ensuring that he is not laid against any wires or tubing which could both be uncomfortable and create pressure, while respecting his need for comfort and contact.

Mouth care

Any infant who is not having oral feeds benefits from having his mouth cleaned with cotton buds and sterile water (which he may enjoy sucking), not only to refresh the mouth but, by keeping the mucus membranes moist, avoiding a potential route of infection. Oral candidosis is common with antibiotic therapy, and so the compromised preterm baby will require treatment with an antifungal agent (both oral suspension and topical application to the buttocks may be prescribed).

Promoting rest and sleep

The LFD infant may have no additional problems with regard to rest and sleep requirements except for needing plenty (about 20 hours a day). Chapter 14 discusses ways in which the neonatal nurse can promote rest and sleep. Unfortunately, this is a problem for the preterm baby, who requires plenty of rest and sleep to conserve energy and develop normally but his often critical condition supersedes this requirement. A preterm baby may require short periods of rest between nursing interventions so that he can recuperate and stabilize oxygen levels (Speidel, 1978) and, if very sick, a continuous infusion of analgesia will alleviate suffering associated with handling.

Positioning

The preterm baby is at risk of craniofacial deformity because of the tendency to nurse these babies prone, with their head to the side, resting on the firm mattress. In this position the infant is unable to turn his head and the pressure of the rapidly developing brain exerts a flattening effect on the immature, poorly mineralized bone. This scenario is the opposite of that found *in utero*, where the head is supported by the amniotic fluid and can develop spherically as the brain grows. Resting the baby's head on a soft waterbed, beanbag or pillow, instead of a hard mattress, may reduce the amount of bilateral flattening of the head as a soft pliable support moulds around the head. Likewise, nursing the preterm infant in a supported supine position so that it is the back of the head that takes the weight of the brain rather than the sides, as occurs when the baby is nursed prone with the head to one side, have been suggested and investigated to reduce the elongated head of the preterm infant (Chubby, 1991). If the head is elevated on a soft support, then consideration needs to be made as to the degree of flexion to the neck. This can be overcome by laying all of the baby on the waterbed, beanbag or pillow, or placing additional sheepskins and blankets under the baby's body.

The preterm baby has very poor muscle control and, due to his early birth, has not experienced natural flexion, as occurs in the womb (Turrill, 1992), so that normal development may be impaired. The full-term light-for-dates infant does not have these disadvantages, although all babies will respond to proper positioning and handling so that the body is kept in alignment, as discussed in Chapter 15 (Rushton, 1986; Turrill, 1992).

A baby should be nursed in supported positions, maintaining symmetrical flexion with the head in the midline when possible, thereby promoting comfort and security. These positions can be maintained by bedding rolls and soft toys (Rushton, 1986; Turrill, 1992) and should be planned according to the baby's needs and development. A baby lying on his side will appreciate a support in the form of a rolled blanket or suitably sized soft toy behind his back and head, and something interesting in front of him to flex towards and gain tactile stimulation. No one position should be used extensively, as it can cause skeletal deformities and fixed positioning (Turrill, 1992), but rotating with care procedures and the exercising of the joints through their full range of movement, as the baby's condition allows, is good nursing care.

The preterm baby has to undergo a rapid and early adaptation to extrauterine life, requiring changes in all the systems, some of which may still be relatively immature and unable to function adequately. The baby born too small may not experience fuctional disturbances due to immaturity, but reduced growth *in utero* may predispose the baby to imbalances and problems in the newborn period.

REFERENCES

Bain, J. (1993) Umbilical cord care. *The Neonatal Nurses Year Book 1993*, Neonatal Nurses Association.

Brooke, O.G., Anderson, H.R., Bland, J.M. *et al.* (1989) Effects on birth weight of smoking, alcohol, caffeine, socioeconomic factors and psychological stress. *British Medical Journal*, **498**, 795–801.

Cabal, L.A., Larrazabal, C. and Siassi, B. (1986) Hemodynamic variables in infants weighing less than 1000 grams. *Clinics in Perinatology* **13**(2), 327–38.

Chubby, C. (1991) Craniofacial deformation in premature infants. *Paediatric Nursing* **3**(2), 19–21.

Dubowitz, L.M.S., Dubowitz, V. and Goldberg, C. (1970) Clinical assessment of gestational age in the newborn infant. *Journal of Pediatrics* **77**(1), 1–10.

Fleming, P.J., Speidel, B.D. and Dunn, P.M. (1986) *A Neonatal Vade-Mecum*, Lloyd-Luke (Medical Books) Ltd, London.

Guignard, J.P. and John, E.G. (1986) Renal function in the tiny premature infant. *Clinics in Perinatology* **13**(2), 377–401.

Kelnar, C.J.H. and Harvey, D. (1987) *The Sick Newborn Baby*, 2nd edn, Baillière Tindall, London.

Kling, P. (1989) Nursing interventions to decrease the risk of periventricular intraventricular hemorrhage. *Journal of Obstetrics, Gynaecology and Neonatal Nursing* **18**(6), 457–64.

Korones, S.B. (1986) High Risk Newborn Infants, 4th edn, Mosby, St Louis, Mo., Chapter 13.

Levene, M.I., Tudehope, D. and Thearle, J. (1987) *Essentials of Neonatal Medicine*, Blackwell Scientific Publications, Oxford.

Pildes, R.S. and Pyati, S.P. (1986) Hypoglycaemia and hyperglycaemia in tiny infants. *Clinics in Perinatology* **13**(2), 351–75.

Redshaw, M.E., Rivers, R.P.A. and Rosenblatt, D.B. (1985) *Born Too Early*, Oxford University Press, Oxford.

Richardson, K. (1991) Renal function in the neonate: an overview. *Neonatal Network* **10**(4), 17–23.

Roberton, N.R.C. (1986) *A Manual of Neonatal Intensive Care*, 2nd edn, Edward Arnold, London.

Roberton, N.R.C. (1987) Top up transfusions in neonates. *Archives of Diseases in Childhood* **62**, 984–6.

Roberton, N.R.C. (1993) *A Manual of Neonatal Intensive Care*, 3rd edn, Edward Arnold, London.

Rushton, C.H. (1986) Promoting normal growth and development in the hospital environment. *Neonatal Network* **4**(6), 21–30.

Speidel, B.D. (1978) Adverse effects of routine procedures on preterm infants. *Lancet* **1**, 864–5.

Turner, T.L., Douglas, J. and Cockburn, F. (1988) (eds) *Craig's Care of the Newly Born Infant*, 8th edn, Churchill Livingstone, Edinburgh.

Turrill, S. (1992) Neonatal nursing: supported positioning in intensive care. *Paediatric Nursing* **4**(4), 24–7.

World Health Organization (1977) *Manual of International Statistical Classification of Diseases, Injuries and Causes of Death*, Vol 1, WHO, Geneva.

6

Nursing care of a baby with a disorder of the gastrointestinal system

Maryke Morris

Many gastrointestinal disorders are congenital malformations and some of these can be identified antenatally by ultrasound scan. In these cases, parents can prepare for the events that will occur immediately after delivery. For others, the defect is not suspected until after the birth and comes as a major shock. Table 6.1 gives the major conditions which can occur.

Table 6.1 Major gastrointestinal disorders in the newborn

Upper GI disorders
Oesophageal atresia (with or without tracheo-oesophageal fistula)
Pyloric stenosis
Lower GI disorders
Imperforate anus
Necrotizing enterocolitis (NEC)
Rectal Fistula
Hirschprung's disease
Middle GI disorders
Diaphragmatic hernia
Small/large bowel atresia
Meconium ileus
Volvulus
Malrotation
Necrotizing enterocolitis (NEC)
Gastroschisis
Omphalocele
Inguinal hernia
Duodenal obstruction
Intussusception

Space prevents the discussion of all gastrointestinal disturbances, and so three have been chosen: oesophageal atresia and tracheo-oesophageal fistula, necrotizing enterocolitis and gastroschisis, as these effectively cover a wide range of nursing care.

NURSING CARE OF A BABY UNDERGOING SURGERY

The baby (and his family) need preparing for surgery, ensuring that the safety and wellbeing of the baby is maintained, unit policies are adhered to and informed consent is obtained from the parents.

Nursing observations

The infant is weighed and baseline observations, including level of respiratory support required, are made and these are recorded in the notes to act as a reference after surgery. Monitoring the vital signs continues with hourly recordings; any deviations from the baby's usual parameters should be reported to the medical staff.

Assessing haematological status

The baby's haemoglobin, urea and electrolyte status is assessed and recorded before surgery. Maternal blood may be required for cross-matching (Wallis, 1982). Most units still recommend the administration of vitamin K to all newborn babies as prophylaxis, but there is some debate that vitamin K, given in the first week of life, is associated with an increased incidence of childhood cancer (Golding, Paterson and Kinlen, 1990). Conversely, not giving vitamin K can increase the risk of haemorrhagic disease and intraventricular haemorrhage (Kelsall, 1992) and, therefore high-risk babies (including those undergoing surgery) should be given it.

Meeting nutritional requirements

The last enteral feed should be given not less than 4 hours prior to surgery, with the time and amount of feed recorded in the notes. An intravenous infusion of dextrose is started to maintain hydration and blood sugars. This is calculated according to the baby's weight, age and fluid requirements. The rate, volume infused and condition of the cannula site need checking and recording hourly. Blood sugar levels are checked with a blood glucose stick and recorded, both to give a preoperative baseline and to check tolerance to the dextrose.

Parental consent and knowledge

Obtaining informed consent is the doctor's responsibility, explanations are reinforced and appropriate leaflets are given when necessary. The parents may be in a state of shock after the birth and the discovery that there was something wrong with their child (Klaus and Fanaroff, 1986). Chapter 1 discusses the care of the family and the parental responses expected when a baby is admitted to a neonatal unit.

Transportation to and from theatre

The principles of transfer described in Chapter 4 apply to ensure the warmth and safety of the infant going to theatre.

NURSING CARE OF A BABY AFTER SURGERY

Supporting respiration

Many babies require ventilatory assistance for the first few hours due to the effects of surgery, the wound and to control pain. Once the baby is stable and making effective respiratory efforts, weaning off the ventilator into headbox oxygen, if necessary, can commence. Discussion of the care of a ventilated baby is given in Chapter 8.

Care of the operation site

The wound site should be checked hourly and the dressing should be visible at all times, to enable any bleeding or serious leakage to be noted. Any drainage should be measured and charted and its character noted. Some drainage, e.g. gastric aspirate, may need to be replaced to prevent the loss of valuable electrolytes.

Nursing observations

Observations, including blood pressure and temperature, should be recorded hourly. All vital signs should be continuously monitored and alarm limits appropriately set. Any deviations from the normal parameters should be recorded as they occur and investigated. Indications of haemorrhage (increased heart rate, falling blood pressure and pallor) and infection (raised temperature, widening temperature gap, bradycardia etc.) should be further investigated.

Altered gut function

To help minimize abdominal distension after abdominal surgery and to aid decompression, a nasogastric tube is passed and left on free drainage with 4 hourly aspiration of the stomach contents. Nasogastric aspirates are often replaced by intravenous infusion of 0.9% sodium chloride ml for ml. Conventionally, this is calculated by totalling the nasogastric loss from free drainage and aspiration for the last 4 hours and replacing the same amount with normal saline over the next 4 hours.

Before enteral feeding is considered drainage from the nasogastric tube should be minimal and not bile stained. Bowel sounds and activity should have returned.

Meeting nutritional requirements

After major surgery, the baby should not be fed orally but by intravenous infusion. Blood glucose levels should be performed 4–8 hourly. Gastric feeding normally begins with the return of normal gut activity and function. It is usually started slowly via a nasogastric tube (see Chapter 7). The volume of feed can be increased, depending on the baby's condition and the i.v. rate reduced accordingly. Some units have a policy of giving clear fluids first and quickly graduating to milk (Wallis, 1982).

If the baby has had stomach or bowel surgery, then it may be several weeks before enteral feeds can be recommenced. In these situations, a long line/central line is sited and total parenteral nutrition (TPN) prescribed. The patency and sterility of this line must be maintained and fluids changed daily using an aseptic technique.

Assessment of fluid balance

Urine and bowel activity are recorded in the nursing documentation. If urine has not been passed 4–6 hours after surgery, or is less than 1 ml/kg/h, then a doctor should be informed.

Maintaining warmth and comfort

Nursing the baby in a warmed incubator or heated cot, set at the thermoneutral environment (Appendix 3) will allow for full visualization as well as reducing energy and oxygen requirements. Bedding rolls can be used to provide support and comfort in the position most suited to the baby and his condition.

As the need for continuous observation decreases and the wound is healing satisfactorily, the baby can be dressed and, once he is maintaining his own temperature, can be transferred to a cot.

Control of pain and discomfort

Controlling pain should be foremost in the nurse's mind and actions while providing routine care or specific procedures, e.g. removal of dressings and sutures or Steristrips. The baby should have a continuous infusion of pain-relieving drugs. Discomfort should be minimized using the methods detailed in Chapter 14, and the effectiveness of pain management documented.

Psychological support of the family

The emotional and psychosocial needs of the baby cannot be ignored and are important at every stage of care, from admission to discharge (Chapters 1 and 14).

Parents should be informed when their baby returns from theatre, once his immediate needs have been met.

Once the baby has responded to the immediate post-operative period, then rehabilitation can begin.

OESOPHAGEAL ATRESIA AND TRACHEO-OESOPHAGEAL FISTULA

Aetiology

This occurs when there is a failure in the differentiation of the foregut into the trachea and oesophagus during the middle of the first trimester. There are five types identified, of which the most common consists of oesophageal atresia and a distal tracheo-oesophageal fistula (TOF). The oesophagus from the pharynx ends in a blind pouch, and below this atresia the oesophagus restarts as a tract attached to the trachea. Variations exist in which the fistula can occur on either side of the atresia and, rarely, there is no joining tract. TOF occurs once in every 3000 live births (Fleming, Speidel and Dunn, 1986).

Diagnosis

Diagnosis can be made antenatally due to polyhydramnios (the fetus is unable to swallow because of the oesophageal atresia), but is usually noticed in the newborn who has a lot of frothy saliva which is constantly regurgitated. If the condition is not identified before the baby is fed, then the baby coughs and chokes on his feed and may become cyanosed if milk is aspirated into the lungs.

To confirm the diagnosis, a large radio-opaque nasogastric tube (size 8 or 10 Fr) is passed as far as possible (about 8–10 cm) (Castellette, 1979). The aspirate from this tube is usually not gastric. An X-ray is performed to identify the level of the atresia. Contrast medium is contraindicated because of the risks of aspiration into the lungs (Reyes, Meller and Loeff, 1989).

Immediate nursing care

A double-lumen or Replogle tube is passed into the pouch or oropharynx and continuous low suction, less than 50 cm H_2O (Castellette, 1979), started. The tube requires aspiration every 15–30 min and irrigation with either 2 ml of air or 0.5 ml of normal saline (depending on the unit policy) to prevent obstruction with secretions. The tube must be securely attached and every care taken to prevent it dislodging. If additional oral suction is required, it should be performed very gently.

The infant may require additional oxygen, which can be given by headbox if full ventilation is not required. Chest physiotherapy to improve pulmonary function may be performed if surgery is delayed and when aspiration of saliva or milk is likely. Physiotherapy is discussed in Chapter 8.

The baby will have nil given by mouth and a dextrose infusion is started.

Nursing the baby undressed in the lateral position with the head tilted at an angle of 45° (Castellette, 1979) provides the optimum position, avoiding aspiration of the stomach contents into the lungs and maximizing the position of the Replogle tube.

Surgical approach

Surgery is usually performed by a right thoracotomy and access to the trachea gained by deflating the right lung. The fistula is ligated and an anastomosis of the oesophagus performed. If it is not possible to join the ends of the oesophagus, then an oesophagostomy can be performed and a gastrostomy tube inserted for feeding.

An extrapleural chest drain is inserted (to aid reinflation of the lung) and a large nasogastric tube is passed across the anastomosis into the stomach.

Postoperative nursing care

Suction should be performed with care because of the sutured trachea. The catheter should be passed very gently and not through the repair. Chest physiotherapy is required to help the right lung to reinflate and to prevent complications. This is usually performed 4-hourly (Castellette, 1979).

The underwater drainage bottles from the chest drain are suspended securely below the level of the chest. The amount and colour of any drainage should be noted, along with any bubbling or swinging in the reservoir. In case of accidental disconnection, a spare pair of forceps should be kept nearby. The chest drain is removed when there is no drainage apparent and the water has stopped 'swinging' and bubbling, usually 48–72 hours postoperatively. The tubing should be clamped for a day, prior to removal of the drain.

Bedding rolls can be used to support the lateral position, wound site uppermost, to aid reinflation and facilitate drainage.

Every precaution and care must be taken to prevent the trans-anastomotic tube from falling out. If this occurs, the tube should be repassed by the doctor. The tube is left on free drainage to aid gastric decompression and aspirated 4-hourly, with the colour, consistency and amount of drainage recorded. Large amounts of drainage may need to be replaced intravenously.

A barium swallow is performed before the baby begins breast or bottle feeding to assess the efficiency of the anastomosis. Any leaks that could cause aspiration of feeds into the lungs, or strictures that may require dilatation, will be detected. If the X-ray is satisfactory, then oral feeding may commence. If aspiration occurs the baby may choke and go blue, and milk may be found in the chest drain. A stricture can cause the baby to choke and have difficulty swallowing his feeds, and there may be more oral secretions than would normally be expected.

Before introducing oral feeds, if the gastric aspirate is minimal, nasogastric feeds may be commenced with the surgeon's permission.

In the rare instance of a leak occurring at the site of anastomosis, the baby will require antibiotics and remain 'nil by mouth' until the anastomosis has healed. If the breakdown is severe, the repair is resutured or a cervical thoracotomy performed, with the distal portion of the oesophagus closed, until correction is possible. If fluid has seeped into the lung a chest drain may be needed (Reyes, Meller and Loeff, 1989).

If a stricture forms at the anastomosis, dilatation may be necessary, starting 1 month after surgery and performed weekly until resolved (Reyes, Meller and Loeff, 1989).

If the proximal end of the oesophagus was too short to allow primary repair of the defect, then a cervical oesophagostomy will be created, allowing the drainage of oropharyngeal secretions. To enable gastric feeds to commence, a gastrostomy is created. Gastrostomy feeds need to be given over 20 minutes (Harjo, 1988, p. 100) to prevent gastric distension, vomiting and aspiration. While gastrostomy feeding is taking place, 'sham' feeding from the breast or bottle is given so that the baby associates sucking with satiety. The milk drains at the oesophagostomy. The oesophagus is then repaired at 8–12 months of age. Parents should be instructed how to perform these feeds and also in the care of the gastrotomy tube, so that the baby can be discharged home.

NECROTIZING ENTEROCOLITIS

Aetiology

The incidence of necrotizing enterocolitis (NEC) suggests a multifactorial origin; it is mainly associated with the seriously ill baby who weighs less than 1500 g, and occurs 6–7 days after enteral feeding (Fetterman, 1971; Rushton, 1990). There is an increased risk associated with many of the procedures which are performed during intensive therapy, for example, intermittent positive pressure ventilation and umbilical catheterization. Other factors, such as blood transfusions, polycythaemia, patent ductus arteriosus and early enteral feeding in the very sick baby (Pearse and Roberton, 1988; Koloske and Musemeche, 1989) and *in utero* complications of infection, third trimester bleeding, multiple birth and maternal diabetes (Filston and Izant, 1985), have been linked to NEC but there is no proven causative factor.

The important point to note is that the preterm baby responds to perinatal stress, hypotension and hypoxia by shunting too much blood to the vital organs, reducing the mesenteric circulation and thus causing necrosis and damage. Damaged intestinal mucosa allows the entry of the gas-producing bacteria which normally reside in the intestine. Bacterial proliferation is enhanced by formula milk, acting as a food source and gas is formed by the bacteria in the sub-mucosal wall, causing the bowel to distend, luminal pressure to increase and the blood flow through the mucosa to decrease. The result of these processes, if left undetected, is bowel perforation or infarction, which may be localized or general (Pearse and Roberton, 1988; Koloske and Musemeche, 1989; Rushton, 1990a).

Diagnosis

In the early stages of NEC, a baby may have a distended, tense abdomen and an increasing volume of possibly bile-stained aspirates from the nasogastric tube. As the bowel obstructs the distended abdomen becomes hard, red and shiny, with loops of bowel identifiable. Occult or frank blood may be present in the faeces and a Clinitest of the stool will detect the presence of reducing sugars. Vomiting and diarrhoea (loose, seedy and yellowy green stools) may occur. The baby may also show non-specific symptoms of lethargy, temperature instability and poor colour. As the necrosis progresses he will show the classic neonatal symptoms of infection and a shocked appearance, i.e. apnoea, bradycardia, oliguria, pallor with poor peripheral perfusion and possibly mottling of the skin. He may become jaundiced and hypoglycaemic (Pearse and Roberton, 1988; Koloske and Musemeche, 1989; Rushton, 1990a). Abdominal X-ray will show gas in the bowel wall along with dilated, thickened portions of bowel, which may be perforated. This necrosis can be in any part of the gastrointestinal tract but is most commonly in the terminal ileum, ileocaecal region, appendix or colon (Pearse and Roberton, 1988).

Nursing measures to help prevent NEC

Meticulous attention should be paid to the site around any umbilical catheters and the perfusion to the lower limbs. If there appears to be any thrombosis around the tip, or impairment of the blood supply to the legs during infusion, or problems in taking specimens, then the line should be removed immediately (Pearse and Roberton, 1988). All infusions should be carefully calculated and rates and volumes monitored to prevent fluid overload.

Enteral feeds may not be commenced in the ill baby who weighs less than 1.5 kg until bowel signs are present, meconium is passed and the abdomen soft (Pearse and Roberton, 1988). Once nasogastric feeds are started, the stomach contents should be aspirated 4–6 hourly to ensure the feeds are being absorbed and, if in doubt, feeds stopped.

In sick, low birth weight babies preference should be given to expressed breast milk and the avoidance of high-osmolarity milk and oral drugs (Pearse and Roberton, 1988). Delaying enteral feeding for the first week of life and then introducing milk slowly, while nutrition is maintained using TPN, is thought to prevent the occurrence of NEC (Brown and Sweet, 1978).

Nursing care associated with conservative management of NEC

The aim of conservative management of NEC is to rest the gut, allowing the inflammation to resolve while treating infection and maintaining the baby's life (Pearse and Roberton, 1988). Any indwelling umbilical catheters must be removed if NEC is suspected and enteral feeding discontinued.

Assisted ventilation may be required due to the very sick state of the baby. The effect of the disease causes splinting of the abdomen, making breathing difficult, and the sepsis can cause recurrent apnoea and bradycardia (Pearse and Roberton, 1988).

Regular observation is necessary, with 4–6 hourly recording of the state of the abdomen with respect to the overall appearance, tenseness, colour, turgor of the skin, palpable masses and amount of distension. Depending on unit policy, the distension can be measured with a tape measure around the area of maximum distension (usually the midriff). This position should be marked on the baby with a pen, so that the same place is measured each time. Any sudden increase in girth may indicate perforation or ascites (Pearse and Roberton, 1988).

To help minimize abdominal distension and aspiration and aid decompression, a nasogastric tube needs to be passed for free drainage with 4 hourly aspiration of the stomach contents. These losses are replaced intravenously.

A stool specimen and a gastric aspirate are sent for microbiological examination. A ward test, for reducing substances and the presence of blood, is performed on all faeces. Continuous monitoring of all vital signs and skin colour should be undertaken and recorded hourly. Any trends that show deviations from normal parameters need identifying to assess the process of the disease. The baby may need medical intervention to maintain any of these vital signs.

A peripheral arterial line may be sited for ease of obtaining blood specimens and assisting in monitoring. Perfusion to the peripheries of the limb in which the line is situated requires hourly observation, and any blanching of the cannulated artery should be reported and the line removed immediately.

Enteral feeding must be discontinued at the first indication of NEC and may not be tolerated for a few weeks.

Hydration is maintained with an i.v. infusion and a long line/central line is sited so that TPN can commence (Chapter 7).

Extremes of blood sugar may occur as a result of stress, infection, dehydration and poor nutrition. Blood sugar estimates need to be repeated hourly until stable and then the time between readings may be lengthened. Levels of less than 1 mmol/l or greater than 8 mmol/l (Fleming, Speidel and Dunn, 1986) are unacceptable and should be reported.

Haematological and electrolyte disturbances may occur and require intervention. Hypotension (see Chapter 9 for minimum systolic pressure), poor tissue perfusion, ascites and oliguria may indicate the need for an infusion of plasma (Kliegman and Fanaroff, 1984) and anaemia indicates the possible need for a blood transfusion (Perkins, McFee and Andrassy, 1985). Additives may be prescribed to correct electrolyte imbalances and their compatibility with other infusions must be defined. Careful regulation of fluid balance is required to prevent fluid overload, and electrolyte levels of both serum and urine need measuring. A catheter may be passed into the bladder (a nasogastric tube is suitable) so that urine output can be accurately monitored, especially if it is less than 1.5–2 ml/kg/h (Rushton, 1990b), and colloids may be prescribed. Specimens of urine are sent for urea and electrolyte levels daily. Ward analysis of pH, specific gravity and content is performed 4-hourly and recorded.

The baby is nursed naked in the lateral or supine position in an incubator or open heated cot to allow continuous assessment of the abdomen, with early identifications of changes without disturbance.

Pain must be effectively controlled, both by pharmacological and nursing interventions (Pearse and Roberton, 1988). The neonatal nurse, with a knowledge of a baby's reactions to pain and discomfort (Chapter 14) can respond to his needs and monitor and evaluate the effectiveness of treatment. An appropriate antibiotic schedule will be instituted and will last until 10–14 days after resolution of the NEC (Pearse and Roberton, 1988).

Nursing care after the critical period

If the baby responds to the nursing and medical measures positively, as shown by the resolution of gas in the bowel wall, reduction of abdominal distension, clear gastric aspirates and normal bowel movements, along with increasing stability of the vital signs and less reliance on pharmacological and mechanical intervention (Pearse and Roberton, 1988), then the next stage of nursing care can be introduced. Medical approval must be given and the nurse should remain observant for any signs of relapse or intolerance, with particular attention to signs of obstruction.

Girth measurements need to be continued and all stool specimens tested for blood and reducing substances. Any positive specimens should be noted and feeding discontinued. Antibiotic therapy is continued for 10–14 days from the first clear X-ray (Pearse and Roberton, 1988).

Nasogastric tube feeding is recommenced, starting at a rate of 1 ml/h and increasing slowly. Free drainage is discontinued. The intravenous feeding regimen is weaned down at the same rate. If any of the aspirate is bile stained, feeding should be immediately discontinued and full parenteral therapy instituted.

Nursing care with the surgical management of NEC

If there are signs of obstruction, as evidenced by recurrent abdominal distension, bile-stained aspirate or vomiting, blood or reducing substances in the stool, and the baby has not responded to conservative management, then surgery may be necessary. Continuing deterioration after 72 h (Rushton, 1990b), or if the bowel was perforated or obstructed when the disease was identified, also requires surgical intervention (Pearse and Roberton, 1988).

Surgical approach

The operation is a laparotomy with resection of the necrotic bowel and anastomosis of the ends. Alternatively, the two ends are sutured to the abdominal wall forming an active stoma and a distal stoma. With surgically treated NEC, general pre- and postoperative care are as detailed at the start of this chapter.

Postoperative nursing care

Nursing care is the same as for the conservative management of NEC and the nurse needs to be aware of deterioration, as evidenced by abdominal distension, vomiting, no return of bowel activity and any of the identifying characteristics of NEC as previously described. Enteral feeding must be delayed until normal gut motility has returned, which may take several weeks.

Care of a baby with a stoma

The baby will return from theatre with an abdominal wound and the formation of two stomas from the proximal and distal ends of the resected bowel. The type of stoma depends on the area excised, i.e. ileostomy or colostomy.

Initially, the wound and stomas may be dressed with gauze, which may be left *in situ* until it becomes soiled from stomal discharge.

The stoma needs checking every 4–6 h for colour, perfusion and activity. A healthy stoma is initially dark and may bleed easily immediately after the operation, and then becomes red or pink in colour and is slightly raised above the skin. The abdominal skin around the stoma should show no signs of irritation from the stoma, the sutures or the stomal appliance.

With very small babies, non-adherent gauze dressings may be all that is necessary until the stoma begins to function, which should be within 5–7 days when, if the stoma has healed, an appropriate appliance or a stoma bag can be put on. This bag can be kept *in situ* for as long as it is not leaking and the stoma and surrounding skin are in a satisfactory condition.

The bag is emptied 8-hourly and the amount, consistency, colour and ward analysis of the contents charted. Output should be less than half of the food intake (Harjo, 1988) and any excessive loss reported to prevent dehydration. A reducing sugar result greater than 0.5% needs to be reported as intolerance is common because of the damage to the intestinal mucosa and decreased intestinal absorption (Harjo, 1988).

Stomas created from the jejunum or first part of the ileum cause excessive sodium and nutrient losses, resulting in a metabolic acidosis and 'failure to thrive' (Bower, Pringle and Soper, 1988). Oral supplementation with sodium and high-calorie additives are required.

Feeding can begin once the bowel has recovered from surgery and the gastric aspirate is clear, which usually takes

7–10 days. Tube feeding is started, possibly using a quarter-strength formula preparation or an elemental formula to aid absorption.

The paediatric stoma nurse will provide information on appropriate appliances, skin care and educate parents.

Closure of the stoma, if possible, will be considered once the infant has recovered from the neonatal insults, from 4 weeks of age onwards, especially if the stoma is formed from the jejunum (Bower, Pringle and Soper, 1988).

GASTROSCHISIS

Aetiology

During the formation and differentiation of the embryo, the bowel spends some time in the umbilical cord before returning to the abdomen during the first trimester. Gastroschisis occurs when the base of the umbilical cord tears and bowel herniates through the defect (Meller, Reyes and Loeff, 1989). This tear is always to the right of the umbilicus, on the abdominal wall, and the space between the cord and the tear becomes covered by skin. An infant with gastroschisis is usually growth retarded *in utero* but is rarely associated with other anomalies; incidence is approximately 1 in every 6000 deliveries (Fleming, Speidel and Dunn, 19867; Meller, Reyes and Loeff, 1989; Swift *et al.*, 1992).

Diagnosis

Diagnosis of gastroschisis can be made in the second trimester of pregnancy by the presence of intra-amniotic fronds which are seen on ultrasound scan (Roberton, 1988; Swift *et al.*, 1992) or by the appearance of uncovered prolapsed bowel at birth.

The herniated bowel is exposed to the amniotic fluid and can become matted and, as adhesions form, the individual loops are inseparable. Stenosis and atresia can occur if the bowel twists around the hole in the abdominal wall (Roberton, 1988; Meller, Reyes and Loeff, 1989). Gangrene and perforation occur if the bowel is damaged or becomes ischaemic (Fleming, Speidel and Dunn, 1986).

Immediate nursing care

The choice of delivery is often by planned caesarean section to prevent trauma to the externalized bowel and colonization with the vaginal flora (Swift *et al.*, 1992). At birth the baby's lower body, including his legs, should be placed in a sterile plastic 'bowel' bag. This is drawn up over the herniated bowel and secured underneath the arms. This is to keep the exposed bowel sterile and reduce water and heat losses from evaporation. This is not removed until the baby is in theatre.

Respiratory assistance by additional headbox oxygen or intubation and ventilation may be required, depending on the baby's blood gas report.

The baby will be unable to take enteral feeds, so a dextrose infusion is commenced. The infant may need up to twice the usual maintenance volume to ensure adequate hydration, depending on the insensible fluid losses from the exposed bowel and serum electrolyte status. This must be given in the form of an osmotic fluid, e.g. 5% dextrose and Ringer's lactate (Harjo, 1988) to maintain the fluid and electrolyte balance as hypotonic solutions will only further exaggerate the fluid shift.

Hypotension and hypovolaemic shock resulting from the insensible fluid and plasma losses can occur quickly and dramatically. Extra fluids or an infusion of colloid, e.g. plasma protein fraction (10–20 ml/kg) may be required (Stringer, Brereton and Wright, 1991). Blood pressure readings need to be taken and recorded hourly along with all the other vital signs.

Accurate fluid balance charting of all input and output is essential. Insensible losses from the gastroschisis can be estimated from how much free fluid is in the bag, but no attempt should be made to measure this loss accurately. Urine production of less than 1 ml/kg/h (Harjo, 1988) should be reported and, if possible, tested by dipstick and measured. Renal failure can occur as a result of dehydration or compromised circulation. If urine production is low yet blood pressure acceptable, then changing the baby's position may help to relieve the pressure of the defect compromising the renal blood flow (Harjo, 1988).

A large-bore nasogastric tube (size 8 or 10 Fr) is passed to aid decompression of the bowel and prevent bilious vomiting. This tube is left on free drainage and aspirated every 15 min (Harjo, 1988; Stringer, Brereton and Wright, 1991) and aspirates replaced intravenously.

The baby is nursed naked in an incubator or heated cot set in the thermoneutral range (Appendix 3) so that the bowel is visible. The baby's axilla temperature is recorded hourly. A skin temperature probe may be attached as near to the abdomen as possible without entering the sterile bag.

The exposed bowel represents a large surface area that will lose heat quickly and severely. Additional clingfilm or bubble wrap can be placed over the abdomen to reduce excessive fluid loss and preserve the central temperature. Warm saline-soaked gauze swabs should not be placed around the bowel as they occlude visualization, preventing early detection of ischaemic changes and, when cooled, contribute to a reduction in core temperature (Stringer, Brereton and Wright, 1991).

The appearance of the bowel is assessed hourly. Nursing the baby in the lateral position allows good visualization and reduces the pressure that the gastroschisis can have on the abdominal contents. If the circulation to any area is compromised, shown by a blue discoloration of the bowel, then his position needs to be changed and medical staff informed. If he is nursed supine, observations must be made to ensure that the defect is not impairing circulation to the kidneys and legs.

Broad-spectrum antibiotic therapy is commenced immediately, as the exposed bowel is susceptible to contamination and infection.

The parents must be allowed to see and touch their baby as soon as possible, as their imaginings may be worse than the reality of the defect (Klaus and Fanaroff, 1986).

Surgical approach

Surgery should commence within 6 hours of birth because of the vulnerability of the exposed bowel (Meller, Reyes and Loeff, 1989) and the baby requires the usual preparation for theatre. The aim of surgery is to return the bowel to the abdomen without compromising abdominal ciculation or the functioning of the bowel. Primary (and complete) closure can be achieved if the abdominal wall will stretch over the bowel sufficiently but, where this cannot happen or the bowel is very oedematous, a silastic patch is attached to the skin surrounding the bowel and primary closure is delayed until the skin has stretched and oedema resolved.

If the bowel has suffered ischaemic insults, stenosis or stricture formation, the affected area is resected and an end-to-end anastomosis or stoma formation performed (Meller, Reyes and Loeff, 1989; Swift *et al.*, 1992). Removal of the silastic patch and closure of the skin usually occurs within the week because of problems associated with infection, suture line dihescence and epithelialization on to the silastic (Meller, Reyes and Loeff, 1989).

Postoperative nursing care

The baby will require the usual postoperative nursing care. Assistance with breathing may be prolonged (longer than 72 h) due to any of the following factors reducing the efficiency of the baby's respiratory effort (Meller, Reyes and Loeff, 1989; de Lorimier, Adzick and Harrison, 1991):

- Intra-abdominal pressure can be raised.
- The diaphragm may be displaced upwards.
- The silastic patch embarrasses respiration.
- Analgesic infusions are necessary and the baby may need paralysing.

Respiratory support will, in most instances, be necessary until after the patch has been removed.

The suture line is inspected daily for signs of infection (redness, inflammation, tenderness), septic areas or tissue breakdown. Abnormal findings are recorded, likewise if there appears to be any infection or ischaemia of the encased bowel. If the baby has a silastic patch, the suture line may be treated with a topical antibacterial agent and dressed daily, using an aseptic technique, with dry gauze to absorb any serous drainage (Harjo, 1988; de Lorimier, Adzick and Harrison, 1991). The amount and colour of the drainage is recorded on the fluid balance chart.

If a silastic pouch has been created, it is then suspended from the incubator (using the ties which were attached in theatre) so that tension is placed on the skin, stretching it so that it will eventually cover the bowel. The size of the pouch is reduced daily over the next week, until the skin has sufficiently stretched and all the bowel can be returned to the abdomen (Meller, Reyes and Loeff, 1989; de Lorimier, Adzick and Harrison, 1991). During handling of the baby, the tension on the silastic pouch needs to be maintained by another person.

Intra-abdominal pressure can be increased with repair of the defect (de Lorimier, Adzick and Harrison, 1991). The lower limbs should not be covered with blankets (bubble wrap or clingfilm can be used) so that the legs can be observed for signs of discoloration, oedema and impaired perfusion (decreased pulses, blanching, coolness and capillary return can be tested by applying slight pressure to the feet). Central venous pressure (CVP) may be monitored to detect inadequate venous return or impaired intra-abdominal perfusion (Harjo, 1988, de Lorimier, Adzick and Harrison, 1991).

Renal impairment and poor urine production may occur due to hypotension, large fluid and plasma losses from the herniated bowel and as a side effect of replacing the bowel into a tight abdomen (Stringer, Brereton and Wright, 1991). Urine production needs to be greater than 1 ml/kg/h (de Lorimier, Adzick and Harrison, 1991), with all specimens measured and urinalysis performed and recorded. A specific gravity of greater than 1.015 may indicate dehydration.

Fluid balance is important and extra fluids may need to be prescribed. Gastric losses from the nasogastric tube require intravenous replacement. Plasma expanders may be necessary to maintain a systolic BP above 40–50 mmHg (Harjo, 1988).

Until enteral feeding can commence, nutritional requirements must be met by total parenteral nutrition (Roberton, 1988; Meller, Reyes and Loeff, 1989). Commencement of enteral feeding may take a few weeks or months, depending on the condition of the bowel, as the return of gut motility may be slow. Before considering feeding, drainage from the nasogastric tube has to be minimal, clear fluid only (no evidence of bile), bowel sounds and activity should have returned and the silastic patch removed (Meller, Reyes and Loeff, 1989; de Lorimier, Adzick and Harrison, 1991; Shah and Wolley, 1991).

Tube feeding begins using small infusions of milk (preferably breast milk) or semielemental isomolar preparations. Tolerance is shown by bowel activity and the volume and composition (pH greater than 5, absence of reducing substances and blood) of stool passed. Signs of intolerance include gastric aspirates greater than half of the volume of milk fed or bile-stained, abdominal distension, stools that are of increasing volume, or testing positive for reducing substances (greater than 0.5%) and a pH less than 6 (Harjo, 1988). If an elemental solution is being absorbed, then the infant can slowly graduate to milk feeds (Goulet *et al.*, 1991).

The baby with a silastic patch is still prone to additional heat loss and consequently hypothermia because of the large area of exposed bowel. The use of an incubator or open heated cot is continued. Skin temperature probes may be used to provide continuous temperature readings and detect a fall in temperature associated with poor perfusion to the legs or a rising core temperature, which may indicate infection. The effectiveness of pain control is assessed and analgesia is given by continuous infusion or as required. Antibiotic therapy is continued after surgery because of the risk of peritoneal contamination. Systemic candidiasis is a potential problem because of antibiotic therapy and slow gut transit times (Roberton, 1988) and may require therapy.

Prognosis

Gastroschisis no longer represents long-term morbidity and normal recovery is usually expected once closure of the defect is achieved and the baby tolerates enteral feeds. Complications of intestinal infarction, stoma formation and resistant constipation may occur (Roberton, 1988; Stringer, Brereton and Wright, 1991).

In utero transfer to a centre that has both surgical and intensive care facilities shortens ventilation times and the baby is discharged home sooner, thereby avoiding the increased incidence of hypothermia, hypovolaemia and inadequate gastric drainage during neonatal transfer (Stringer, Brereton and Wright, 1991).

REFERENCES

Bower, T.R., Pringle, K.C. and Soper, R.T. (1988) Sodium deficit causing decreased weight gain and metabolic acidosis in infants with ileostomy. *Journal of Pediatric Surgery* **23**, 567–72.

Brown, E.G. and Sweet, A.Y. (1978) Preventing necrotising enter-colitis in neonates. *Journal of the American Medical Association* **240**, 2452–4.

Castellette, P. (1979) Baby with oesophageal atresia. *Nursing* 1st. series **7**(2), 330–5.

Fetterman, G.H. (1971) Neonatal necrotising enterocolitis: old pitfall or new problem. *Pediatrics* **48**, 345–8.

Filtson, H.C. and Izant, R.J. (1985) *The Surgical Neonate: Evaluation and Care*, 2nd edn, Appleton-Century-Crofts, Norwalk, pp. 222–7.

Fleming, P.J., Speidel, B.D. and Dunn, P.M. (1986) *A Neonatal Vade-Mecum*, Lloyd-Luke (Medical Books) Ltd, London.

Golding, J., Pateron, M. and Kinlen, L.J. (1990) Factors associated with childhood cancer in a national cohort study. *British Journal of Cancer* **62**, 304–8.

Goulet, O.J., Revillou, Y., Jau, D. *et al.* (1991) Neonatal short bowel syndrome. *Journal of Pediatrics* **119** (part 1), 18–23.

Harjo, J. (1988) Alterations in the gastrointestinal system, in *Neonatal Surgery, A Nursing Perspective*, (eds C. Kenner, J. Harjo and A. Brueggemeyer), Harcourt Brace Jovanovich, London, pp. 121–90.

Kelsall, A.W.R. (1992) Vitamin K and childhood cancer. *British Medical Journal* **305** (6860), 1016–7.

Klaus, M. and Fanaroff, A. (1986) Care of the parents, in *Care of the High Risk Neonate*, Admore Medical Books, W.B. Saunders Company, Philadelphia, pp. 147–69.

Kliegman, R.M. and Fanaroff, A.A. (1984) Necrotising enterocolitis. *New England Journal of Medicine* **310**(17), 1093–1103.

Koloske, A.M. and Musemeche, C.A. (1989) Necrotising enterocolitis of the neonate. *Clinics in Perinatology* **16**(1), 97–111.

de Lorimier, A.A., Adzick, N.S. and Harrison, M.R. (1991) Amnion inversion in the treatment of giant omphalocele. *Journal of Paediatric Surgery* **26**(7), 804–7.

Meller, J.L., Reyes, H.M. and Loeff, D.S. (1989) Gastrochisis and omphalocele. *Clinics in Perinatology* **16**(1), 113–22.

Pearse, R.G. and Roberton, N.R.C. (1988) Infection in the newborn, in *Textbook of Neonatology* (ed N.R.C. Roberton), Churchill Livingstone, Edinburgh, pp. 753–9.

Perkins, M., McFee, A.S. and Andrassy, R.J. (1985) Neonatal necro-tising enterocolitis: an overview. *Contemporary Surgery* **182**, 57–74.

Reyes, H.M., Meller, J.L. and Loeff, D. (1989) Management of esophageal atresia and tracheosophageal fistula. *Clinics in Perinatology* **16**(1), 79–84.

Roberton, N.R.C. (1988) (ed) *Textbook of Neonatology*, Churchill Livingstone, Edinburgh.

Rushton, C.H. (1990a) Necrotising enterocolitis Part 1: Pathogenesis and diagnosis. *Maternal and Child Nursing* **15**, 296–300.
Rushton, C.H. (1990b) Necrotising enterocolitis part 2: Treatment and nursing care. *Maternal and Child Nursing* **15**, 309–313.
Shah, R. and Wolley, M.M. (1991) Gastroschisis and intestinal atresia. *Journal of Pediatric Surgery* **26**(7), 788–90.
Stringer, M.D., Brereton, R.S. and Wright, V.M. (1991) Controversies in the management of gastroschisis: a study of 40 patients. *Archives of Diseases in Childhood* **66**(1), 34–6.
Swift, R.I., Singh, M.P., Ziderman, D.A. *et al.* (1992) A regime in the management of gastroschisis. *Journal of Paediatric Surgery* **27**(1), 61–3.
Wallis, M. (1982) Emergency surgery for the newborn. *Nursing Mirror* **6**, 22–4.

7

Feeding low birth weight infants in today's neonatal environment

Helen Gardiner

Optimal nutrition is critical in the management of the increasing number of very immature infants in today's neonatal environment. Meeting their nutritional needs is important in ensuring their survival and subsequent growth and development.

Although there is some controversy in defining the most appropriate goal for nutritional management of the low birth weight infant, 'achieving a postnatal growth that approximates the *in utero* growth of normal fetus at the same post conception age . . .' (American Academy of Pediatrics, 1985) is often adopted as an aim of feeding these infants. In the short term, it is also important that the diet allows the infant to adapt properly to extrauterine life. Recently there has been mounting interest in the effects of early nutrition on the long-term clinical outcome of these infants, including neurological development and morbidity in later life.

A wide range of problems may be encountered in the nutritional management of low birth weight infants. The main nutritional problems will be discussed in the first section of this chapter.

Feeding low birth weight infants of varying levels of immaturity and size poses a real challenge to those involved in their care. Careful assessment of the nutritional needs of each individual infant is required to ensure that the most appropriate feeding regimen is chosen. Subsequently, close monitoring is essential to ensure the infant reaches his or her full potential. The nutritional requirements of low birth weight infants and the various means of nutritional management, including the use of breast milk, the use of formula and methods of feeding, will be discussed.

NUTRITION-RELATED PROBLEMS

The causes of the nutritional problems seen in low birth weight infants are summarized below.

- Limited nutrient stores
- Physiological immaturity
- High nutrient requirements for growth
- High risk of morbidity

Limited nutrient stores

These infants are often born before the deposition of the relatively large amounts of nutrients that occurs *in utero* during the last trimester of gestation. It is because of this severely limited supply of endogenous nutrients that prematurely born infants have an increased requirement for many nutrients compared with larger infants born at term. The infant of less than 28 weeks' gestation has less than 3% fat, compared with 16% in the term infant, and will survive less than a week if no food is provided. Morgan (1992) quotes survival reserves of only 2 days for infants weighing 500 g.

One nutrient of special interest is iron. Preterm infants have limited reserves of iron and stores are exhausted after 6–8 weeks in infants less than 1400 g and between 8 and 12 weeks in those greater than 1400 g, resulting in anaemia.

Physiological immaturity

The nutritional requirements of these infants and their ability to tolerate certain nutrients is affected by the immaturity of certain body systems, including the gastrointestinal tract, protein metabolism, renal function and skin.

Gastrointestinal tract

Infants of less than 34 weeks' gestation have poorly co-ordinated sucking and swallowing reflexes. They are prone to regurgitation of feeds and have a reduced gastric volume. Tolerance is further reduced as many have a slower rate of gastric emptying and a decreased intestinal motility, which will affect their feeding.

In very immature infants parenteral feeding will often be indicated initially, and in others feeding via a suitable enteral tube is necessary until the infant can be fed orally. Occasionally in enterally-fed infants digestion and absorption of fat is impaired by reduced bile salt secretion and low pancreatic lipase activity.

Protein metabolism

These infants have an increased need for protein for growth but a reduced ability to synthesize and excrete urea. This must be taken into account in assessing the optimum protein intake. Excess dietary protein may result in hyperammonaemia and aminoacidaemia, which could adversely affect later development. Certain amino acids, known as essential amino acids, are required in increased amounts to allow for the high rate of body protein turnover. There are 11 essential amino acids for premature infants, including taurine and cystine which, although not normally essential, are essential in young babies due to the deficiency of certain enzymes which enable the body to synthesize them from methionine.

Renal function

In addition to the reduced ability to excrete urea, the kidneys of a premature infant are not capable of forming a concentrated urine and conserving sodium. Hence the premature infant has a higher requirement for water and sodium compared to a full-term infant.

Skin

Water loss through the thin uncornified skin of infants

under 28 weeks' gestation may be extremely high. These losses are increased if the infant is nursed under a radiant heater or phototherapy unit.

High nutrient requirements for growth

The aim of feeding is to achieve a weight gain approximating that usually seen during the last trimester of pregnancy, i.e. 14–17 g/kg/day. In some infants the rate of postnatal growth is less than the intrauterine rate, and catch-up growth is necessary if they are to continue to grow along the same centile chart as they were born on.

Some tissues, notably bone, develop differently in preterm infants compared with *in utero*, and so the body composition of these infants differs in some respects from that of full-term infants.

High risk of morbidity

Very immature infants are at particular risk of cardiorespiratory disease. Sick infants with severe respiratory distress syndrome (RDS) tolerate enteral feeds poorly and will usually require parenteral feeding initially. Bronchopulmonary dysplasia is a major cause of poor growth because of the associated high energy expenditure.

Necrotizing enterocolitis (NEC), is a condition in which the bowel wall suffers ischaemic damage, and is most often seen in enterally-fed infants. Exclusively formula-fed infants are more likely to develop NEC than infants fed breast milk alone. It has been suggested that supplementing formula-fed infants with small amounts of breast milk reduces the risk of these infants developing NEC (Lucas and Cole, 1990). On diagnosis, all enteral feeds must stop and parenteral feeds be started. Surgical removal of necrotic sections of the gut is often necessary, and parenteral feeding may need to continue for extended periods while the gut recovers.

NUTRITIONAL REQUIREMENTS

Nutritional requirements vary between individuals depending on their stage of development and state of health. In 1987 the European Society for Paediatric Gastroenterology and

Nutrition (ESPGAN) published their guidelines for the nutrition and feeding of preterm infants (Wharton, 1987). These guidelines were formulated following a review of the world's literature. As always, the opinions expressed are not universally shared by experts in nutrition and this accounts for individual variations between neonatal units.

Water

Water is quantitatively and qualitatively the single most important nutrient in all humans. In the very low birth weight infant water requirements are extremely variable and depend on the age of the infant (gestational and postnatal) and environmental conditions. Insensible water losses are very high for the preterm infant (30–60 ml/kg/day) and are further increased by the use of radiant warmers and phototherapy; 150–200 ml/kg/day is the usual amount of fluid recommended, although higher or lower intakes may be recommended in certain clinical conditions, for example:

- Higher intakes may be required in infants who have high insensible losses of water through the lungs and skin.
- Infants with high energy requirements, such as small for gestational age infants who are receiving low-energy formula or human milk, and who will require higher intakes of feed in order to achieve adequate weight gain.
- Lower intakes may sometimes be necessary, e.g. in renal failure, heart failure and patent ductus arteriosus.

Energy

Energy requirements are also extremely variable, but an intake of 130 kcal/kg/day (range 110–165 kcal/kg/day) is estimated to meet the needs of most low birth weight infants under normal circumstances. About 40% of non-protein energy should come from carbohydrate and 60% from fat.

Protein

The amount and type of protein should be sufficient to achieve normal growth and body composition while taking into consideration the metabolic capacity of the liver and the excretory powers of the kidneys. Protein intakes of between 2.9 and 4 g/kg/day have been recommended for formula-fed infants. This may not, however, be achieved in infants receiving human milk, because of its low protein content, and protein supplementation may be necessary to achieve optimal growth in these infants.

Fat

Dietary fat is an important source of energy and essential fatty acids, the latter being an essential component of all tissues, including the central nervous system. As previously mentioned, the preterm infant has a reduced ability to digest and absorb dietary fat and steatorrhoea is a common problem in low birth weight infants. These losses of dietary fat will impair calcium and fat-soluble vitamin absorption.

Preterm infants may be more vulnerable than full-term infants to essential fatty acid (EFA) deficiency as a result of this fat malabsorption. Other factors, such as the more rapid rate of growth and low body stores of these infants, will put them at greater risk of deficiency.

The two most common essential fatty acids are linoleic (C18:2n6) and α-linolenic (C18:3n3) acids. The information shown in the brackets refers to the structure of the fatty acids, indicating the number of carbon (C) atoms, the number of double bonds and the position of the first of these double bonds (n-6 or n-3) in the fatty acid chain. These fatty acids play an important role as the precursors of the n-6 and n-3 long-chain polyunsaturated fatty acids (LCPs), respectively. The synthesis of LCPs from linoleic and α-linolenic acids by a series of desaturation and chain elongation reactions is, however, impaired in preterm infants.

Full-term infants are born with LCP stores deposited during the last trimester of pregnancy. Preterm infants are often born before this deposition of LCPs occurs, and are therefore more prone to LCP deficiency. Because of their reduced ability to synthesize LCPs and inadequate LCP stores, preterm infants require a dietary supply of LCPs. Phospholipids of the central nervous system and of retinal receptor cells in the eye are particularly rich in the LCPs arachidonic acid, or AA (C20:4n6) and docosahexaenoic acid, or DHA (C22: 6n3). Dietary deficiency of n-3 LCPs, including DHA, has been shown to impair retinal function in preterm infants (Uauy *et al.*, 1990). It has been suggested that arachidonic acid may be a specific growth-stimulating factor during early human development, and therefore a dietary deficiency of n-6 LCPs should be avoided (Koletzko, 1990). Research by Leaf *et al.* (1992) has demonstrated a strong positive correlation between plasma choline phosphoglyceride n-6 LCP levels and weight and head circumference measurements in 22 preterm infants. They also showed that n-3 LCP levels in these infants correlated positively with length of gestation. All these considerations are important when deciding the amount and type of fat to give to the preterm infant.

Type of fat

Unsaturated fats are better absorbed than saturated fats, and this explains why the fat in human milk is so well absorbed by the infant. For the same reason vegetable oils, which contain a high proportion of unsaturated fats, are better absorbed than cow's milk fat, which has a high proportion of saturated fats.

The degree of fat digestion with human milk is further aided by the presence of milk lipases, although this effect is reduced if the milk undergoes heat treatment.

To guard against EFA deficiency it is important that the diet provides at least 4.5% of total calories as α-linoleic acid and at least 0.5% of total calories as linolenic acid.

Breast milk has an optimal fat blend and is able to provide preterm infants with sufficient essential fatty acids, including LCPs, to match intrauterine accretion rates of both n-6 and n-3 fatty acids.

Until recently, low birth weight formulas provided adequate amounts of linoleic and α-linolenic acids, but no LCPs. In 1991, the ESPGAN Committee on Nutrition published guidelines on the lipid composition of formulas, recommending that those for low birth weight infants should be supplemented with LCPs in similar quantities to those found in breast milk. Following these guidelines, Prematil with Milupan (Milupa) has become available, which provides n-6 and n-3 LCPs in a ratio of about 2:1, as seen in breast milk.

Amount of fat

The amount of fat given will be determined by the individual infant's fat tolerance. The recommended intakes for fat range from about 4 to 9 g/kg/day, depending on the capacity for fat absorption.

Sodium

Hyponatraemia arising in the first week of life is usually secondary to inappropriate secretion of antidiuretic hormone leading to water retention. After about the 7th day of life, hyponatraemia may develop as a result of poor renal concentration ability and insufficient sodium intake. This 'late hyponatraemia' is particularly common in infants born before 32–34 weeks gestation.

To maintain the plasma sodium concentration above 130 mmol/l and to provide sufficient sodium for growth, the estimated daily sodium requirement is 3–5 mmol/kg (69–115 mg/kg) for infants weighing less than 1500 g with late hyponatraemia during the first 4–6 weeks of life (up to 32–34 weeks' gestation). From then until full term the requirement will fall to between 1.5 and 2.5 mmol/kg (34.5–57.5 mg/kg) per day. Regular monitoring of plasma sodium concentration is necessary and a supplement (sodium chloride) should be given when necessary.

Calcium, phosphorus and vitamin D

Hypomineralization of bone (osteopenia) and rickets of prematurity are problems commonly encountered in these infants. An incidence of rickets as high as 50% has been reported in preterm infants weighing less than 1000 g (McIntosh, Livesey and Brooke, 1982). It is very difficult to mimic the *in utero* levels of bone mineralization in preterm infants. This is partly due to the poor solubility of calcium and phosphorus in milk and parenteral solutions in the amounts required to achieve these accretion rates. In fact, too high an intake of phosphorus may lead to hyperphosphataemia, which leads to hypocalcaemia. Very high intakes of calcium can impede fat absorption and induce metabolic acidosis and, if taken for long periods without additional phosphorus, can cause renal calculi.

Having said this, calcium and phosphorus intakes should be increased above the levels indicated for term infants to improve bone mineralization. Whichever method of feeding is used the amounts of calcium and phosphorus and the ratio between these nutrients should be monitored and additional supplements supplied when appropriate.

Breast milk contains inadequate calcium and phosphorus (about 30 mg/100 ml and 15 mg/100 ml, respectively) for very low birth weight infants and requires supplementation. Whitelaw (1986) recommends that if the plasma phosphate level falls below 1.6 mmol/l, 1 mmol of phosphate in the form of potassium hydrogen phosphate should be provided. If the plasma calcium level falls below 2.0 mmol/l or the plasma alkaline phosphatase rises above 425 iu/l, 1 mmol of calcium as calcium gluconate should be given daily. These supplements should be added to the milk at different times of the day to avoid precipitation of calcium phosphate in the feeding vessel.

Formula-fed infants benefit from receiving one of the special low birth weight formulas with their higher calcium and phosphorus contents than with standard formulas. Currently available low birth weight formulas provide between 70 and 110 mg calcium and 41–63 mg phosphorus per 100 ml, with calcium:phosphorus ratios similar to breast milk of 1.7:2. In very sick babies and those that have received total parenteral nutrition for long periods, it may be necessary to supplement low birth weight formulas with extra calcium and phosphate to prevent bone disease.

Vitamin D requirements are higher in preterm infants than in full-term infants. Body stores at birth are lower in preterm infants due to the shorter gestation period, and these are further influenced by the mother's dietary intake and exposure to sunlight. Supplementation with Vitamin D (chole- or ergocalciferol) is recommended to provide a total intake of between 800 and 1600 iu (20–40 μg) per day.

Iron

Preterm infants are born with reduced iron stores and, unless iron supplements are given, stores become exhausted from about 2 months of age. A total intake of between 2 and 2.5 mg/kg/day prevents anaemia. However, babies receiving regular blood transfusions will have their iron stores and blood haemoglobin concentration preserved beyond these age limits and thus the provision of dietary iron or supplements can be delayed until after the transfusions are stopped.

Dietary iron may be an aetiological factor in Gram-negative infections (Bullen, Rogers and Leigh, 1972), and so preterm infants may benefit from avoiding dietary iron in the first 6–8 weeks of life, especially the extremely low birth weight infants.

Vitamins

Multivitamin preparations are often given to low birth weight infants and usually provide vitamins A, D, E, K, B_1, B_6 and C. Folic acid may be added or supplied separately. Although not all low birth weight infants will have increased requirements for all these vitamins, they are usually given routinely to prevent deficiencies.

NUTRITIONAL MANAGEMENT

The way nutritional requirements are met will depend on the age, size and health of the infant. The best method of feeding and the most appropriate nutritional source will be decided by the staff caring for the infant, together with the infant's parents.

Parenteral (i.v.) feeding

Although enteral feeding should be chosen whenever possible, some infants, notably those of less than 28 weeks' gestation and sick preterm infants, will require total parenteral nutrition (TPN) in the early days or weeks. Clinical indications for parenteral feeding include an inability to tolerate enteral feeding due to gut immaturity or morbidity, established gut pathology, such as NEC, and the need for surgery (Dear, 1992). Since complications with parenteral feeding are not uncommon, careful monitoring of blood chemistry and regular clinical assessment are essential.

Nutrient sources in parenteral feeding

The aim of TPN is to provide a balanced mixture of carbohydrates, amino acids, fat, minerals, trace elements and vitamins in a well tolerated form which will promote growth without metabolic overload. In assessing the nutrient requirements of the parenterally fed infant it is important to remember that the gut is being bypassed, so no allowances need to be made for intestinal losses through impaired digestion and absorption. The daily recommended allowances will be less overall for the parenterally fed infant than the recommendations made by ESPGAN for the enterally fed infant. However, the recommendations provide useful guidelines.

In addition, the health of the infant may influence the nutrient intake. In severe respiratory distress with patent ductus arteriosus or renal disease, for example, fluid restriction may limit the delivery of energy and nutrients.

Protein

It has been estimated that the parenterally fed infant should receive about 3.2 g protein/kg/day, and currently this is provided by crystalline amino acid solutions. Previously, protein hydrolysate solutions were used although these showed lower levels of nitrogen retention and a higher incidence of hyperammonaemia. Since the neonate is not able to fully metabolize certain amino acids, particularly threonine, phenylalanine, glycine and methionine, special paediatric amino acid solutions have recently been developed, e.g. Vaminolact (Pharmacia), and these should be used in preference to those designed primarily for adults.

Energy

Reasonable growth and nitrogen retention is seen in neonates with parenteral energy intakes of about 90 kcal/kg/day (Nose *et al.*, 1987; Kovar, Saini and Morgan, 1989; Kovar and Morgan, 1990). The energy supply in a parenteral nutrition regimen should ideally come from a combination of fat and the carbohydrate glucose (dextrose). A mixture of these two energy sources results in improved nitrogen retention compared with a high carbohydrate energy source (Nose *et al.*, 1987).

Carbohydrate

Glucose is the carbohydrate of choice and is readily utilized by red blood cells, the brain and cardiac muscle. Alternative sources, such as fructose, which may induce a severe lactic acidosis, are not recommended. The amount of glucose infused will depend on the infant's glucose tolerance, which improves with increasing maturity and postnatal age. Glucose will provide between one-third and two-thirds of the total energy requirement. More than this may give rise to glucose overload (hyperglycaemia and glycosuria).

Fat (lipid)

Parenteral lipid emulsions, e.g. Intralipid (Pharmacia), are a very useful and concentrated source of energy and provide essential fatty acids. However, there is a reduced tolerance to lipid emulsions in preterm infants and this is further reduced in infants who are small for gestational age (Andrew, Chan and Schiff, 1976). Parenteral lipid emulsions should therefore be introduced cautiously: 1–4 g/kg/day over 3–4 days is usually safe, even in the sickest of infants (Kovar and Morgan, 1990). In the presence of sepsis the dose should not exceed 2 g/kg/day due to the impaired utilization of parenteral lipid in these situations (Park *et al*, 1986).

Vitamins, minerals and trace elements

There is little information on the optimal requirements of these nutrients in the parenterally fed infant, but it can be assumed that they are marginally less than with the enterally fed infant. Clinical deficiencies of calcium and phosphorus (osteopenia, convulsions, muscle weakness), zinc (growth retardation, skin rashes) and copper (fractures, osteoporosis, anaemia) are recognized in the parenterally fed preterm infant. By providing these minerals and trace elements in the parenteral feed the incidence of these conditions can be reduced.

Parenteral nutrition regimens

The parenteral nutrition regimen should be tailored to the needs of the individual. This will depend upon a detailed evaluation of the infant's condition, any abnormal fluid and electrolyte losses, concurrent infusion therapy and enteral nutrition. The nutrient requirements should be calculated by an experienced clinician who will then pass these on to the pharmacy department. The pharmacy will interpret these requirements into specific amounts of commercially available parenteral solutions and will aseptically prepare the appropriate mixtures.

Before starting the regimen any disturbances of electrolyte and acid–base balance should be corrected. Parenteral feeding can be introduced gradually over a period of 3–6 days, depending on the size and age of the infant. Due to problems of stability when trying to supply all the nutrients in one solution, the lipid emulsion is supplied separately from the amino acids and glucose mixture. The minerals and trace elements are added to the amino acid/glucose mixture, whereas the vitamin supplements are often added to the lipid emulsion.

Administration of parenteral nutrition mixtures

Parenteral nutrition may be administered peripherally, or centrally via a silastic catheter inserted percutaneously or surgically, threaded through the jugular or venal caval systems to the right atrium. The umbilical arterial catheter can also be used. Central venous feeding is preferred because of the problems of phlebitis seen with peripheral administration. This is a result of the hyperosmolar and acidic nature of the solutions.

A wide range of giving sets, filters and infusion pumps is available for the administration of the parenteral nutrition solutions. The management of these lines is not difficult: the most common problems are sepsis or mechanical problems owing to blockage of the small lumen. Sepsis is possible in lines that are damaged, leaking or cracked. Blocking can occur if there is stasis in the line, e.g. in infusions of less than 2 ml/hr, or if blood is allowed to flow back in the line during routine fluid changes (Leick-Rude, 1990).

Complications of parenteral nutrition

- Infusion-related sepsis
- Parenteral nutrition-associated cholestasis
- Glucose intolerance
- Abnormal plasma amino acid profiles
- Hyperammonaemia
- Electrolyte disturbances
- Hypophosphataemia
- Osteopenia and rickets
- Essential fatty acid deficiency
- Metabolic acidosis
- Trace element deficiencies
- Thrombocyte and neutrophil dysfunction
- Aluminium toxicity

The incidence of parenteral nutrition-associated cholestasis can be reduced by the supply of a small volume of enteral feed in infants on TPN, even if the nutrients supplied via this route are nutritionally insignificant at first. This minimal enteral feeding stimulates the production of several gastrointestinal hormones which play a major role in the development of the gut and adaption to extrauterine life (Hughes *et al.*, 1983; Lucas, Bloom and Aynsley-Green, 1986). Obviously, such management would not include infants with gut pathology.

Aluminium toxicity has been a problem in low birth weight infants fed parenterally due to the high aluminium content of some solutions. This complication arises less frequently nowadays with the newer preparations containing crystalline amino acids than with the older protein hydrolysate-containing solutions.

Enteral feeding

Whenever possible feeds should be given to the low birth weight infant to provide all or part of his daily nutritional requirements. For the infant previously receiving TPN, the changeover to enteral feeding should be a very gradual one. It may take a baby weighing less than 1000 g 2–3 weeks to tolerate nutritionally adequate quantities of enteral feeds.

Tube feeding

In the early stages enteral feeds are often better tolerated if they are passed through a tube into the stomach, jejunum or duodenum, particularly if the infant also has respiratory problems. The feeding tube may be passed through the nose or the mouth. Nasal tubes are easier to stabilize than oral ones (Price, 1989), although occlusion of part of the nasal airway may interfere with respiration of the very tiny infant since infants are obligatory nose breathers. Success with the use of dental plate feeding tube fixation has been reported, and small infants are described as tolerating this method well (Leach, 1991). Larger infants with a better-developed gag reflex are more likely to displace oral tubes and will therefore tolerate a nasal tube better.

Gastric feeding

The chosen enteral feed can be given slowly by intermittent gavage or continuous infusion. Intermittent gavage is commonly used, with feeds spaced 1–3 hours apart depending on the infant's condition. Sick and small infants may need feeding by continuous infusion.

One drawback with continuous infusion of feeds is that they are more prone to bacterial contamination (Schreiner *et al.*, 1979). This necessitates the implementation of strict hygiene practices when handling and administering enteral feeds, and great attention must be paid to the initial bacteriological content of the milk given (Anderton, 1983).

With gastric feeding it is important to assess the gastric emptying capacity of the infant by aspirating at regular intervals, usually before each meal with intermittent feeding. Inadequate gastric emptying, relatively competent lower oesophageal sphincter mechanism and small stomach capacity give rise to problems such as regurgitation and increase the risk of aspiration and apnoea. Feeding in the prone position with the head elevated may help to improve the rate of gastric emptying in tube-fed infants.

Problems are minimized by continuous infusion rather than intermittent gavage, although the former method may have adverse metabolic and endocrine effects on the infant.

Continuous infusion is further complicated by the loss of nutrients, especially fat, within the syringes and connecting tubing (Brooke and Barley, 1978; Stocks *et al.*, 1985). This nutrient loss is greater with breast milk than with formula due to its relative instability.

Transpyloric feeding

This method of feeding is usually reserved for very small and sick infants who may show better feed tolerance than with gastric feeding. Complications seen in infants fed in this way include fat malabsorption, diarrhoea, bilious vomiting and, since transpyloric feeds are given continuously, problems with feed contamination. The risks of feed contamination increase with the amount of time the feeds are kept at room temperature before giving: many hospitals stipulate that enteral feeds should be used within 4 hours.

Oral feeding

Since the sucking and swallowing reflexes of low birth weight infants are often poorly developed, oral feeding is rarely possible initially. It is important to check the sucking ability of preterm infants frequently and introduce them to the breast or a bottle when possible. Sucking patterns differ not only between infants of different gestational ages, but between breast- and bottle-feeding infants, the non-nutritive sucking pattern being more rapid than nutritive sucking behaviour (VandenBerg, 1991). Non-nutritive sucking is thought to accelerate the maturation of the sucking reflex, thus allowing the earlier introduction of breast- or bottle-feeding (Kimble, 1992).

Successful breast- and/or bottle-feeding can be achieved in infants with a mean body weight of 1300 g and a mean postnatal age of 11 days (Pearce and Buchanan, 1979). Because of possible breathing impairment, orally fed infants should be closely watched.

Breast milk of formula?

For enterally fed infants the ideal food should supply all the energy, amino acids, essential fatty acids, minerals, trace elements and vitamins the baby needs in balanced quantities. It should not introduce infection, stimulate an allergic response or provoke vomiting, constipation or diarrhoea (Whitelaw, 1986). The options for feeding the enterally fed low birth weight infant include the mother's own breast milk, donated human milk, low birth weight (preterm) milk formula or standard infant formula. The advantages and disadvantages (nutritional and non-nutritional) of the different feeds will now be discussed.

Mother's own breast milk

The mother's own fresh breast milk contains a number of protective substances, including immunoglobin A (IgA), lactoferrin, lysozyme, folate-binding protein, white cells and complement, all giving the breastfed infant greater protection against infections. Other non-nutritional components of fresh breast milk, including enzymes, hormones and growth factors, may convey further benefits to the low birth weight infant.

Most neonatal units encourage mothers to breastfeed or to provide their infants with expressed milk as the sole diet or in conjunction with formula or donated human milk. Many factors may influence a mother's choice to provide for her premature infant, and work by Lucas and colleagues (1988) suggested that hospital staff are unlikely to play a major part in influencing her decision.

Milk from mothers of preterm infants, especially during the first month after delivery, contains more protein, sodium and chloride than milk from mothers of term infants (Hamosh and Hamosh, 1987). If fed at 180–200 ml/kg/day, preterm breast milk may often provide adequate nutrition. However, the composition of human milk shows considerable variation between different individuals and in the same individual at different times of lactation, and the production of these volumes is not often achieved, so supplementation is usually necessary. Supplements of calcium, phosphate, sodium, energy and protein may be required. There are now commercially available breast milk fortifiers (eg. Eoprotin, Milupa Limited) which can be added to breast milk to improve its nutritional composition whilst still providing the benefits of breast milk.

Donated human milk

Until recently it was common for infants whose mothers were not able or willing to feed their babies themselves to receive donated milk from a milk bank. This was used to give the babies some of the non-nutritional advantages and better tolerance of breast milk. Very low birth weight infants have been reported to regurgitate less and have less constipation, abdominal distension and better gastric emptying on breast milk than with any artificial milk formula (Whitelaw, 1986).

Donated breast milk is inferior to mother's milk both immunologically and nutritionally. All donor milk undergoes heat treatment, which destroys about half of the protective substances in breast milk. The pasteurization process may also result in significant losses of some vitamins, notably B_6, C and folic acid (Van Zoeren-Grobben *et al.*, 1987), and inactivates milk lipases, thus affecting fat absorption (Wardell *et al.*, 1984). Donated milk nearly always requires supplementation with sodium, phosphate and, sometimes, energy, protein and calcium.

Because of concerns over the transmission of viral infections, including HIV, from donated human milk, milk banks are not as common as they once were and only a few hospitals now offer this facility. During 1988 and 1989 the Department of Health and Social Security issued recommendations that donors of human milk should be screened for HIV monthly, with all deposits of milk frozen until the donor tests negative. The controversy over breastfeeding and HIV infection has not been resolved. Advice given to women who test HIV-positive in the western world differs from the advice given to HIV-positive women in developing countries because of the economic burden of artificial feeding on poor families and where the availability of clean water and formula milk is less certain. The risk to the infant from breast milk which may contain HIV and cause seroconversion is less than the risk to the infant from bottle feeding (Claxton and Harrison, 1991).

Storage of human milk

Expressed mother's own milk can be stored by refrigeration or freezing. Donated human milk should be frozen as described above. A major problem in the storage of expressed milk is its contamination by bacteria such as *Staphylococcus albus* and

Streptococcus viridans. Hygiene therefore plays an extremely important role in the collection of human milk supplies, and refrigerated milk should be consumed within 24 hours of being expressed.

When storage is required for longer than 1 day, supplies must be frozen at about −20°C, usually for a maximum of 3 months. As with pasteurization, freezing is accompanied by loss of some vitamins (Bank *et al.*, 1985).

If frozen milk does not undergo heat treatment first there can be problems with free fatty acids in stored samples. Milk lipases remain active during freezing at −20°C, which results in the lipolysis of human milk triglycerides. As free fatty acids have been associated with the development of breast-milk jaundice, (Poland, Schultz and Garg, 1980), this is an important consideration. Freezing and thawing can also cause disruption of fat globules and a significant decrease in the percentage of essential polyunsaturated fatty acids (Wardell, Hill and D'Souza, 1981).

Milk formulas

If inadequate breast milk supplies are available, or it is decided that an infant should be formula fed, there are two choices available: either a standard infant formula or a special low birth weight (preterm) formula can be given. The list below shows which formulas are currently available in each category.

Standard infant formulas are available in dried and ready-to-feed form

Whey dominant

- Aptamil with Milupan (Milupa Limited)
- Cow & Gate Nutrilon Premium (Nutricia)
- SMA Gold (Wyeth Laboratories)
- First Milk (Farleys)

Casein dominant (not normally used in low birth weight infants)

- Milumil (Milupa Limited)
- Cow & Gate Nutrilon Plus (Nutricia)
- SMA White (Wyeth Laboratories)
- Second Milk 2 (Farleys)

Low birth weight formulas are available in ready-to-feed form only

- Prematil with Milupan (Milupa Limited) (also available in dried form)
- Cow & Gate Nutriprem (Nutricia)
- SMA LBW Formula (Wyeth Laboratories)
- Osterprem (Farleys)
- Premcare (Farleys) (also available in dried form)

Standard infant formulas are designed for full-term infants and do not meet specific nutritional needs of low birth weight infants, especially those weighing less than 1800 g. If standard milk formulas are used supplements will invariably be required.

On the other hand, the special low birth weight formulas have been specially developed for low birth weight (preterm) infants and thus require minimal or no supplementation. Low birth weight formulas have increased protein, sodium, calcium, phosphate and energy contents, compared with breast milk and standard infant formulas, and have been shown to produce better growth (weight, length and head circumference) than other methods of feeding (Brooke, Wood and Barley, 1982; Curran *et al.*, 1982; Lucas *et al.*, 1984; Spencer, Stammers and Hull, 1986). Despite these advantages, neonates fed on cow's milk-based formulas show an increased incidence of gastro-intestinal disturbances and become latently sensitized to cow's milk protein. Although this does not appear to increase the overall risk of allergy in the long term for most infants, if there is a family history of atopy, early exposure to cow's milk increases the risk of allergic reactions, especially eczema (Lucas *et al.*, 1990).

If a low birth weight formula is being used it should ideally be given until body weight reaches 2000–2500g, or until discharge from the neonatal unit, whichever is sooner.

Composition of low birth weight formulas

The ESPGAN Committee on Nutrition of the Preterm Infant have issued guidelines (1987, 1991) on the composition of milk formulas intended for preterm infants. The composition

Table 7.1 Low birth weight formulas - Nutritional Composition

		Typical analysis per 100 ml ready to feed formulation					
		ESPGAN		Prematil with Milupan (Milupa)	SMA LBW formula (Wyeth)	Nutri-prem (Cow & Gate)	Oster-prem (Farleys)
		min	max				
Protein	g	1.5	2.6	2.0	2.0	2.2	2.0
Casein: whey		NS		40:60	NA	40:60	40:60
Taurine	mg	NS		6.0	4.8	1.5	5.1
Fat							
Total	g	2.9	5.1	3.5	4.4	4.4	4.6
Linoleic acid	g	0.325	1.2	0.38	0.7	0.57	0.51
AA	g	NS		0.016	-	0.001	-
DHA	g	NS		0.011	-	0.014	-
Sat/Unsat		NS		53/47	48.2/51.8	41/59	42.3/57.7
Carbohydrate							
Total	g	4.55	11.9	7.7	8.6	8.0	7.65
Lactose	g	2.1	10.2	5.0	4.3	4.0	6.0
Maltodextrin	g	NS		2.7	4.3	-	1.65
Glucose syrup	g	NS		-	-	4.0	-
Minerals							
Sodium	mg	15	45	27	33	32	42
Potassium	mg	46	126	71	74	71	72
Chloride	mg	30	75	38	54	45	60
Calcium	mg	46	119	70	77	108	110
Magnesium	mg	3.9	10.2	6.0	7.0	8.0	5.0
Phosphorus	mg	33	77	42	41	54	63
Iron	mg	NS		0.1	0.67	0.9	0.04
Ca/P		1.4	2.0	1.7	1.88	2.0	1.8
Trace elements							
Zinc	mg	0.36	0.9⁺	0.39	0.82	0.7	0.88
Copper	µg	59	102	64	74	80	96
Manganese	µg	1.4	6.4⁺	13	6.0	14	3.0
Iodine	µg	6.5	38	10	8.2	20	8.0
Vitamins							
Vitamin A	µg	59	128	63	74	100	100
Vitamin D_3	µg	-	2.6	2.1	1.2	2.4	2.4
Vitamin E	mg	0.4	8.5	2.0	1.1	1.0	10
Vitamin K_1	µg	2.6	17⁺	2.8	7.1	9.0	7.0
Vitamin B_1	µg	13	213⁺	40	82	100	95
Vitamin B_2	µg	39	510⁺	140	131	160	180
Niacin	mg	0.52	4.21⁺	0.55	0.65	1.55	0.99
Vitamin B_6	µg	23	213⁺	90	49	80	100
Vitamin B_{12}	µg	0.1	-	0.15	0.25	0.2	0.2
Folic acid	µg	39	-	43	49	48	50
Pantothenic acid	µg	195	-	266	369	500	500
Biotin	µg	1.0	-	1.1	1.8	3.0	2.0
Vitamin C	mg	4.6	34	15	7.0	28	28
Energy	kJ	272	356	298	335	336	334
	kcal	65	85	70	80	80	80
Osmolality	mosmol/kg			280	268	246	300
Potential renal solute load	mosmol/l			121	128	133	134

These analytical values are subject to slight variations normally accepted with natural products. NS = Not specified ⁺ = Tentative guidelines of the currently available formulas and the ESPGAN guidelines are shown in Table 7.1. Although these low birth weight formulas are very similar in composition, in many respects there are differences in the fat blends used and the degree of iron supplementation.

Fat blend

As mentioned earlier, n-6 and n-3 LCPs are now considered essential nutrients for preterm infants and therefore it may be beneficial to choose a formula which has been supplemented with LCPs.

Iron

If a low birth weight formula is to be used, the choice can be made between using one that is supplemented with iron or one that is not. As previously discussed, it may be advantageous to avoid dietary iron before the age of 6–8 weeks (later in babies receiving regular blood transfusions) because of the risk of Gram-negative infections. Whichever formula is used, iron supplements should be given from not later than 8 weeks to achieve a total iron intake of 2–2.5 mg/kg/day (maximum 15 mg/day).

Other formulas

Infants showing poor tolerance of certain nutritional components of standard or low birth weight formulas may benefit from the use of one of the other special formulas available for infants with special dietary needs. For example, if an infant shows an allergic response to the whole cow's milk protein found in standard and low birth weight formulas, a protein hydrolysate feed, e.g. Prejomin (Milupa), Pregestimil (Mead Johnson), may be indicated. These 'hypoallergenic' feeds are also free from lactose, galactose, sucrose and fructose, making them suitable for infants with intolerance to these sugars. Because of their 'semi-elemental' nature, these formulas are generally well absorbed and may therefore be appropriate for feeding the infant with short bowel syndrome and other malabsorption syndromes.

Infants with any of the inborn errors of amino acid metabolism, such as phenylketonuria, will only be able to tolerate small amounts of breast milk or standard/low birth weight formulas and will require a specially designed feed to provide them with their nutritional requirements. In the case of phenylketonuria, a phenylalanine-free or phenylalanine-low formula will be required, e.g. Analog (SHS) or Minafen (Nutricia). Several other products for infants with special dietary needs are available, and details of these can be obtained from the hospital dietitian.

Enteral feeding regimens

The well preterm infant should be fed within 2 hours of birth. Sick and very low birth weight infants will require intravenous dextrose for the first 24 h, before enteral feeding is tried. The feed should be introduced with quantities of 40–60 ml/kg/day. This volume is increased by 20–30 ml/kg daily until a level of 150–200 ml/kg/day is achieved. Small for gestational age infants will need to receive the upper limit of these volume ranges in order to consume adequate energy and thus avoid hypoglycaemia.

Whichever method of feeding is chosen, the parents are integral partners in care and are encouraged to play an active role. In many units this active role may extend to tube feeding and, with education, help and support, some parents can learn to pass the feeding tube itself.

Some infants are very difficult and frustrating to feed. These include infants who have been intubated and ventilated for a long time, those who have developed oral hypersensitivity (Harris, 1986) and those who have survived but have residual chronic lung disease. These infants have little spare energy and they quickly tire and lose their sucking and swallowing co-ordination. They then choke and panic, causing feeding to become a negative experience.

The infant who is squirming, fussing and refusing the teat is not enjoying his feed. Feeding should be a comfortable, pleasurable experience, happily associated with warm and gentle handling, preferably by the family. VandenBerg (1990) suggests a flexible approach to feeding, trying several types of teat and not remaining entrenched with one type. Teats come in many different shapes, sizes, flow rates and textures. Some look quite bizarre but are really effective. One recently developed teat has been very successful in the feeding of infants with poorly developed lower jaws (Haberman, 1988). Several small holes are better than one large one. Thickening the feed can result in greater swallowing control but this means that the infant has to suck harder to complete the feed. Experimentation with feeding times, temperature of the feed and, unless contraindicated, flavouring an unpalatable formula may result in a routine which suits the uncooperative feeder. In feeding, as in other aspects of care, staff have different handling patterns and it helps if the number of caregivers can be minimized.

Meier (1988) questioned the dogma that surrounds many infant feeding practices and points out that the practice of not allowing the mother who wants to breastfeed her infant to do so until the infant is feeding satisfactorily by bottle, is unfounded. If the infant is thought to be sufficiently well to attempt an oral feed by mouth then, arguably, this is also the case with breastfeeding. Some research suggests that sucking, swallowing and breathing are better coordinated during breastfeeding (Meier and Anderson, 1987) and the beneficial spinoffs are that infants remain warmer and have better oxygen saturation levels.

Infants being fed intermittently should have gastric pH and residue levels checked before each successive feed to ensure that they are tolerating the feed. This is important since increasing gastric aspirate volumes, which may be bile-stained, can indicate the development of NEC.

Effects of feeding choice on development and clinical outcome

There is a great variety of feeding regimens, differing in nutritional and non-nutritional content, used in neonatology today. Besides meeting the immediate needs of the low birth weight infant for survival, the chosen feeding regimen should give the infant the best opportunity to grow and develop normally.

There have been very few studies on the effect of diet on clinical outcome, but since 1982 a large multicentre study in the UK has attempted to answer some of the questions asked. Does early diet affect later growth in preterm infants? Does feeding choice influence long-term neurological development? In this study developmental differences between preterm infants receiving preterm formula, standard formula or banked human milk as the sole source of nutrition or as a supplement to expressed mother's breast milk, have been measured. In a 9-month follow-up of some infants in the study mean development quotients were lower in infants receiving unfortified banked human milk than in those receiving a preterm formula, particularly in small for gestational age infants (Lucas *et al.*, 1989).

At the 18-month post-term follow-up, infants who had received a preterm formula in the postpartum period were shown to have higher mental and psychomotor developmental scores (Bayley scales of infant development) and social quotients (Vineland social maturity scale) and a lower frequency of moderate developmental impairment than infants fed a standard formula. This beneficial effect of preterm formula was significantly greater for small for gestational age than for appropriate for gestational age infants and for males more than females (Lucas *et al.*, 1990b).

Follow-up of the same children at 7.5–8 years of age has shown that children who had consumed mother's milk in the early weeks of life had a significantly higher intelligence quotient (IQ) than those children who received no mother's milk (Lucas *et al.*, 1992). Although these results could be explained by differences in parenting skills or genetic potential (even after adjustment for mother's education and social class), it appears that breast milk has beneficial effects on the neurological development of the preterm infant.

Breast milk is known to contain LCPs which are important for the structural development of the nervous system (Koletzko *et al.*, 1989). Numerous hormones and trophic factors in human milk might also influence brain development. Further research is needed to determine whether the advantage of feeding preterm infants with human milk is due to parenting or genetic factors, or to factors in the milk itself.

REFERENCES

American Academy of Pediatrics Committee on Nutrition (1985) Nutritional needs of low birth weight infants. *Pediatrics* **75**(5), 976–86.

Anderton, A. (1983) Microbiological aspects of the preparation and administration of naso-gastric and naso-enteric tube feeds in hospitals – a review. *Human Nutrition: Applied Nutrition* **37A**, 426–40.

Andrew, G., Chan, G. and Schiff, D. (1976) Lipid metabolism in the neonate. 1. The effects of Intralipid infusion on plasma triglyceride and free fatty acid concentrations in the neonate. *Journal of Pediatrics* **88**(2), 273–8.

Bank, M., Kirksey, A., West, K. and Giacoia, G. (1985) Effects of storage time and temperature on folacin and vitamin C levels in term and preterm human milk. *American Journal of Clinical Nutrition* **41**, 235–42.

Brooke, O. and Barley, J. (1978) Loss of energy during continuous infusion of breast milk. *Archives of Disease in Childhood* **53**, 344–5.

Brooke, O., Wood, C. and Barley, J. (1982) Energy balance, nitrogen balance, and growth in preterm infants fed expressed breast milk, a premature infant formula, and two low-solute adapted formulae. *Archives of Disease in Childhood* **57**, 898–904.

Bullen, J., Rogers, H. and Leigh, L. (1972) Iron-binding proteins in milk and resistance to *Escherichia coli* infection in infants. *British Medical Journal* **1**, 69–75.

Claxton, R. and Harrison, T. (1991) *Caring for Children with HIV and Aids*, Edward Arnold, London.

Curran, J.S., Barness, L.A., Brown, D.R., *et al.* (1982) Results of feeding a special formula to very-low-birthweight infants. *Journal of Pediatric Gastroenterology and Nutrition* **1**, 327–32.

Dear, P. (1992) Total parenteral nutrition of the newborn. *Care of the Critically Ill* **8**(6), 252–7.

ESPGAN Committee on Nutrition of the Preterm Infant (1987) Nutrition and feeding of preterm infants. *Acta Paediatrica Scandinavica* **Supplement 336**.

ESPGAN Committee on Nutrition (1991) Committee Report. Comment on the content and composition of lipids in infant formulas. *Acta Paediatrica Scandinavica* **80**, 887–96.

Haberman, M. (1988) A mother of invention. *Nursing Times* **84**(2), 52–3.

Hamosh, P. and Hamosh, M. (1987) Differences in composition of preterm, term and weaning milk, in *New Aspects of Nutrition in Pregnancy, Infancy and Prematurity*, (ed M. Xanthou), Elsevier Science Publishers B.V. (Biomedical Division), Amsterdam, The Netherlands, pp. 129–41.

Harris, M. (1986) Oral motor management of the high risk neonate, in*The High Risk Neonate; Developmental Therapy Perspectives*, (ed. J. Sweeny), Haworth Press, New York, pp. 231–51.

Hughes, C., Talbot, I., Ducker, D. and Harran, M. (1983) Total parenteral nutrition in infancy: effect on the liver and suggested pathogenesis. *Gut* **24**, 241–8.

Kimble, C. (1992) Nonnutritive sucking; adaptation and health for the neonate. *Neonatal Network*, **11**(2), 29–33.

Koletzko, B. (1990) Inproved essential fatty acid status of premature infants by dietary supplementation of both omega-6 and omega-3 long chain polyunsaturates, in *Recent Advances in Infant Feeding, Symposium Leidschendam 1990*, (ed B. Koletzko, A. Okken, J. Rey,

B. Salle, J. Van Biervliet), Georg Thieme Verlag, Stuttgart, pp. 28–32.

Koletzko, B., Schmidt, E., Bremer, H., Haug, M. and Harzer, G. (1989) Effects of dietary long-chain polyunsaturated fatty acids on the essential fatty acid status of premature infants. *European Journal of Pediatrics* **148**, 669–75.

Kovar, I. and Morgan, J. (1990) Parenteral nutrition in the preterm infant. *Clinical Nutrition* **9**, 57–63.

Kovar, I., Saini, J. and Morgan, J. (1989) The sick very low birthweight infant fed by parenteral nutrition: studies of nitrogen and energy. *European Journal of Clinical Nutrition* **43**, 339–46.

Leach, G. (1991) Dental plates for oral feeding. *Nursing Times* **87**(46), 58–9.

Leaf, A., Leighfield, M., Costeloe, K. and Crawford, M. (1992) Long chain polyunsaturated fatty acids and fetal growth. *Early Human Development* **30**, 183–91.

Leick-Rude, M. (1990) Use of percutaneous silastic catheters in high risk neonates. *Neonatal Network* **9**(1), 17–25.

Lucas, A. and Cole, T. (1990) Breast milk and neonatal necrotising enterocolitis. *Lancet* **336**, 1519–23.

Lucas, A., Bloom, S. and Aynsley-Green, A. (1986) Gut hormones and 'minimal enteral feeding'. *Acta Paediatrica Scandinavica* **75**, 719–23.

Lucas, A., Gore, S., Cole, T. *et al*. (1984) Multicentre trial on feeding low birthweight infants: effects of diet on early growth. *Archives of Disease in Childhood* **59**, 722–30.

Lucas, A., Cole, T., Morley, R., *et al*. (1988) Factors associated with maternal choice to provide breast milk for low birthweight infants. *Archives of Disease in Childhood* **63**, 48–52.

Lucas, A., Morley, R., Cole,T. *et al*. (1989) Early diet in preterm babies and developmental status in infancy. *Archives of Disease in Childhood* **64**, 1570–8.

Lucas, A., Brooke, O., Morley, R., Cole, T. and Bamford, M. (1990a) Early diet of preterm infants and development of allergic or atopic disease: randomised prospective study. *British Medical Journal* **300**, 837–40.

Lucas, A., Morley, R., Cole, T. *et al*. (1990b) Early diet in preterm babies and developmental status at 18 months. *Lancet* **335**, 1477–81.

Lucas, A., Morley, R., Cole, T., Lister, G. and Leeson-Payne, C. (1992) Breast milk and subsequent intelligence quotient in children born preterm. *Lancet* **339**, 261–4.

McIntosh, N., Livesey, A. and Brooke, O. (1982) Plasma 25-hydroxyvitamin D and rickets in infants of extremely low birthweight. *Archives of Disease in Childhood* **57**, 848–50.

Meier, P. (1988) Bottle and breast feeding: effects on transcutaneous oxygen pressure and temperature in preterm infants. *Nursing Research* **37**(1), 36–41.

Meier, P. and Anderson, G. (1987) Responses of small preterm infants to bottle and breast feeding. *American Journal of Maternal and Child Nursing* **12**, 97–105.

Morgan, J. (1992) Nutrition of the very low birthweight infant. *Care of the Critically Ill* **8**(3), 122–4.
Nose, O., Tipton, J., Ament, M. and Yabuuchi, H. (1987) Effect of the energy source on changes in energy expenditure, respiratory quotient, and nitrogen balance during total parenteral nutrition in children. *Pediatric Research* **21**(6), 538–41.
Park, W., Paust, H., Brosicke, H., Knoblach, G. and Helge, H. (1986) Impaired fat utilization in parenterally fed low-birthweight infants suffering from sepsis. *Journal of Parenteral and Enteral Nutrition* **10**(6), 627–30.
Pearce, J. and Buchanan, L. (1979) Breast milk and breast feeding in very low birthweight infants. *Archives of Disease in Childhood* **54**, 897–9.
Price, B. (1989) Making sense of nasogastric intubation. *Nursing Times* **85**(13), 50–2.
Poland, R., Schultz, G. and Garg, G. (1980) High milk lipase activity associated with breast milk jaundice. *Pediatric Research* **14**, 1328–31.
Schreiner, R.L., Eitzen, H., Gfell, M.A. *et al.* (1979) Environmental contamination of continuous drip feedings. *Pediatrics* **63**(2), 232–7.
Spencer, S., Stammers, J. and Hull, D. (1986) Evaluation of a special low-birthweight formula, with and without the use of medium-chain triglycerides. *Early Human Development* **13**, 87–95.
Stocks, R.J., Davied, D.P., Allen, F. and Sewell, D. (1985) Loss of breast milk nutrients during tube feeding. *Archives of Disease in Childhood* **60**, 164–6.
Uauy, R., Birch, D., Birch, E., Tyson, J. and Hoffman, D. (1990) Are omega-3 fatty acids required for normal eye and brain development of the very low birth weight infant? in *Recent Advances in Infant Feeding, Symposium Leidschendam 1990* (eds B. Koletzko, A. Okken, J. Rey, B. Salle, J. Van Biervliet), Georg Thieme Verlag, Stuttgart, 13–21.
VandenBerg, K. (1990) Nippling management of the sick neonate in the NICU. The disorganized feeder. *Neonatal Network* **9**(1), 9–16.
Van Zoeren-Grobben, D., Schrijver, J., Van den Berg, H. and Berger, H. (1987) Human milk vitamin content after pasteurisation, storage, or tube feeding. *Archives of Disease in Childhood* **62**, 161–5.
Wardell, J., Hill, C. and D'Souza, S. (1981) Effect of pasteurization and of freezing and thawing human milk on its triglyceride content. *Acta Paediatrica Scandinavica* **70**, 467–71.
Wardell, J., Wright, A., Bardsley, W. and D'Souza, S. (1984) Bile salt-stimulated lipase and esterase activity in human milk after collection, storage and heating: nutritional implications. *Pediatric Research* **18**(4), 382–6.
Wharton, B. (ed.) (1987) *Nutrition and Feeding of Preterm Infants*, Blackwell Scientific Publications, Oxford.
Whitelaw, A. (1986) Feeding the very-low-birthweight infant. *Human Nutrition: Applied Nutrition* **40A** (Supplement 1), 19–26.

8

Nursing care of a baby with a disorder of the respiratory system

Doreen Crawford

Respiratory problems are the commonest cause of morbidity and mortality in the neonatal period. Each infant has individual differences in the rate of respiration, although the average is approximately 40 breaths per minute. Efficient and effective respiration, with adequate gas exchange, never results in laboured respiration. What constitutes tachypnoea may be defined differently between units; Roberton (1986) considers the average to be between 35 and 45 breaths per minute, and Levene (1987) states that a respiratory rate of 60 breaths per minute or over is tachypnoeic.

The collection of clinical symptoms indicating respiratory difficulties remains fairly constant across a wide range of diseases and disorders. The main ones are as follows:

- The extra effort required to meet the infant's respiratory needs causes retraction of the intercostal and subcostal muscles. This makes him look as if his chest wall is caving in.
- The use of accessory muscles, such as the ali nasi, makes the nose flare.
- Combined use of neck and shoulder muscles gives the infant a tense distorted look and the chest may look too big for him.
- Hypoxia leads to pallor or cyanosis of the skin and mucous membrane tissues.

- Respiratory muscle failure, including the diaphragm, leads to exhaustion and apnoea, especially in the premature infant.
- Initially, the infant may be restless but the sicker he is the more lethargic he will become, conserving all his energy in a desperate struggle to breathe and stay alive.

ANATOMY AND PHYSIOLOGY OF THE RESPIRATORY SYSTEM

Knowledge of the development of the respiratory system and of the transition from uterine to extrauterine life will enhance the neonatal nurse's understanding of when life is actually feasible, and of the complications which can occur in term, as well as premature, infants.

Table 8.1 Summary of respiratory tract development

Time from fertilization	*Developmental aspects*
Days 15–21	Ectoderm, endoderm and mesoderm formation. Diaphragm development begins
Day 24	Laryngotracheal groove develops
Days 26–28	Bronchial buds form
Day 28+	Primary nasal cavity, tongue and pharynx formation. Phrenic nerve originates
Day 35+	Pseudoglandular phase lobar bronchi present, pulmonary artery and vein develop. Lungs bud into pleural canals
Day 42+	Arytenoid swellings (precursor to formation of larynx)
Day 49+	Oropharynx develops. Tracheal cartilage. Smooth muscle of bronchi present
Day 56+	Vocal cords develop
Day 63+	Bronchial arteries develop. Secondary palate forms, mucous glands appear
11 weeks	Lymphatic tissue appears, cilia develop. Tracheal cartilage
13 weeks	Goblet cells appear
16 weeks	Canalicular phase begins, preacinar bronchial branches complete
22 weeks	System for synthesis of lecithin
24 weeks	Alveolar phase begins; respiratory bronchioles develop, terminal sacs develop
26–28 weeks	Alveolar–capillary surface now sufficient to support life
36 weeks	Mature alveoli present
After birth	Additional conductive airways form (respiratory bronchioles, alveoli, ducts and sacs)
Age 8 years	Respiratory tract now complete

The lungs develop to a relatively fixed timetable late in fetal life. They are often referred to as non-functional organs until after birth, i.e. they grow and mature independently of the needs of the gowing embryo and fetus (Table 8.1).

Upper respiratory tract

The development of this is complex and inextricably intertwined with that of the face. It is completed fairly early and all the major structures are recognizable by 12 weeks' gestation.

Lower respiratory tract

Airway and lung development may be divided into three parts:

- Glandular stage: 5–15 weeks
- Canalicular stage: 16–24 weeks
- Alveolar stage: 24+ weeks

Glandular stage

This includes the tracheobronchial development which, after birth, is vital to the conduction of air into the lungs. If the fetus is born at this stage there is no hope for independent existence, as respiration is not possible. The airways have blind ends and are not yet joined to the precursors to the alveoli. Gas exchange cannot occur.

Canalicular stage

During this stage, the formation of the alveoli and associated capillary network is developed to a point at which it is possible to exchange gas. Each terminal bronchiole has given rise to two or more respiratory bronchioles. The alveoli have formed and are lined with a continuous sheet of specialized epithelium. Two kinds of highly specialized cells (type 1 and type 2 alveolar cells) can be identified.

Type 1 cells are thought to have a structural supporting role in the alveoli and type 2 cells are thought to play a role in the synthesis of surfactant. Surfactant is a complex fat and protein substance which first appears in the lungs at 22–24 weeks' gestation, and the concentration of this greatly increases as the lungs mature. Surfactant plays a crucial role in lowering surface tension in the alveoli: a deficit gives rise to alveolar instability, which may lead to collapse during expiration and cause respiratory distress. Respiratory distress syndrome is discussed later in this chapter. In a few cases, life is possible towards the end of this stage.

It is just possible that the chances of survival in the preterm infant could be enhanced if our resuscitation methods were to be revised (Chapter 4). Animal studies (Kolobow, 1988) have shown that, if a higher inflatory pressure is sustained for several seconds with the first gasp, then further lung units are cannulated and these remain in use with subsequent ventilation. Full clinical trials would need to be performed to ensure that this would be of long-lasting benefit and that the underdeveloped air sacs cannulated by force were valuable gas-exchanging units.

Alveolar stage

During this stage the alveoli multiply, thus increasing the gas exchange area available to support life. At birth this stage is incomplete and continues until the 8th year of life. The fact that the fetus makes breathing motions while *in utero* is not disputed, and the ratios of surfactant found in the amniotic fluid give us a clue as to how advanced development actually is. It is not known at what stage of gestation these breathing movements actually commence. It is probable that the lungs need to be sufficiently mature for expansion to occur.

In cases of threatening preterm labour, the development of the lungs is said to be enhanced by giving steroids to the mother (Liggings and Howie, 1972), although there is some debate about this. The maturation of the lungs after birth can be retarded by acidosis and hypothermia.

TRANSITION FROM INTRAUTERINE LIFE TO INDEPENDENT EXISTENCE

Prior to birth the lungs are full of fluid. They have had no contact with air. During the process of birth, this fluid is partly squeezed out by the extra thoracic pressure exerted on the on the baby's chest wall by the maternal birth canal. Under normal circumstances, the fluid remaining in the lungs is removed by increased lymph drainage and swallowing after coughing and sneezing.

The first breath does not expand both lungs fully and it is probable that minutes, perhaps even hours, elapse until the lungs are fully ventilated and evenly expanded. Vital capacity and residual volume will also increase as the pattern of breathing becomes established. Chest circumference has a rapid increase in the first 24–48 h after birth. Marieb (1992) states that it is nearly 2 weeks before the infant's lungs are fully expanded, and that at birth the infant has only a sixth of the adult number of alveoli.

Occasionally, in an otherwise well, mature, term baby, these mechanisms fail to clear and expand the lungs and the infant suffers a temporary respiratory problem called transient tachypnoea of the newborn.

STRUCTURAL DIFFERENCES IN ANATOMY BETWEEN THE INFANT AND THE ADULT

Differences exist in the anatomy of the infant's respiratory system compared to that of the adult. The main differences are:

- the smaller diameter of the infant's airway;
- the relative immaturity and inelasticity of the lungs;
- the cough reflex is absent until 32–34 weeks' gestation;
- the infant has a high larynx, protected by the epiglottis. This has the effect of producing a direct airway from the nasal cavity to the lungs. The infant is therefore an obligatory nose breather.
- the ribs of the newborn are positioned horizontally and the intercostal muscles are weak;
- the thoracic wall is compliant. The net effect of this is that the mode of lung ventilation is essentially a diaphragmatic one and, if difficulties occur, the thoracic wall may 'cave in' and give rise to sternal and intercostal retractions with the extra strain of breathing;
- the premature and sick newborn is highly susceptible to diaphragmatic fatigue and, up to a point, compensates for this by increasing the rate of respiration rather than the tidal volume. This is, in effect, a vicious cycle and the sick newborn comes closer to respiratory failure.

The lungs, which are relatively inactive during fetal life, have no role in keeping the infant oxygenated because prior to birth the placenta and the membranes perform the functions of protecting, respiring, nurturing and excreting for the infant until an independent status is reached. Without an efficient system for the above functions there would have been severe fetal insult and death.

Under normal circumstances, maternal and fetal circulations never mix and the fetus receives materials for transfer courtesy of a difference in pressure between the high-pressure maternal side and the lower-pressure fetal side. Oxygen and carbon dioxide are transferred by simple diffusion and the fetal haemoglobin has a greater affinity to oxygen and so makes the most of a limited saturation. Certain maternal factors also limit the saturation of oxygen available to the fetus. Active or passive smoking is incriminated in a smaller birth weight than would otherwise be expected. High maternal blood pressure causes damage to the placenta and maternal hypotensive incidents limit the placental circulation and hence the circulation available to the fetus.

CARE OF THE INFANT WITH BREATHING DIFFICULTIES

Some causes of infant breathing difficulties are:

- meconium inhalation;
- congenital pneumonia;
- aspiration pneumonia;
- pulmonary hypertension;
- transient tachypnoea of the newborn;
- respiratory distress syndrome;
- chronic lung disease;
- hypoplastic lungs;
- choanal atresia;
- diaphragmatic hernia;
- tracheo-oesophageal fistula;
- tracheomalacia;
- drug-induced respiratory depression.

The subject of breathing difficulties is too vast to be easily condensed into a single chapter. As this is a nursing text and not a medical encyclopaedia, three different respiratory conditions, each with differing severity and requiring different levels of care, will be discussed. These are transient tachypnoea of the newborn, severe respiratory distress syndrome needing ventilation with intermittent positive pressure ventilation, and the surgical condition of severe diaphragmatic hernia.

Transient tachypnoea of the newborn

Aetiology

This condition commonly affects the large, otherwise well, term infant but it can also affect the premature (Roberton, 1986). It is thought to arise from delayed clearance of fetal lung fluid. Typically the infant develops increasing respiratory distress within an hour or two of birth. There may be grunting, nasal flaring, sternal and rib retractions, and the respiratory rate is greatly elevated. Infants with this condition are satisfying to nurse as they are quickly ill, demanding of one's nursing skill for a period of about 48 hours, and then they are quickly better.

Differential diagnosis

It is difficult to distinguish the respiratory difficulties of transient tachpynoea of the newborn from pneumonia, other infections or respiratory distress syndrome, especially in the early stages. Blood and, occasionally, gastric aspirates are cultured. Chest X-rays are performed, but at such an early stage they are rarely helpful. Later, they may show large hyperinflated lungs and increased pulmonary vascularity. Free fluid may be present in the horizontal fissure. Because of the difficulty of distinguishing this condition from congenital pneumonia, intravenous antibiotics are often given until negative cultures come back from the laboratory.

Care of the parents

Sudden admission or transfer to a neonatal unit is a shock: parents tend to feel less at ease on the unit, as their infant is usually the biggest one there and looks so out of place in an incubator, among the small and premature.

Nursing care and management

The nursing diagnosis is one of 'breathing difficulties and distress' and the aim would be to 'support the infant, to provide relief, to ease the work of breathing and to closely monitor the baby to detect signs of deterioration'. The care plan would take into account the infant's individual needs but would include:

- Consideration of the infant's position. Position him prone or supported on either side, head elevated on an apnoea mattress which should be covered in a warm soft sheet, duvet or sheepskin to provide tactile comfort, warmth and support (Chapter 14).
- Monitor and observe the infant. He should be fully monitored to ensure continuous readings of cardiac trace, oxygen saturation and rate of respiration. Non-invasive methods are used whenever possible (Paige, 1990). The advantage of continuous readings is that the baby is less handled and stressed. He is able to rest, conserve energy and recover. The disadvantage is that parents focus on the monitors and may become anxious. This is less likely if the reason for using the monitors is explained and reassurance given that these are all very temporary and will be removed as soon as he starts to improve.
- Provide oxygen according to the infant's needs. Warm and humidified oxygen should be given as prescribed, probably via a headbox. This is a clear plastic dome which is placed over the infant's head. Into it flows oxygen and air which has been warmed and humidified by allowing it to flow over a hot-water tank. The amount of gas needed is regulated by a flowmeter. The concentration that the baby is actually receiving is checked by having an oxygen analyser at a safe distance from his face. Typically this is about 30–40% but may be more (Halliday, McClure and Reid, 1981). The amount of oxygen that a baby requires is determined by blood gas results. As these infants are typically not very ill, radial samples are probably sufficient, on a 4–6 hourly basis, with the frequency decreasing as the condition stabilizes. Arterial catheterization is rarely warranted unless the infant is very unstable or there is serious doubt about the cause of the tachypnoea.

Once he is clinically stable and the respiratory rate settling and blood gas results improving, the amount of oxygen should be weaned down (according to the level of SaO_2 recorded by non-invasive pulse oximetry).

- Keep the infant warm and comfortable. The infant is nursed exposed, for ease of observation, in an incubator or under an overhead heater, which should be set at an appropriate temperature. A term infant typically needs less support in assisting temperature control and may become hot and sweaty due to the high environmental temperature of the unit. Skill is needed to keep the infant (and the parents) cool. His basic hygiene needs are the same as for any big normal infant except that he will initially tolerate less handling.
- The infant's need for stable blood glucose. On admission a blood glucose level should be checked by blood glucose stick. If this is satisfactory (4–6 mmol/l), random levels can be checked whenever he is being disturbed for handling. Normal blood glucose is maintained by intravenous dextrose.
- The infant's need for hydration and nutrition. He needs fluid and nutrition but is unable to suck because of the tachypnoea and respiratory distress. Typically an intravenous line is established and he would receive intravenous fluids, calculated according to weight and local protocol. Fluid needs may vary as sick infants retain fluid and may not tolerate the calculated requirements. The disadvantage of keeping him 'nil by mouth' is that once he starts to feel better he may become hungry and quite cross. He can be offered a soother, if the parents consent. A distressed, cross and hungry infant results in an elevated respiratory rate and a vicious cycle begins.

Feeding by nasogastric tube can be tried until he is able to feed by mouth. The nasogastric tube would be passed and taped securely in place, then left for an hour to see if the placing of the tube and the narrowing of the infant's airway compromise the respiratory function. Once milk feeding is commenced, the intravenous infusion is decreased. Typically he will improve rapidly and can be introduced to the breast or bottle (whatever the parents choose) when it becomes apparent that he is ready to feed. Feeding techniques and the management of hydration and nutrition are discussed elsewhere (Chapter 7), as is the care and support of the parents (Chapter 3).

Respiratory distress syndrome

Aetiology

Respiratory distress syndrome (RDS) is still the commonest cause of neonatal mortality in the UK (Roberton, 1993). It affects 20% of low birth weight infants and 60–70% of very low birth weight infants. Improvement of these mortality figures will depend on improved socioeconomic factors to improve infant birth weight, as well as high standards of nursing care and medical treatment.

The disease is characterized by a typical 'ground-glass' chest X-ray with air bronchograms. The clinical picture is one of multiple signs of respiratory distress:

- Grunting: the sound of exhaling against a closed glottis. This maintains a high residual air volume in the lungs to prevent functional collapse.
- Nasal flaring, tachypnoea and cyanosis may be present soon after birth, or within 4 hours.
- Severe rib and sternal retractions may be present in the preterm infant with a highly compliant chest wall.

Classically RDS follows an acute course with deterioration for the first 2–3 days of life, a period of supported stability and then, often, dramatic improvement.

RDS affects infants who are born too early and have immature lungs. Other causes include perinatal asphyxia, birth by caesarean section and maternal diabetes. The disease is not yet fully understood; why some infants born at 28 weeks' gestation do not develop the disease and others born at 36 weeks do, is not known (Roberton, 1986).

The level of surfactant plays a major role in the aetiology of the disease. The higher the surfactant levels before birth, the less likely the infant is to develop the disease. Infants with low surfactant levels are said to have 'stiff lungs': the alveoli tend to collapse on expiration and a high inspiratory pressure is needed to reinflate them (Bhutani *et al.*, 1992). Medical treatment of this condition includes the use of artificial surfactant, although there is some debate as to the most effective preparation (Cummings *et al.*, 1992), frequency and dosage to use (Speer *et al.*, 1992), and whether to give it prophylactically or therapeutically (Hoekstra *et al.*, 1991). Surfactant has given encouraging results and will, in some cases, support the infant until he can produce his own natural surfactant. Gortner (1992) suggested that infants appropriately treated with surfactant are less likely to develop bronchopulmonary dysplasia (BPD). This is encouraging as the expense of surfactant is often given as one reason for not using it, yet the cost of caring for a baby with BPD may mitigate this argument. Production of the infant's own surfactant is impeded by cold, stress and metabolic disturbances.

The mainstay of treatment is to keep the baby alive by supporting his respiratory function and keeping him well oxygenated until the condition improves and allows for independent existence. Infants with severe respiratory distress are often ventilated soon after birth. In order to ventilate effectively, an endotracheal tube is passed through either the nose or the mouth, into the trachea and secured. In order to keep him well oxygenated, the use of an indwelling arterial line is highly desirable, as this allows easy access for sampling with minimal disturbance and, in the case of a umbilical arterial line, also for continuous blood gas monitoring.

Methods of respiratory support

- Warm and humidified headbox oxygen;
- Continuous positive airway pressure (CPAP);
- Intermittent mandatory volume (IMV);
- Intermittent positive pressure ventilation (IPPV);
- Continuous negative extrathoracic pressure (CNEP).

Ventilatory support

The headbox technique has been already described.

Ventilation is a commonly used technique in neonatal units. Today's ventilators are flexible and allow the rate, ratio and pressures to be tailored to suit the individual. Ventilators may be either volume- or pressure-controlled. In volume control, a measured amount of gas is delivered to the patient. In the very small baby with stiff lungs volume ventilation is not easy. Most paediatricians use pressure-controlled ventilators, with the cycle being controlled by time: a set pressure of gas is given and maintained for a set time. This causes a rapid rise in pressure which then maintains a plateau for the preset inspiratory (PIP) time, gives the stiff lungs chance to inflate and, once inflated, this inspiratory time allows gas exchange to occur by molecular diffusion across the alveolar membrane. In order to remove waste gas, the pressure is allowed to drop to a preset positive end-expiratory pressure (PEEP) which prevents alveolar collapse. Displayed on a graph this sequence would be seen as a series of square waves (Milner and Field, 1985).

The closed circuit of a continuous-flow ventilator ensures that fresh gas is always available with the start of each cycle. This is important as many small infants, unless heavily sedated, will continue to make some respiratory effort between ventilator breaths and the rebreathing of used gas is not desirable. The continuous-flow ventilator is flexible and infants can be weaned off it by gradually decreasing the amount of ventilator support given to them. Trigger ventilators which detect the infant's own attempts at initiating a breath have been described by Mehta, Callan *et al* (1986). Ventilation is triggered by changes in the infant's abdominal expansion or changes in airway or oesophageal pressures, and works by either reinforcing the infant's inspiratory effort or synchronizing with the infant while also delivering a predetermined number of breaths. These ventilator developments are proving valuable, especially in the clinical management of difficult ventilator-dependent infants.

Complications of ventilator therapy

The use of mechanical ventilation to care for sick infants with respiratory failure has been responsible for saving lives. The pressures that are sometimes needed have been associated with the development of severe barotrauma. Pulmonary air leaks and bronchopulmonary dysplasia are recognized as major consequences of conventional management (White *et al.*, 1990).

Specific care of an infant who is mechanically ventilated

Some infants who are mechanically ventilated tolerate the treatment surprisingly well, but others fight the ventilator. All infants who are being artificially ventilated should be sedated. A diamorphine infusion is becoming more and more popular and, if correctly titrated, the balance between optimum sedation and prevention of depression of the respiratory system can be achieved. Sedation can be weaned down slowly as the ventilation is reduced prior to extubation.

Synchrony with the ventilator can also be useful in helping the infant to tolerate the treatment. This can be achieved by close observation of his respiratory rate and adjustment of the ventilator rate and rhythm.

Alternative ventilation methods

High-frequency positive-pressure ventilation techniques are gaining interest and popularity. The term 'high-frequency ventilation' covers a myriad of respiratory support strategies, which commonly involve ventilation rates in excess of physiological respiratory patterns and may use tidal volumes which approximate to the dead airspace volume. Complete understanding of the way that these techniques work is yet to be achieved, but the techniques have been efficient in the rescue of infants who would otherwise have died. With enhanced clinical understanding and improving technology, this technique may become more common in the near future (Robert *et al.*, 1990).

Currently, continuous negative pressure ventilation/ respiratory support is enjoying a comeback. This is modelled on the old 'iron lung' device which supported polio victims during the 1950s and 1960s. Extensive remodelling of the device has taken place and it is much more friendly to both the user and the patient than its predecessor. It now looks similar to an incubator, and those available for preterm infants are efficiently heated. Trials are taking place to assess the effectiveness of this method of management of chronic lung disease (Samuels and Southall, 1989; Noyes, 1990).

Care of an intubated infant

Babies are ventilated via endotracheal tubes (ETT) which allow effective access to the lower airways. Endotracheal intubation impairs the natural ability to clear lung secretions, owing to the impediment of the mucociliary function and an ineffective cough reflex (the result of a permanently open glottis). Tubes can be inserted orally, nasally or, in some cases where long-term ventilation is being considered, via a tracheostomy. Each method has its advantages and disadvantages. Parents seem to prefer oral intubation but this is difficult to stabilize as movement can cause tracheal abrasion and dislodgement. Long-term oral intubation can distort the soft palate, causing feeding and orthodontic problems.

To stabilize the endotracheal tube, it is stitched to a tube holder, which is supported in position by tying the distal ends of the holder to a small bonnet. Foam rectangles take the pressure of the holder and the ties off the face. There are a number of other methods of fixation. The best is probably the familiar, secure method you already have confidence in.

Nasal intubation is more secure but can result in a lot of tape on the infant's face, which can distress the parents as they cannot see what he looks like. Pressure necrosis on the anterior nares (from a badly positioned tube) can result in quite severe deformity, necessitating plastic surgery.

Both nasotracheal and endotracheal methods of intubation can cause ear infection. The presence of an artificial airway can cause epithelial erosion and inflammation. The mucus and debris which builds up on the tube provides an excellent culture medium which can then be colonized by opportunistic pathogens, providing a focus for infection which can then track through the eustachian tube to the middle ear.

Tracheostomy has the advantage that it cuts down dead air-space, making ventilation more efficient, but as with the other methods the infant cannot communicate by crying. The longer the tracheostomy is present, the longer verbal skills are retarded and introduction to a speech therapist is recommended.

Suctioning of the artificial airway

There is controversy concerning the frequency and technique used in suctioning. Each unit has its own guidelines regarding suction method, frequency and instillation of irrigating fluid. There are no national recommendations to aid the nurse. The purpose of endotracheal suctioning is to remove secretions and prevent obstructions, and it is an important aspect of neonatal nursing care.

Deep ETT suction can cause tissue damage to the trachea, so the length of the tube and the connector is measured and this is the length to which the suction catheter is inserted. This ensures that the catheter does not go beyond the tube. Suction is applied only during withdrawal of the catheter and should last approximately 5–10 seconds. Each catheter is only used once and a sterile technique prevents the introduction of infection.

Suggested diameter of catheter/ETT ratio

Diameter of ET tube (mm)	*Catheter size (Fr)*
2.5–3.5	6
4–5	8
6.5	10

An inappropriately sized catheter can result in the generation of a negative pressure when suction is applied if the catheter snugly fits the lumen of the tube, thereby occluding the entire artifical airway. The instillation of irrigation fluid is contentious and arguments in favour of the use of saline instillation include thinning the mucus within the tube and making it easier to aspirate. How much to use is debated: the smaller the infant the less he will tolerate (Shorten *et al.*, 1991).

Suggested suction strength and fluid instillation

Current weight (g)	*Suction pressure (mmHg)*	*Saline instillation (ml)*
$\leq$1500	40	0.25
>1500	60	0.50

The deleterious effects of the procedure include bradycardia and stress tachycardia (Shorter *et al.*, 1991), trauma to the delicate bronchial mucosa (Runton, 1992), fluctuations in cerebral oxygenation and increases in intracranial pressure

(Shah *et al.*, 1992). Continuous observations of vital signs are made during suction and the infant is allowed to recover between each pass.

Controversy also surrounds the use of presuction hyperoxygenation, hyperventilation and hyperinflation. It is suggested that these practices reduce the likelihood of dangerous fluctuations of the cerebral oxygenation during suctioning of the preterm infant (Tolles and Stone, 1991), but could be dangerous in unskilled hands. The science of infant ventilatory care is a recent one and much study remains to be done. In the absence of guidelines and an extended nursing role (as a neonatal respiratory therapist), all changes to ventilation must be prescribed by the clinician. Each infant has his care planned according to his unique needs.

Physiotherapy

Debate also exists as to the timing, frequency and duration of physiotherapy and by whom it should be performed. It is a vital part of the care of an infant with breathing difficulties as it loosens secretions prior to suctioning, so preventing the accumulation of secretions and reducing the risk of hypostatic infection. Preventing mucus buildup helps to maintain patent airways and prevents localized collapse and consolidation. Few units have full physiotherapy cover, although such resources would be ideal. Neonatal nurses need to work in partnership with the physiotherapist to become skilled in the techniques of chest physiotherapy.

The techniques of percussion and vibration to loosen secretions are the most favoured, with postural drainage to aid the removal of secretions being selectively used and prescribed on an individual basis. Methods used include:

- Laerdal face masks size 00;
- specially designed palm cups;
- electric toothbrushes for small infants.

These aids can be applied to the chest wall. Palm cups are used rhythmically, intermittently and gently. As face masks and palm cups make contact with the chest wall they trap air and provide the benefit of movement, force and contact without the trauma of repeatedly hitting the infant's chest with a flat surface. With the electric toothbrush, vibration is continuous. The need for physiotherapy is assessed with each shift change and, whenever possible, the treatment is given to coincide with handling. For infants who are positioned on their side, physiotherapy starts at the anterior apex on the most accessible lung, working towards the base and gradually round under the arm to work on the posterior aspects of the lung fields. The infant is then turned and the treatment repeated on the opposite lung. Suction is applied to remove loosened secretions during or after treatments. Indications for suction would be visible or audible secretions (Runton, 1992). Fluctuations from the infant's physiological baseline may be an indication for suctioning but could equally be a response to handling.

During treatment the infant's condition is carefully observed and full emergency equipment (previously checked) is on standby. Suction should be switched on and set at an appropriate predetermined pressure. Oxygenation is continually monitored and, if fluctuations occur, time is allowed for recovery. Preoxygenation may be prescribed with or without manual bagging. There is a paucity of studies available for guidance (Downs and Parker, 1991). A review of physiotherapy technique is given by Bertone (1988).

Nursing care plan

The nursing diagnosis would be 'failure to self ventilate in room air'. The aims would include 'maintain clear airway, provide respiratory support and comfort until able to self ventilate in air with ease'. The infant's individualized care plan would include:

- Position of comfort and rest. The infant needs to be supported on his side with the head elevated to prevent movement of the endotracheal tube, which has been incriminated in tracheal necrosis and subglottic stenosis. Anglepoise, sandbags, beanbags, rolled sheets and limb restrainers all help to keep the tubing in the correct position.
- Management of indwelling arterial line. Owing to the critical instability of an infant with severe respiratory distress syndrome, an indwelling arterial catheter is necessary.

Preferably this should be an umbilical line through which blood can be sampled, the PO_2 continuously monitored and blood pressure measured with minimal disturbance. Like other invasive procedures, the use of arterial lines is not without risk, e.g. haemorrhage, local or systemic infection and vascular complications. Vascular complications may arise from trauma, thrombus formation, embolus formation, vasospasm and hypertension. The true incidence of umbilical line complications may never be known, as many remain asymptomatic.

Vasospasm is perhaps the most common vascular complication. It may be caused by the initial catheter placement, manipulation, sampling or removal of the catheter. Vasospasm causes blanching or cyanosis of the distal area. To prevent further damage, removal is recommended (Bryant, 1990).

Thrombus formation in the umbilical artery is potentially very serious as it may result in emboli, which can lodge in and occlude blood vessels, impairing the circulation and resulting in distal tissue hypoxia and necrosis. Loss of toes and necrotic buttocks and limbs have all been seen in neonatal units throughout the world.

Care of an indwelling arterial line involves aseptic installation, secure splintage and ease of visiblity of the catheter site and potentially affected extremities. The location of the catheter is confirmed by X-ray; a high placement is between thoracic vertebrae 6 and 10, and a low placement is between lumbar vertebrae 3 and 4. Different policies exist regarding the infusion of fluids through these lines. Some are conservative, with use restricted to the slow infusion of heparinized saline and blood sampling. Others use the line to administer drugs and infuse all fluid requirements. Whichever policy is in force, the maintenance of strict fluid balance remains of primary importance. There is some suspicion that the presence of an umbilical arterial catheter is associated with an increased risk of necrotizing enterocolitis (see Chapter 6).

- Feeding and nutrition. The infant with severe respiratory distress syndrome cannot tolerate enteral feeding owing to a combination of factors, such as instability of clinical condition and immaturity of the gastrointestinal system.

Feeding is discussed in Chapter 7; however, the following points will be made here. The preterm infant has limited reserves. Intravenous hydration and correction of electrolyte imbalance is insufficent for longer than 3 days. If enteral feeding is not going to be introduced or if there is doubt that it will be tolerated, a long feeding line should be placed and total parenteral nutrition commenced.

- The maintenance of a thermoneutral environment. The infant with RDS needs warmth and there are two ways of maintaining optimal temperature, the closed incubator and the cot with a radiant heater. Other aids to maintain warmth include heat shields to cut down on the amount of heat loss, bubble wrap plastic and clear clingfilm for insulation and good visibility. As soon as his condition improves, the baby should be dressed and wrapped. This is satisfying for the parents, who can choose his clothing. It is equally satisfying for the infant, who feels more secure when cosily dressed. Once his condition is stable and temperature control is satisfactory, he can be transferred to a small crib in a low-dependency area to establish feeding and to grow.

Care of the family

The care of a ventilated infant is a rewarding challenge, as the infant and family have multiple needs. So much information is given to the parents in so short a time that it is worth checking later that it has all sunk in. An idea which was introduced in Leicester some time ago was the issue of a leaflet to parents which describes their infant's condition (Crawford, 1992).

Withdrawing care

For the majority of infants with RDS, recovery is assured. For some, usually the questionably viable, there is no improvement despite support, and they sink inextricably into a chronic state and multisystem failure.

Withdrawing care is a difficult ethical issue. The legal position is clear: no steps can be taken to hasten the demise of an infant but no officious measures need to be taken to resuscitate in the event of a collapse. Between these two extremes there is a large and potentially dangerous minefield to be negotiated in the amount of support which should be offered to hopeless cases.

The nursing perspectives include the viewpoint that the hopeless infant does not suddenly become unloved. As always, the family is nursed and not just the infant. The family's views and wishes are as important and perhaps even more so than our own.

Congenital diaphragmatic hernia

This condition occurs in approximately 1 in 2200 live births. There is a 70–80% mortality but this is not evenly distributed geographically (Theorell, 1990). The infants who collapse immediately after birth are the most seriously affected and tend to do badly. Infants who present days or weeks later, or are routinely found by chance X-ray, do very well.

Aetiology

The anatomical defect is a simple one. The most common and the most severe is the left-sided defect resulting in a failure of the diaphragm to develop and fuse. Technically this is described as a posterolateral Bochdalek-type hernia. The less severe and occasionally symptomless type is an anteromedial defect below the sternum, the Morgagni type.

A severe diaphragmatic defect results in the herniation of abdominal contents through the gap in the diaphragm into the thorax, causing mediastinal shift which in turn compresses the developing lung tissue. Although this defect is potentially surgically correctable, the hypoplasia of the lung tissue often makes the infant difficult to ventilate.

Initial resuscitation

An infant who has collapsed in the delivery room with a diaphragmatic hernia is one of the most sudden and acute emergencies which the midwife or neonatal nurse will ever face. In the worst-case scenario, typically and sadly, these are term or near-term babies with whom no difficulty had been anticipated. The infant is born normally, gasps and then fails to establish a normal respiratory pattern and becomes cyanosed.

Diaphragmatic hernia should be suspected if the heart sounds are heard on the right and if the abdomen appears to be scaphoid. Definitive diagnosis is by chest X-ray, showing bowel in the chest and a displaced heart but, unless the infant is properly resuscitated, such a diagnosis is likely to be of academic interest only. Resuscitation by traditional methods of bag and mask inflation of the lungs, is undesirable as the misplaced abdominal contents also become inflated, compounding pulmonary embarassment. Initial resuscitation includes the passage of a wide-bore oral/nasogastric tube, left on free drainage after aspiration. This decompresses the inflated bowel and allows the expansion of existing lung tissue. Ventilation should be commenced via an endotracheal tube.

All senior midwives should be trained to perform emergency intubation (Whitten, 1989) as expert paediatric help can take time to arrive, especially in the middle of the night. The minimum possible pressures which keep the baby pink should be used to prevent lung damage. The infant will be shocked, so warmth, gentle handling and correction of metabolic abnormalities are important.

The neonatal unit's workload needs to be fully appraised and individual nurses need to be allocated to look after such critically ill infants.

Initial care of the parents

The culmination of an uneventful pregnancy and a normal labour should result in a beautiful healthy child. In contrast, the arrival of a pale, shocked infant who cannot breathe and is removed for resuscitation must seem the material of a nightmare. At some point during resuscitation, photographs of the infant should be taken, as tastefully as possible, as well as hand or foot prints. These should be sent to the parents as soon as possible, with an update on his condition. The parents should not be left alone – someone quiet, calm and sympathetic should stay and help them to keep a hold on the situation.

The parents should see their child as soon as possible, and be offered honest explanations of the condition by the team responsible for his care. This is especially important as many maternity units do not have the facilities for neonatal intensive care or surgery, and the infant will need to be transferred away from the parents to another hospital. The needs of every family are different and the management of the family is planned to meet those needs. Sometimes access to a telephone is all that is required.

Transfer

The receiving centre's flying squad will usually be responsible for the transfer. This can sometimes be quite tricky, as it is dangerous to move an unstable infant, but time is of the essence and it is vital to get the patient to a fully equipped hospital as quickly as possible and in the best possible condition. General flying squad management is discussed in Chapter 4; however, the infant with diaphragmatic hernia is best transported with the contralateral lung upwards to avoid further compression by the weight of the bowel.

Traditional management

This is both medical and surgical. The decision whether to go for early or deferred surgery is made on the clinical condition and the responses to treatment of each individual infant.

Observation of vital signs and clinical condition is constant. The ventilation management of a big, term infant typically involves sedation and muscle relaxants as large vigorous term infants can be very difficult to ventilate. Hypoplastic lung tissue can be stiff and high inspiratory pressure may be needed to inflate them; this means that a pneumothorax is a very real danger, especially if the infant is fighting the ventilator. To prevent this, a muscle relaxant is used and the infant is effectively paralysed. This muscle relaxant is often based on curare and may be given by bolus, although continuous infusion is preferred. The immobile infant can still be an infant who is frightened and in pain (Noerr, 1992), so sedation and analgesia should also be given.

Deliberate respiratory alkalosis may be induced by hyperventilation in order to break the vicious cycle of right-to-left shunting and pulmonary hypertension. A reduction of CO_2 levels may reduce shunting.

Pharmacological support may involve the use of tolazoline (Noerr, 1988) for the management of secondary pulmonary hypertension. Tolazoline is a direct peripheral vasodilator which acts by blocking α-adrenergic action, but because of its ability to decrease peripheral resistance, systemic hypotension can result. Circulatory supportive measures may also include dopamine and the infusion of human albumin or whole-blood products. Major vessel access is preferable.

Specific nursing management of the paralysed infant

The transmission of nerve impulses to muscles blocked by relaxant prohibits movement and the infant becomes very dependent on the nurse. Secretions in the oropharynx build up as he is unable to swallow, limbs can become overstretched and sore, and skin breakdown becomes a possibility. Bowel and bladder function may be impaired.

Oropharyngeal suction

Suction technique has already been described and should be carried out frequently to prevent the aspiration of saliva.

Subluxation of limbs and skin care

Positioning and supporting the limbs in a neutral position of comfort is vital and the limbs should be moved through a full range of normal movement. This practice is called passive limb physiotherapy and should be performed when the infant has his cares. Followed cares, the infant's position should be changed and pressure areas inspected. How frequently this is done depends on how handling is tolerated. If his toleration is limited, the nurse could try making a net bed or a waterbed with litre bags of i.v. infusion fluids. Soft miniature pressure-relieving mattresses are commercially available and mattresses that move, such as electric ripple, are an excellent idea, but should be used with caution for fear of displacing the ETT.

Risk of urinary stasis and constipation

The paralysed infant may retain urine in his bladder. A large bladder containing stagnant urine, apart from being uncomfortable, may cause a urinary tract infection. In infants who do not have a catheter, suprapubic presure may be needed to void this urine. Prolonged use of muscle relaxant may mean that the infant has to have a small suppository to evacuate the bowel.

Surgery

There are two approaches to surgical repair, the transthoracic and the transabdominal. Both are successful and each has particular advantages. The method of choice differs with the severity of the hernia, the experience of the surgeon and the condition of the baby. The transthoracic approach allows for the quickest decompression of the embarrassed pulmonary function and the diaphragmatic defect is repaired from above. However, if there is insufficient abdominal space to contain the herniated bowel an abdominal incision and the formation of a silastic pouch may have to be performed and the abdomen repaired in stages.

The transabdominal approach is felt by some to be less traumatic, and the associated malrotation of the bowel can be repaired at the same time.

Postoperatively no attempt is usually made to expand the compressed lung with suction decompression of the intrapleural space or selective intubation of the bronchi and positive-pressure ventilation. The compressed lung naturally and gradually expands on its own and the mediastinal shift will return to a midline position with passive management. Passive lung expansion and air leak are managed by underwater seal drainage.

Underwater seal drainage

Intercostal drains are sited to allow fluid and air to escape from the pleural cavity and to allow the lung to expand. This is a closed and airtight method of management. The drainage end of the system is submerged below a measured amount of sterile water. The water bottles are suspended below the level of the patient and never lifted above this level. Expansion of the chest wall on inspiration increases the intrapleural tension and reflux of the fluid from the bottle occurs. On expiration, normal presures are established and the level of fluid in the tube falls. These drains are said to 'swing'. Constant bubbling of the fluid in the drains suggests a continuing air leak. Intercostal drains are never routinely clamped off while active. Emergency clamping, as close to the chest wall as possible, is performed if accidental disconnection occurs.

Frequent observation of drain activity for patency is vital. Drains stop swinging if kinked, clogged or clotted. Excessive length of tubing can cause fluid to become trapped in bends, effectively blocking the flow of air down the tube.

Active drains will stop swinging when the lung is fully expanded and a chest X-ray will be taken to confirmn this. Provided that the clinical condition is stable, the chest drains are removed and an airtight occlusive dressing is applied (Walsh, 1989).

Alternative management methods for congenital diaphragmatic hernia

Extracorporeal membrane oxygenation (ECMO) is gaining popularity. The infant's circulation is accessed via major vessels and a small amount of deoxygenated blood removed and run through a circuit containing a membrane lung, which oxygenates the blood and this is returned to the infant (Crawford, 1991). Trials with postoperative ECMO management for infants who are deteriorating, on full ventilation and pharmacological support, show promise. Basically it buys time and allows the lungs to rest and recover to a level compatible with survival.

This method is not without some risk as, unfortunately, the technique is not available in every neonatal unit and the infant would need to be transferred to a centre where this facility is available. An additional risk for the infant who has undergone surgery for the repair of a diaphragmatic hernia is that he has to be heparinized to prevent systemic and circuit coagulation.

Prenatal diagnosis of congenital diaphragmatic hernia

This is increasingly available as scanning techniques improve. It is valuable, as it means that affected infants can be fully assessed and safely transferred, while still in the uterus, for delivery in a unit with facilities to manage this condition. In future, it is probable that early diagnosis will become even more important as midtrimester surgical techniques are improved (the diaphragmatic hernia could be repaired at about 24–30 weeks' gestation). Successful intrauterine repair has the advantage of allowing subsequent pulmonary development (Harrison *et al.*, 1990).

COMMON INVESTIGATIONS

Respiratory management would be impossible without some routine investigations that we take for granted. Blood gas analysis has been available since the late 1950s, and although interpretation is still debated current ventilator management would be unthinkable without it.

Blood gases explained

Homeostasis is of vital importance to the maintenance of life and operates within strict limits. If the body is subjected to repeated or prolonged deviation, serious organ damage or death can follow.

The transport of oxygen and carbon dioxide in the blood relies on healthy erythrocytes, good haemoglobin levels and amounts of bicarbonate ions within the plasma. Blood gases can be defined as a measure of oxygen and carbon dioxide levels within the blood, which is commonly referred to as the partial pressure or PO_2 and PCO_2. The balance is finely maintained by a chain of reversible biochemical events.

Oxygen diffuses across the alveolar membrane into the blood and combines reversibly with haemoglobin. Only a small amount is dissolved in the plasma. The haemoglobin carries the oxygen from the alveolar capillaries to the tissue capillaries, where it is released and diffuses across the cell membranes. The oxygen is used by the tissue cells. During aerobic respiration carbon dioxide is released as a waste product. The carbon dioxide diffuses from the cells into the capillaries and is carried dissolved in the plasma, in combination with haemoglobin or as bicarbonate ions:

$$\begin{array}{ccccccccc} CO_2 & + & H_2O & \rightleftharpoons & H_2CO_3 & \underset{\text{anhydrase}}{\overset{\text{Carbonic}}{\rightleftharpoons}} & H^+ & + & HCO_3 \\ \text{Carbon dioxide} & + & \text{Water} & \rightleftharpoons & \text{Carbonic acid} & \rightleftharpoons & \text{Hydrogen ion} & + & \text{Bicarbonate ion} \end{array}$$

Acidosis is generally regarded as being below pH 7.25 and alkalosis as above pH 7.45.

Saturation monitoring

Approximately 97% of the oxygen carried in the blood is transported in combination with haemoglobin and the remaining 3% is dissolved in the plasma. The oxygen–haemoglobin dissociation curve demonstrates the percentage of haemoglobin saturated with oxygen at any given PO_2. Haemoglobin is saturated when an oxygen molecule is bound to each of its four haem groups. At any PO_2 above 70 mmHg, nearly 100% of the haemoglobin is saturated with oxygen.

It is important to note that fetal haemoglobin changes to adult haemoglobin by about 4 months. At birth, an infant's Hb is approximately 16–20 g/dl. This is important because, when monitoring an infant's saturation and PO_2 levels, the oxygen dissociation curve shifts to the left. This means that at a lower PO_2, the relative saturation is higher. Toxic oxygen levels must not be reached, due to the risk of retinopathy of prematurity developing.

Chest X-ray

The lung fields of a neonate have a uniform radiolucent appearance: the hilar and perihilar regions appear dense because of the bronchi and vascular structures (Grossglauser, 1992). The spine should lie in the middle of the chest X-ray, actually dividing the chest in two, and there should be symmetry between each hemithorax. This is a useful guide to assessing whether or not there is significant rotation. Other useful landmarks are the nasogastric tube and the endotracheal tube if in place.

It is possible to shoot a good film through the perspex hood of an incubator, but shadows and artefacts are possible with open portholes and the hole in the top of an incubator The infant's cooperation can be enhanced by covering the cold X-ray film plate with soft tissue or cloth. To avoid lordotic positioning, the infant should not be stretched to give a good position but can remain comfortably supported by a towel roll below the buttocks.

REFERENCES

Aloan, C. (1987) *Respiratory Care of the Newborn*, J.B. Lippincott Company, Philadelphia.

Bertone, B. (1988) The role of physiotherapy in the neonatal intensive care unit. *Australian Journal of Physiotherapy* **34**(1), 27–34.

Bhutani, V., Abbasi, S., Walker, A. and Gendes, J. (1992) Pulmonary mechanics and energetics in preterm infants who had respiratory distress and were treated by surfactant. *Journal of Pediatrics* **120**(2), 18–24.

Bryant, B. (1990) Drug, fluid and blood products administered through the umbilical artery catheter; complication experiences. *Neonatal Network* **9**(1), 27–43.

Carlo, W. and Chatburn, R. (1990) *Neonatal Respiratory Care*, 2nd edn, Year Book Medical Publishers, Chicago.

Crawford, D. (1991) A boost to the chances of survival: extra corporeal membrane oxygenation in neonatal care. *Professional Nurse* **6**(8), 426–30.

Crawford, D. (1992) Putting parents in the picture. *Nursing Times* **88**(2), 41–2.

Cummings, J., Holm, B., Hudak, M. *et al.* (1992) A controlled clinical comparison of four different surfactant preparations in surfactant deficient preterm lambs. *American Review of Respiratory Diseases* **145**(5), 999–1004.

Downes, J. and Parker, A. (1991) Chest physiotherapy for preterm infants. *Pediatric Nursing* **3**(2), 14–17.

Gortner, L., Bernsau, U., Hellwege, H. *et al.* (1992) Early treatment of respiratory distress syndrome with bovine surfactant in very preterm infants: a multi centre controlled clinical trial. *Pediatric Pulmonology* **14**(1), 1–3.

Grossglauser, L. (1992) Neonatal radiology: assessment of the quality of the neonatal X ray film. *Neonatal Network* **11**(7), 69–72.

Halliday, H., McClure, G. and Reid, M. (1981) Transient tachypnoea of the newborn: two distinct clinical entities. *Archives of Disease in Childhood* **56**, 322–5.

Harrison, R., Langen, J., Adzick, N. *et al.* (1990) Correction of congenital diaphragmatic hernia in utero. Initial clinical experience. *Journal of Pediatric Surgery* **25**(1), 47–57.

Hoekstra, R., Jackson, J. and Myers, T. (1991) Improved neonatal survival following multiple doses of bovine surfactant in very premature infants at risk of respiratory distress syndrome. *Pediatrics* **88**(1), 8–10.

Kolobow, T. (1988) *Acute Respiratory Failure,* XXXIV. Transactions American Society Artificial Internal Organs **XXXIV**, 31–4.

Levene, M., Tudenhope, D. and Thearle, J. (1987) *Essentials of Neonatal Medicine,* Blackwell Scientific Publications, Oxford.

Liggings, G. and Howie, R. (1972) Controlled trial of antepartum glucocorticoid treatment for the prevention of respiratory distress syndrome in premature infants. *Pediatrics* **50**, 515.

Marieb, E. (1992) *Human Anatomy and Physiology,* 2nd edn, Benjamin Cummings Publishing Company, California.

Mehta, A., Callan, K., Wright, B. and Stacey, T. (1986) Patient triggered ventilation in the newborn. *Lancet* **ii**, 706–12.

Milner, T. and Field, D. (1985) Ventilation in the neonatal period. *Care of the Critically Ill* **1**(6), 14–15.

Noerr, B. (1988) Pointers in practical pharmacology. Tolazoline. *Neonatal Nework* **8**(12), 74–5.

Noerr, B. (1992) Pointers in practical pharmacology. Pancuronium bromide. *Neonatal Network* **11**(2), 77–9.

Noyes, J. (1990) Respiratory failure in infants. *Nursing Standard* **4**(49), 28–30.

Paige, P. (1990) Non-invasive monitoring of the neonatal respiratory system. *American Association for Critical Nursing* **1**(2), 409–21.

Robert, E. and Lefrak, S. (1990) Alternative modes of mechanical ventilation. *American Association for Critical Nursing* **1**(2), 248–59.

Roberton, N. (1986) *A Manual of Neonatal Intensive Care,* 2nd edn, Edward Arnold, London.

Roberton, N. (1993) *A Manual of Neonatal Intensive Care,* 3rd edn, Edward Arnold, London.

Runton, N. (1992) Suctioning artificial airways in children: appropriate technique. *Pediatric Nursing* **2**(2), 115–8.

Samuels, M. and Southall, D. (1989) Negative extra thoracic pressure in treatment of respiratory failure in infants and young children. *British Medical Journal* **229**, 1253–7.

Shah, A., Kurth, C., Gwiazdowski, S. *et al.* (1992) Fluctuations in cerebral oxygenation and blood volume during endotracheal suctioning in premature infants. *Journal of Pediatrics* **120**(5), 769–74.

Shorten, D., Byrne, P. and Jones, R. (1991) Infant Responses to Saline Instillation and Endotracheal Suctioning. *Journal of Obstetrics, Gynaecology and Neonatal Nursing* **6**(2), 464–69.

Speer, C., Robertson, B., Curstedt, T. *et al.*(1992) Randomised European multi centre trial of surfactant replacement therapy for severe neonatal respiratory distress syndrome. Single versus multiple doses of Cureosurf. *Pediatrics* **89**(1), 13–20.

Theorell, C. (1990) Congenital diaphragmatic hernia: a physiological approach to management. *Journal of Perinatal and Neonatal Nursing* **3**(3), 66–79.

Tolles, C. and Stone, K. (1991) National survey of neonatal endotracheal suctioning practices. *Neonatal Network* **9**(2), 7–14.

Walsh, M. (1989) Making sense of chest drains. *Nursing Times* **85**(24), 40–1.
White, C., Richardson, C. *et al.* (1990) High frequency ventilation and extracorporeal membrane oxygenation. *American Association for Critical Nursing* **1**(2), 427–44.
Whitten, C. (1989) *Anyone Can Intubate: A Practical, Step by Step, Guide for Health Professionals,* Medical Arts Press, K-W Publications, San Diego, California.

FURTHER READING

Tortora, G. and Anagnostakos, N. (1990) *Principles of Anatomy and Physiology,* 6th edn, Harper and Row, New York.
Williams, P. and Warwick, R. (1980) *Gray's Anatomy,* 36th edn, Churchill Livingstone, Edinburgh.

ACKNOWLEDGEMENT

The author wishes to thank Marie-Claire Turrell for the contribution of blood gas analysis to this chapter.

9

Nursing care of a baby with a disorder of the cardiovascular system

Marie-Claire Turrall, Doreen Crawford and Maryke Morris

Few branches of nursing can be as challenging as neonatal cardiology. Nursing an infant with a cardiac defect requires limitless creativity and skill as well as excellent nursing standards. Small deviations from the infant's usual baseline may herald a significant deterioration in condition. Nurses are uniquely placed to monitor these deviations by close observation and, coupled with intuition based on experience, can then alert the medical team. Early intervention is often the key to a successful outcome.

ANATOMY AND PHYSIOLOGY

Embryogenesis

In order to comprehend cardiac anomalies, it is useful to have a basic understanding of early development. The human heart derives from the mesoderm, which forms two endothelial tubes that quickly become a single functioning chamber. As this chamber twists and contorts major structural changes cause the formation of four chambers, which eventually become recognizable as the heart. Any malformation or adverse developmental occurrence, such as maternal infection, at this early stage, may lead to life-threatening cardiac lesions.

Congenital heart defect (CHD) is now the commonest cause of major congenital abnormality in the UK (Levene, Tudehope and Thearle, 1987). In the uterus, the fetal heart is functional by the 28th day of gestation and, for many, it never skips a beat throughout a lifetime (Marieb, 1992).

Fetal circulation

The purpose of fetal circulation is to optimize fetal growth in the uterus and also to supply oxygen, from the maternal circulation via the placenta, to the fetus. Three modifications are present to protect the lungs:

- The patent ductus arteriosus connects the aorta and pulmonary arteries; this prevents the lung fields being flooded with too much blood.
- The foramen ovale; this is a gap in the septum between the two atria, and allows blood to bypass the right ventricle.
- The ductus venosus allows the blood to enter the fetal circulation from the umbilical arteries into the portal vein.

The first two modifications are important to enable blood to mix and circulate to the body effectively, via the aorta (Figure 9.1).

Changes at birth

The fetal circulation has to adapt, at birth, to support extrauterine existence and these changes result in a recognizably mature circulatory pattern. The first few breaths are of vital importance and initiate the alteration of the circulation. These changes are brought about by:

- the onset of respiration in air;
- an increase in capillary Po_2;
- increased extrathoracic pressure and blood pressure;

and are as follows:

- The ductus venosus closes.
- The foramen ovale closes.

- The patent ductus arteriosus closes.
- The ductus venosus becomes the ligamentum teres.
- The patent ductus becomes the ligamentus arteriosus.
- The foramen ovale closes to form the septum between the two atria.

If these changes do not occur then complications may result and need correcting (Roberts, 1990).

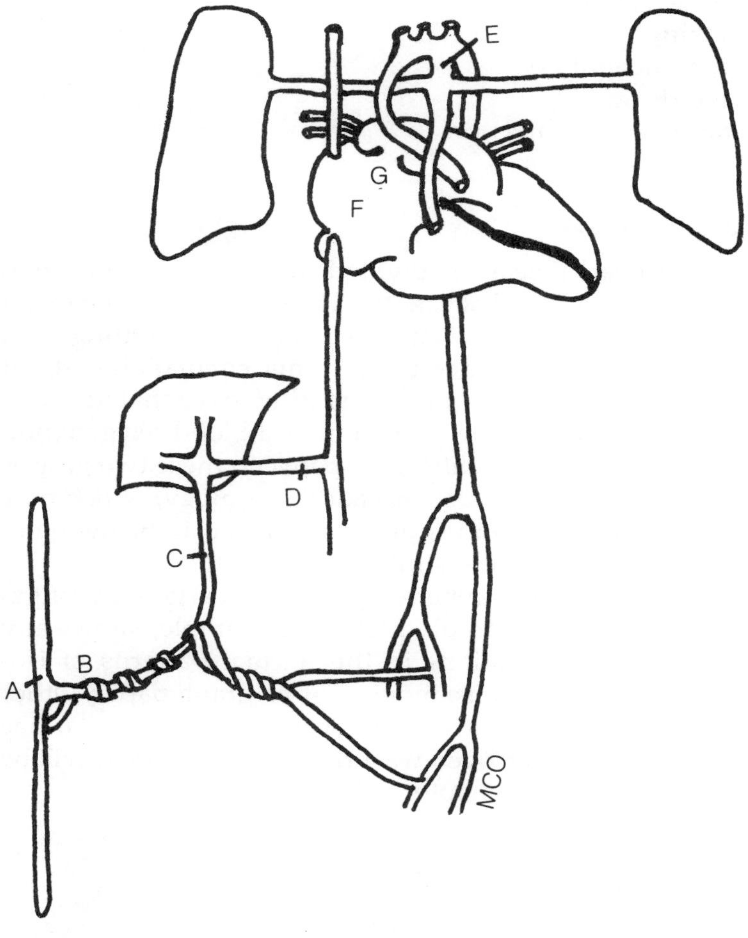

Figure 9.1 Fetal circulation. Key: A: Placenta, B: Umbilical vessels, C: Umbilical vein, D: Ductus venosus, E: Patent ductus arteriosus, F: Right atria and G: Formen ovales.

CAUSES OF CONGENITAL HEART DISEASE

The exact cause of most heart defects is not known as the heart has undergone major development, usually before the woman realizes that she is pregnant.

Possible aetiology

- Genetic inheritance
- Poor diet
- Environmental factors
- Smoking
- Excess alcohol
- Some drugs
- Fetal/maternal infection
- Maternal diabetes
- Maternal age
- Gestational age

Congenital heart disease is divided by convention into two categories, cyanotic and acyanotic. The difference is the result of blood mixing. Cyanosis is the result of blood shunting from the pulmonary circulation to the systemic circulation without having perfused through the lungs to be oxygenated. With acyanotic lesions the lung perfusion and blood oxygenation may not be affected. The difference between these two groups is not rigid and a lesion such as Fallot's tetralogy, which may initially present as acyanotic, may become cyanotic owing to a change in the haemodynamics.

An abnormal heart can be recognized by certain investigations. An electrocardiograph (ECG), for example, shows any abnormalities by deviations in the normal patterns of iso-electric lines displayed on a monitor or on graph paper. Other investigations include ultrasound scan, chest X-ray, cardiac catheterization and nitrogen washout. Details of these will be discussed later in the chapter.

Cyanosis

Central

This occurs when venous blood bypasses the lungs so that the arterial oxygen saturation remains low even when high inspiratory oxygen fractions are given. Severe lung disease can present with the same features, and a differential diagnosis must be made (Qureshi, 1989).

Peripheral

This is more common in the neonate and is evidenced by blueness of the hands and feet, with good perfusion and pink colour of the warm parts of the body such as the lips. Arterial oxygen saturations are normal (Qureshi, 1989). Peripheral cyanosis may be caused by poor circulation, often associated with hypothermia, shock or polycythaemia.

Acrocyanosis is a relatively common phenomenon; the characteristic blueness of the palms of the hand and soles of the feet is typically of short duration in the newborn during transitional status.

The infant presenting with cyanosis needs to have his respiratory pattern observed and noted so that lung disease can be excluded as a diagnosis. The heart rate should be continuously monitored and oxygen saturations measured. Further investigations will need to be performed and many of these are discussed below. An infant with no apparent respiratory distress who remains cyanosed in 100% oxygen needs urgent referral to a cardiac unit. Prostaglandin E_2 is prescribed for immediate therapy to maintain a open ductus arteriosus until diagnosis and correct medical or surgical treatment can be given.

CONGESTIVE CARDIAC FAILURE (CCF)

Neonates in cardiac failure commonly present with breathlessness during feeding and may become increasingly lethargic. At rest, the infant may have a characteristic bounding tachycardia of over 180 beats/min. This is owing to ventricular overload and is often called gallop rhythm. In addition, these infants also may have copious, frothy secretions which require frequent suction, and often have a respiratory rate of more than 60 breaths/min. Feeds may be inadequate for the infant's needs or may take longer than 30 min to be completed, leaving the infant exhausted, pale and sweating, but despite this poor feeding, weight gain may be in excess of 30 g/day

(Qureshi, 1989). Hepatomegaly may be detectable on examination.

In later infancy, pulmonary oedema causes a dry cough and leads to respiratory infections. The infant is either lethargic or irritable and is cold, pale and sweaty, with grunting, indrawing and possible cyanosis.

Cardiac failure may be rapid in onset and, if presenting early in life, the cause is more sinister (Qureshi, 1989). Medical therapy may succeed in controlling heart failure for a short time and surgical correction of the cardiac defect, where applicable, may be urgently required. Delays in recognizing and treating heart failure may lead to a rapid deterioration and cardiogenic shock. Cardiac shock may resemble early septicaemia, pneumonia and meningitis.

In full-term infants, from birth to 1 week, left ventricular failure is more common than right ventricular failure. Cardiac failure in later infancy is often combined right- and left-sided failure.

Nursing care of an infant with CCF

Working as a partner with the parents

Explain to the family what all the monitoring equipment is for and what CCF means in simple terminology: back up verbal explanations with written information. There is a set of excellent leaflets produced by the British Heart Foundation which may help. In cardiac care, as in other specialist branches of neonatology, the parents are partners in care and should be aware of any changes in the infant's condition. Changes in the management of a child needs the consent of the parents.

Maintenance of optimal temperature

Nurse the infant in an incubator or under an overhead heater to help maintain a thermoneutral environment. In large infants this may not be required, but temperature should be regularly monitored and the baby should be kept warm and adequately dressed.

Administration of medication

Medication should be administered as prescribed and, where possible, timed to coincide with feeds so that the infant is not disturbed. Some medication, such as digoxin, can be toxic and its effects cumulative. Prior to administration the heart rate and rhythm should be checked; if these are slower than the infant's usual baseline, or if the beats seem to come together, the nurse should withhold the drug until the infant has been assessed by the medical team. Digoxin will be discussed further later.

Importance of comfort and rest

Invasive procedures should be kept to a minimum; rest and sleep periods are sacrosanct and the mother is encouraged to nurse her infant, cuddling and feeding him to keep him settled. Excess crying is detrimental to these infants and they can be offered a soother if the parents consent. The infant's daily care will include a daily weighing, preferably first thing in the morning, before the bath or as the infant has a nappy change. This daily ritual can often become a focus for anxiety and the parents should be realistic about small fluctuations as the general trend and clinical condition is more important.

Adequate hydration and nutrition

Offer small frequent feeds to avoid overtiring the infant and, if the feed is taking longer than 30 min or the infant is becoming dyspnoeic, the feed could be completed via a nasogastric tube. Should the mother wish to breastfeed she should be encouraged to express until she can feed normally; alternatively the infant can have a short, comforting and closely monitored nuzzle at the breast while the nurse delivers the nasogastric feed. Breast milk may be given instead of formula, and will probably be better for the baby (due to lower levels of sodium); This can help prevent oedema. An intake and output chart should be kept and daily recordings of urine specific gravity charted.

Provision of oxygen according to needs and prevention of orthopnoea

Administer oxygen therapy as prescribed and measure saturations regularly, if possible continuously; chart readings and make regular recording of vital signs. It is important to note the trend of oxygen requirements and if this is increasing alert the medical team. Insufficient attention is given to an infant's position by medical and nursing staff (Turrill, 1992). In cardiac nursing, the infant's comfort and his need for boundaries for security are balanced by how functional a position is. To relieve the weight of the abdominal contents and to allow maximum expansion of the diaphragm, a head-up position is often adopted, with the infant supported on his side. When awake, the infant may enjoy from an early age, a cradle chair with suitable support for the back.

Safe environment and prevention of cross-infection

Assist with any tests and investigations necessary, including cardiac catheterization. Stringent hygiene and limiting the number of carers will help to prevent cross-infection which could delay vital operations or retard growth.

CARE OF AN INFANT UNDERGOING DIAGNOSTIC INVESTIGATIONS

Nitrogen washout or hyperoxia test

This test is used as an aid to confirm suspected cyanotic heart disease, and involves measuring the PaO_2 in air and again after 10 min of the infant breathing 100% oxygen. If the post-ductal PaO_2 fails to rise above 19.5 kPa a right-to-left shunt is suspected. This can be due either to congenital heart disease or to severe respiratory disease.

Before the test begins, the neonatal nurse must calibrate the oxygen analyser and, if a headbox is to be used to deliver the oxygen, ensure that a tight seal is achieved around the infant's neck. The infant should be fully monitored throughout the procedure and details and explanations given to parents.

Chest X-ray

Thousands of chest X-rays are taken every day in hospitals (Desai, 1992). Many anomalies have a typical heart shadow with an abnormal cardiac outline clearly defined. Some have very descriptive names such as the 'boot-shaped heart' which is classic Fallot's, and the 'egg on its side', which is said to be indicative of transposition.

No special preparation of the infant is necessary, but he will need to be held in a suitable position to maximize the quality of the film by preventing unwanted rotation (Grossglauser, 1992). In addition, there should be adequate protection for the nurse and the infant's reproductive organs: lead shields must be used.

Ultrasound scan

This non-invasive technique is used to enable visualization of the heart. In the hands of experienced personnel it can be very informative and in some cases may save the infant from futile surgery. No special preparation is needed; many ultrasound scanners, although large, are portable and it may be possible for the infant to have his scan while on the unit. If this is not possible the transport incubator system or a converted pram could be used to transport the infant to the department. The infant's co-operation and chances of immobility during the procedure can be enhanced if the conductive gel is warmed prior to application. Some commercial gels are very difficult to remove once dried on, so every effort should be made to remove the excess while damp.

Cardiac catheterization

This is performed to confirm X-ray findings and assist in diagnosis and therapeutic management, or in evaluating the severity of the defect either pre- or post-operatively. The nursing care of the baby undergoing this invasive and occasionally risky procedure is discussed below.

CARE OF AN INFANT WITH AN ABNORMAL HEART RATE, RHYTHM OR PRESSURE

Monitoring the heart rate

An electrocardiogram (Figure 9.2) is a tracing of the different stages of the heart's activity by means of an electrocardiograph

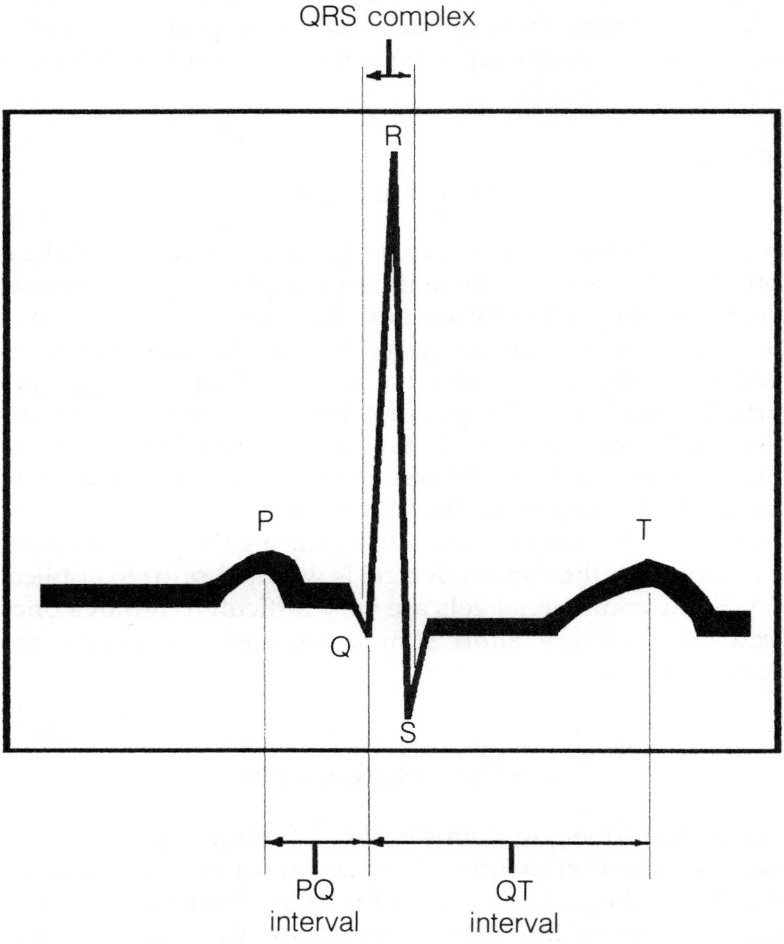

Figure 9.2 Electrocardiogram.

(ECG). The normal ECG comprises of a P wave, a Q, R and S wave (QRS complex), and a T wave. The P wave occurs at the beginning of each contraction of the atria. The QRS complex occurs at the beginning of each contraction of the ventricles. The T wave, in a normal ECG, occurs as the ventricles recover electrically and prepare for the next contraction. The period between these waves is a refractory period. Greater detail can be found in Roberton (1986).

Abnormalities of the heart rhythm can be detected when monitoring the heart rate on a cardiorater or monitor, but a five-lead ECG is required for definitive diagnosis. It is very important to chart all abnormalities in rate and rhythm carefully. As with all equipment, alarms should be set within suitable ranges, responded to if triggered and always switched on.

'Normal' parameters vary tremendously (Catzel and Roberts, 1984), and in the neonatal unit alterations of rate may be influenced by gestational age and clinical condition, so each infant should be individually assessed. Guidelines for the normal parameters are as follows:

	Term infants	*Preterm infants*
Normal	80–160	100–180
Tachycardia	160 >	180 >
Bradycardia	80 <	100 <

Bradycardia

Bradycardia is very common in the premature infant. Most bradycardia are transient and self-resolving, such as those which occur when the infant is in a deep, restful sleep, and require no further action except charting and observation by the neonatal nurse. If the bradycardia is profound (less than 50 beats/min), prolonged (lasting more than 15–30 s) or is accompanied by apnoea, cyanotic attacks, desaturations or unresponsiveness, then immediate action must be taken. Gentle stimulation such as auditory stimulus, gentle touching or stroking is given first, followed by squeezing the heel and patting the bottom; if these interactions have no effect, then more drastic action must be instituted. The baby should be turned supine and the heart rate counted using a stethoscope. If this position change and the invariably cold stethoscope fail to revive the infant and he remains bradycardic, shallow oral, nasopharyngeal or endotracheal suction should be given and resuscitative measures commenced. Assistance should be summoned as necessary and the infant's response to nursing interventions recorded.

Any inferences that can be made pertaining to the bradycardic episode must be documented. These include regurgitation or aspiration of feed, vomiting, vasovagal stimulation caused by deep suctioning or a buildup of secretions, bad positioning and insensitive handling during certain procedures (e.g. lumbar puncture). Other possible triggers of bradycardia include airway compromise, such as a blocked endotracheal tube or a misplaced nasogastric tube, a cerebral event such as an intraventricular haemorrhage or infection, toxicity and hyper- or hypothermia. If there appears to be no presenting cause, then bradycardia of prematurity can be suspected.

Tachycardia

Tachycardia is less common but can be associated with pain and distress or a cardiac dysfunction. A visibly agitated infant, thrashing around his cot, or returning from a traumatic procedure or surgery, may have increased heart rate related to distress and measures to reduce discomfort should be instigated (Chapter 14). In the case of an otherwise settled baby, the tachycardia is most likely caused by an anomaly of heart conduction, for example, supraventricular tachycardia (SVT) which is associated with tachypnoea, pallor and poor feeding. The baby should be monitored, all tachycardia noted and a five-lead ECG performed.

Tachycardia can be reverted by vagal stimulation, either by unilateral massage of the carotid sinus or by initiating the diving reflex. Sreeram and Wren (1990) described a method which involved wrapping the fully monitored baby in a blanket or towel and then immersing the face for 5 s in iced water. Not surprisingly apnoea and bradycardia occur as a reflex and resolve when the infant's normal rhythm returns. Pharmacological intervention may be necessary to maintain an acceptable heart rate, for example digoxin or adenosine to slow down the conduction in the A-V node, or calcium-channel blockers.

Cardioversion may be indicated in some situations. This requires a general anaesthetic and administration of a shock of 0.5–1 J/kg (Sreeram and Wren, 1990).

Wolf–Parkinson–White syndrome can occur after reversion of SVT in some infants and is characterized by ventricular pre-excitation. This lesion is a conductive problem, stemming from an accessory bundle between the atria and the ventricles which causes an abnormal heart rhythm. Wolf–Parkinson–White syndrome is a congenital disorder.

Measurement of blood pressure

In the infant, blood pressure can be monitored continuously and directly by attaching a transducer to an arterial line. If a small-bore peripheral cannula is used a dampened trace may be apparent and readings may not be reliable: as Adelman (1988) reported, some readings may be up to 20 mmHg higher than central blood pressure readings. Accurate non-invasive monitoring can be easily performed using Doppler techniques, with an appropriately sized cuff wrapped neatly around the limb and the pulse located. Doppler techniques allow assessment of the systolic blood pressure only. Oscillometry can measure both systolic and diastolic pressure and some monitors can be programmed to repeat readings at set time intervals. If the cuff is left on the infant to ensure minimal disturbance it needs to be repositioned every 4–6 h to prevent skin damage, nerve palsies and limb ischaemia (Adelman, 1988). The size of the cuff is important, as too large a cuff can give falsely low readings and vice versa (Lum and Jones, 1977).

Blood pressure in the neonate can vary according to the state of arousal of the infant as well as his birth weight and postnatal age. The lowest average blood pressure readings are recorded in the sleeping infant. Wakefulness, suckling, crying and agitation all cause an increase in measurable blood pressure (Adelman, 1988). The effects of extremes of birth weight on blood pressure have not been studied, but it is known that the low birth weight infant has lower readings than the full-term infant (Moss, Duffie and Emmanouilides, 1963). Table 9.1 gives mean arterial blood pressures.

Table 9.1 Mean arterial blood pressure. Reproduced from Stork *et al.* (1984).

Birth weight (kg)	*< 1*	*1–1.5*	*1.5–2*	*> 2.5*
		Blood pressure mm Hg		
Birth	32.9±15.4	39.1±18.2	42.4±19.6	48.8±19.4
7 days	41.4±15.4	47.2±18.2	50.4±19.6	60.2±19.4
14 days	44.6±15.4	50.1±18.2	53.2±19.6	64.2±19.4
28 days	47.6±15.4	53.0±18.2	56.1±19.6	68.3±19.4

SOME COMMON CONGENITAL CARDIAC MALFORMATIONS

Acyanotic

- Pulmonary stenosis
- Coarctation of the aorta
- Aortic valve stenosis
- Atrial septal defect
- Ventricular septal defect

Cyanotic

- Tetralogy of Fallot
- Transposition of great vessels
- Tricuspid atresia

ACYANOTIC CARDIAC MALFORMATIONS

Obstructive lesions

Problems in the development of the heart valves or major arteries lead to obstructive lesions. Pulmonary stenosis restricts blood flow from the right ventricle, whereas aortic stenosis and coarctation of the aorta both restrict blood flow from the left ventricle. Coarctation of the aorta is a constriction of the aorta, and may present as an isolated defect. In infancy it may be associated with a patent ductus arteriosus. Obstruction of the flow from the left ventricle may present as cardiac failure.

Pulmonary stenosis

This may describe any obstruction from the right ventricle. It is generally asymptomatic in the neonatal period but, with severe obstruction, the infant may have dyspnoea and, contrary to the lesion group, may develop general cyanosis. Hepatic enlargement may appear with right ventricular failure and can be associated with tricuspid regurgitation. There may be serious tachycardia and low cardiac output. Sudden death is a great risk. Treatment involves surgery, a valvotomy and, if necessary, aggressive medical management of CCF.

Coarctation of the aorta

This is often asymptomatic unless very severe, particularly in infancy. The most common symptom to be discovered is the reduction in volume or absence of femoral and pedal pulses. Other symptoms include failure to thrive, tachypnoea, dyspnoea, peripheral oedema and severe congestive cardiac failure. Complications can be life-threatening, such as rupture of the aorta. Vigorous management of congestive cardiac failure is essential and surgery is offered to infants who present in the first 6 months with heart failure. An infusion of prostaglandins E_1 or E_2 may be started to increase perfusion of the lower body. Surgery involves the resection of the coarctation and an end-to-end anastomosis or graft performed under partial cardiopulmonary bypass.

Aortic valve stenosis

This condition is rarely symptomatic during infancy but the infant may develop CCF. There may be weak peripheral pulses. Treatment is with an aortic valvotomy; however, bacterial endocarditis is a severe hazard to this condition as it can turn an asymptomatic aortic stenosis into gross aortic regurgitation with severe cardiac failure. Any invasive procedure should be covered by antibiotics to prevent the onset of infection. Medical management with digoxin and diuretics should be tried and, if unsuccessful, valvotomy should be performed promptly. If cardiac failure and poor peripheral perfusion are severe, then a prostaglandin infusion should be started to try to open the ductus and immediate surgical referral made.

Left-to-right shunts

Atrial septal defect (ASD)

This is an abnormal opening in the septum between the right and left atria, of which there are two types: ostium secundum and ostium primum. The former is located in the centre of the atrial septum and the latter is a large gap at the base of the septum, often associated with deformities of the mitral and tricuspid valves; occasionally a ventricular septal defect occurs as an abnormal opening in the septum between the right and left ventricles. An ASD may be asymptomatic, even if the defect is large.

In affected infants there may be slow weight gain, CCF, tiredness, dyspnoea with exertion and severe respiratory infections. If the infant is very sick and suffering frequent infections and/or regular bouts of failure, then surgical closure is advocated, with cardiopulmonary bypass. The defect is repaired with a suture or patch.

Ventricular septal defect (VSD)

These may be asymptomatic and many close spontaneously (Klaus and Fanaroff, 1986). A VSD may be of varying size and may occur in either the membranous or the muscular section of the ventricular septum. Large VSDs may develop symptoms as early as 1–2 months of age. There may be poor weight gain, failure to thrive and feeding difficulties. Often these are pale, delicate-looking infants who have frequent respiratory infections. Other symptoms may include tachypnoea, excessive sweating or CCF, which should be actively treated. If this fails then surgical closure is indicated. Infants who have pulmonary arterial hypertension need early surgery (before 2 years of age) to avoid irreversible pulmonary bed changes.

Patent ductus arteriosus (PDA)

This is the persistence of the fetal connection between the aorta and the pulmonary artery. A considerable and variable blood flow can occur through this channel. As the systemic circulation generates greater pressures the flow through this open duct is in the reverse direction of fetal blood flow and, if undetected or untreated, may result in heart failure. Usually a PDA is detected by the presence of a machine-like murmur.

A PDA, if small, may be asymptomatic. Larger ones may develop symptoms in early infancy and in premature neonates may be the reason for the infant's failure to wean from the ventilator or oxygen. In self-supporting infants there may be bounding pedal pulses, low weight gain, feeding difficulties, frequent respiratory infections or CCF. Medical treatment can be prescribed and is the treatment of choice for many neonates. Indomethacin can be prescribed 8-hourly for three doses but, to be effective, it needs to be given early, preferably in the first 8 days after birth. It is less effective in the very premature (less than 30 weeks) and in those who are more than 3 weeks old, irrespective of gestation. Surgical ligature is recommended for those who do not respond to indomethacin and can be done effectively before 2–3 years of age.

CYANOTIC CARDIAC MALFORMATIONS

Right-to-left shunts

Tetralogy of Fallot

This comprises four abnormalities:

- right ventricular outflow stenosis or atresia
- VSD
- overriding aorta
- right ventricular hypertrophy (gradual onset, not always present at birth).

Occasionally pathology is found which has all of the above plus an ASD. The severity of the lesion is determined by the degree of pulmonary stenosis and the size of the VSD. The extent of the cyanosis depends on the amount of blood shunted from the right to the left, bypassing the lungs.

At birth the infant is not usually cyanosed but this may develop as the infant grows and as the stenosis increases in severity. The infant may be slow to gain weight and be dyspnoeic on exertion, particularly if left crying for long periods of time. The objective of any treatment is to improve the oxygenation of arterial blood, and this can be either palliative or a total correction.

Palliative treatment can be via a Waterston shunt: anastomosis between the posterior lateral aspect of the ascending aorta and the right pulmonary artery; or a Blalock–Taussig shunt: anastomosis between the right or left subclavian artery and the right pulmonary artery. Total correction would involve removal of the palliative shunt (if one had been previously performed) and repair of the ventricular septal defect and relief of the right ventricular outflow obstruction, using cardiopulmonary bypass.

Transposition of the great arteries

This is the most common form of cyanotic heart lesion in infancy (Levene, Tudehope and Thearle, 1987). The aorta arises from the right ventricle and the pulmonary artery from the left. Cyanosis develops shortly after birth and can be very profound. Survival may depend on early diagnosis and infusion of prostaglandins (Silove, 1983) or associated malformations such as a patent ductus arteriosus or a hole in the septum of the heart and effective mixing of pulmonary and systemic blood through this. Surgery can either be palliative or corrective.

Palliative surgery involves:

- the Rashkind procedure: the formation of an ASD with a balloon catheter, which may be performed during cardiac catheterization;
- the Blalock–Hanlon procedure: surgical formation of an ASD;
- pulmonary artery banding, especially for infants who have VSDs with large pulmonary outflow.

Corrective surgery involves:

- the Mustard procedure: using cardiopulmonary bypass, the ASD is closed and the surgeon uses a combination of baffles and pericardium flaps to redirect blood flow through the heart;
- the Rastelli procedure: this is the procedure of choice for transposition when a VSD is present. Facilitated by

cardiopulmonary bypass, the VSD is closed so that the left ventricle communicates with the aorta. The pulmonary artery is ligated and the right ventricle is connected to the distal portion of the pulmonary artery by means of a valve-bearing graft.

Recent surgical techniques have been developed which, in effect, directly switch the transposed vessels. This may become the preferred surgical technique.

Tricuspid atresia

A complete atresia of the tricuspid valve would mean that there was no passage between the right atrium and the right ventricle, so this condition is associated with other anomalies:

- hypoplastic right ventricle
- interatrial septal defect
- ventricular septal defects.

Survival depends on a large atrial septal defect for blood to reach the left ventricle and on the VSD, a PDA or bronchial collaterals for blood to reach the lungs. In a few rare cases, transposition of the great arteries occurs and there may be coexisting anomalies which balance each other.

The condition presents with very severe cyanosis in the neonatal period. There is also respiratory distress, hypoxic spells, delayed weight gain and possibly right-sided heart failure; clubbing of fingers and toes is a later sign and not evident during the neonatal period. Complete surgical correction is not possible at present, but there are palliative procedures to increase pulmonary blood flow:

- The Waterston shunt: anastomosis between the ascending aorta and right pulmonary artery;
- the Glenn procedure: side-to-end anastomosis of the superior vena cava to the right pulmonary artery.

Complications of cyanotic heart lesions

The cyanotic heart lesions discussed previously, notably tetralogy of Fallot, transposition of the great vessels and pulmonary atresia, are the most likely defects to be encountered on a neonatal unit. Complications include:

- congestive cardiac failure, usually in the newborn period;
- infective endocarditis;
- cerebral vascular accident (due to thrombosis or severe hypoxia);
- brain abscess;
- iron-deficiency anaemia;
- death, if the condition is impossible to treat or is undetected.

CARE OF AN INFANT UNDERGOING CARDIAC CATHETERIZATION

This is an invasive procedure which is not without risk, as it involves introducing a radio-opaque catheter into a vein or artery in the groin or in the arm, either by direct insertion as in venepuncture or by cutdown. Venous access (via the groin) is preferred as it allows examination of all four heart chambers (Wakely, 1989). The catheter is passed up into the cardiac chambers and vessels, where pressures are measured and oxygen saturations can be directly obtained. This is usually done in conjunction with angiography, which is the injection of radio-opaque material into the chambers of the heart. This makes it easier to identify anomalies.

The procedure has various functions, both as a diagnostic tool in investigating cardiovascular anomalies and the severity of the defect, and also to evaluate the effects of the defect on the cardiovascular system. As a therapeutic approach, cardiac catheterization can be used to carry out palliative procedures (balloon septostomy) and to locate and close a patent ductus arteriosus using an umbrella device (this prevents the need for surgery and can be done as a day-case).

Preoperative care

Parental anxiety

Give a detailed explanation to parents and check that they understand. Administer any sedation prescribed for the infant, ensure a calm relaxed environment and try to avoid the infant becoming tense and irritable. Try to give the parents time and privacy with their infant, and ensure that they have the support that they need.

Hydration, nutrition and maintenance of blood glucose

Endeavour to keep the infant well hydrated prior to the procedure, and time the investigation to avoid interruption of the feeding regimen. If feeds are going to be missed, ensure that a dextrose infusion is set up to maintain blood glucose and monitor this by using blood glucose sticks. Chart all fluids and send charts to theatre to ensure continuity.

Optimal condition and temperature

Send the infant's baseline observation to theatre with him. Ensure that there is a warm transport incubator available for use with oxygen attached, and all monitoring equipment. Small infants' temperature can drop quickly in theatre, and suitable clothing, such as a warm bonnet, mittens or boots, should be sent to theatre. Quick-release babygros, tops and bottoms fastened by studs or poppers, allow for rapid undressing and redressing. The appropriateness of such clothing depends on the insertion site of the catheter line.

Postoperative care following cardiac catheterization

Safe environment and close observation

Ensure that all emergency equipment is available and functioning. Monitor vital signs frequently as arrhythmias can occur because of cardiac irritability, and check the puncture site for any signs of bleeding. Occasionally damage can be done or infection introduced to the entry vessel, so observe this site for any redness or swelling. Keep the limb exposed and frequently check and record the limb for pallor, decreased temperature, decreased activity, cyanosis or any mottling. Compare the pulses in the affected limb with the unaffected limb, as thrombus formation can be a complication. Absent pulses or a white limb must be reported and acted upon immediately.

Maintenance of the infant's temperature and hydration

Keep the infant warm, comfortable and suitably wrapped to avoid hypothermia and allow him to rest for several hours after the procedure. Ensure that adequate hydration is maintained via an i.v. infusion and check the blood glucose to avoid hypo/hyperglycaemia.

Assessment of urine output

Renal damage can be caused by an overload of contrast medium, so urine output must be recorded and if none has been passed within 4–6 h after surgery, the doctors need to be informed. Sodium overload has been reported as a complication (Wakely, 1989) because of flushing the catheter with saline, and electrolyte levels need to be assessed.

CARE OF AN INFANT UNDERGOING CARDIAC SURGERY

Parental anxiety

Parents of an infant undergoing cardiac surgery are often very vulnerable; many will be away from home living in accommodation which has been provided by the hospital in order to be near their infant, and during this time they may be without the usual support of family and friends and may be worried about other children at home. This is a very emotive time for them; they often feel very guilty and angry at what is happening to their infant, and emotions may run very high. It is important to help them feel involved and that they are doing the right thing. Issues should be freely and fully discussed, not least the chance of their infant dying during or after the procedure. All facts, however unpleasant, must be discussed to avoid conflict later. The neonatal nurse needs to be both compassionate and knowledgeable. Counselling is vital at this point.

One of the major worries is the degree of pain that will be felt by the infant, and reassurance about the use of analgesics can be offered. Where the infant will be nursed is often another major worry, and a trip to the intensive care unit, with introduction to the intensive care area staff who will be involved in their infant's care, is often appreciated. With the correct emphasis on individual variation and needs, a description of how their infant may look after theatre may be helpful in some cases, whereas other parents may prefer to handle one thing at a time.

Warmth and hydration

The infant should be kept warm and well hydrated with an i.v. infusion. Ensure that a transport incubator is available, with all monitoring equipment and full oxygen cylinders.

Prevention of infection

Antibiotic cover is usually given at the start of the procedure to try and prevent sepsis. The most recent weight of the child should be on the prescription chart and sent to theatre with him. If the infant is fit, the parents can enjoy doing the pre-theatre bath. Special skin preparation is usually done in theatre.

Safe environment

Ensure that the infant has his correct hospital number bracelets attached to wrist and ankle. Send all vital sign charts, notes, X-rays and results of investigations (blood tests, ECG, nitrogen washout and cardiac catheterization). Finally, check that there is blood cross-matched and ready should the infant need a transfusion. This might be difficult with some religious groups; if parents do object, then ensure that all staff are aware and make alternative arrangements. Counselling often encourages parents to do what is right for their child, regardless of belief and conviction.

Preoperative care of an infant with PDA

A PDA can pose significant problems to a neonate with respiratory disease, and particularly one who is ventilated on intermittent positive-pressure ventilation. For this reason it is desirable to close the ductus as soon as is clinically possible. In an infant who is ventilated, the clinical signs are a progressive rise in $PaCO_2$, an increasing inspired oxygen requirement and the need for higher inspiratory and expiratory pressures on IPPV. For premature oxygen-dependent infants who are not ventilated, the ductus presents with increasing dyspnoea, increasing oxygen requirements and/or apnoeic episodes. On auscultation, loud machine-like murmurs can be heard and the rhythm is galloping in nature. This murmur may come and go from day to day and neonatal nurses will often hear it when checking the air entry in ventilated infants. Research has shown that the PDA does not close in any neonate until week 33, whether it produces symptoms or not (Rigby, Pickering and Wilkinson, 1984).

Nursing care in the preoperative stage involves keeping the baby warm and stable using the techniques already described. The fluid restriction should be maintained as prescribed and the input continuously balanced with output. In an infant who is not catheterized, the nappies can be weighed before and after use to give an estimation of the amount voided. This is important to detect any signs of CCF and should be recorded on the appropriate chart.

Postoperative care following ligation of PDA

During the immediate postoperative period the infant may be critically unstable and need full ventilatory support and skilled intensive care. Typically these infants get better quickly. Many are rapidly weaned from the ventilator and do very well once extubated and self-supporting in headbox oxygen. Vital signs should be charted as appropriate and blood pressure accurately measured (Jolly, 1991). Any deviation from the infant's norm should be promptly reported to the medical team.

Special observation

Nurse the neonate with the left side uppermost, as the surgical approach is via a left thoracotomy. The lung is collapsed to allow the PDA to be reached and, when it is reinflated, there is a possibility that a pneumothorax, haemothorax or chylothorax could occur. The PDA lies very close to lymphatic vessels and, very rarely, a vessel may be punctured, leading to large amounts of fluid being lost into the thoracic cavity. Chest drains must be kept patent and the colour and quantity of any loss charted. With the wound uppermost it is easier to see any bleeding or oedema developing and the lung is more likely to remain inflated.

Physiotherapy

If physiotherapy is needed it should be very gentle and a non-vibration technique should be used, as vibration could induce a collapse of the lung. The chest drain is usually removed after 24–48 h when a chest X-ray confirms reinflation and a short period of clamping does not result in reaccumulation.

Pain control

This is vital. A thoracotomy is very painful and postoperative recovery will be far quicker if the infant's pain is controlled. Most neonatal units use continuous morphine infusions and then wean them down slowly. This is very effective and keeps the infant very comfortable.

Fluids and blood glucose levels

All intake and output should be noted, and i.v. infusion may be reduced as enteral feeds are reintroduced. The specific gravity of the urine should be checked to ensure normal renal function. Blood glucose levels are checked as appropriate.

COMPLICATIONS OF CONGENITAL HEART DISEASE

Infective endocarditis is an infection of the endocardial surface of the heart or the initial surface of certain atrial vessels. It is a rare condition which is usually found with pre-existing cardiovascular disease (congenital or rheumatic), but can develop in a normal heart during an episode of septicaemia. The infants who are worst at risk are those with:

- VSD, especially a small one
- surgically created shunts
- patent ductus arteriosus

- semilunar valve stenosis
- coarctation of the aorta
- tetralogy of Fallot.

The signs and symptoms are much like any acute infection, but a chest X-ray may reveal vegetative growth within the heart. This is difficult to detect in small infants due to the size of the heart, but if an infection is suspected treatment must be started immediately. The medical management involves administering large doses of intravenous antibiotics over a 4–6-week period. Nursing care should include recording vital signs regularly and encouraging the infant to rest as much as possible. The parents should be encouraged to visit or stay if possible during the long hospitalization, and stringent infection control is essential in both parents and staff.

COMMON DRUGS USED IN CARDIAC MANAGEMENT

Adrenaline

Adrenaline is a vasoconstrictor, prescribed for heart failure, which increases mean arterial and diastolic pressure. Administration can be by bolus, endotracheal, i.v. and occasionally intracardiac injection. Side effects include tachycardia, vasoconstriction and impaired renal and mesenteric perfusion and, if given via an infusion, vasodilator therapy should be concomitant (Keeley and Bohn, 1988).

Atropine

This is an anticholinergic agent which inhibits the action of acetylcholine, a chemical transmitter found in the parasympathetic nervous system. Administration in an arrest situation is to free the heart from the inhibitory effects of the vagus nerve, so increasing heart rate and strength.

Adenosine

Adenosine slows conduction of the A-V node within 10–20 s of intravenous administration (Till and Shinebourne, 1991). Its short half-life of 10–15 s reduces the chances of side effects.

Digoxin

This cardiac glycoside is prescribed to improve the contractility of the myocardium in heart failure and to control ventricular arrhythmias. When commenced on digoxin the infant should be continuously monitored until blood levels are taken and the correct maintenance dose is established for maximum stability. Digoxin may take up to 6 h to work, and may precipitate ventricular fibrillation and increased blood pressure.

Dopamine

Dopamine is a precursor of noradrenaline and has sympathomimetic properties. It is prescribed for the treatment of shock and hypotension associated with cardiovascular surgery, sepsis and severe asphyxia (Keeley and Bohn, 1988). This vasodilator must be given by continuous i.v. infusion because of its short half-life, and not infused with alkali (causes inactivation). It has therapeutic effects by increasing stroke volume and cardiac output, raising the mean arterial pressure and improving urine volume, depending on the dose regimen (Keeley and Bohn, 1988). Dopamine causes blanching of the skin overlying the vein, so central access is preferred.

Dobutamine

This increases the contractility and output of the heart, improving tissue perfusion. The drug has a dose-dependent benefit and has a short half-life, necessitating a continuous i.v. infusion (Keeley and Bohn, 1988). Tachycardia has been reported as a side effect, requiring discontinuation.

Frusemide

This is a powerful diuretic which acts by preventing the reabsorption of sodium in the kidneys.

Indomethacin

Indomethacin is a prostaglandin synthetase inhibitor, and although the pharmacokinetics are not fully known, the drug is thought to block the action of naturally occurring prostaglandin, which has a role in maintaining this unwanted channel. Monitoring of the infant's fluid balance is vital during administration as indomethacin reduces renal blood flow.

Lignocaine

Lignocaine is an antiarrhythmic agent used for serious ventricular arrhythmia. It is given as an initial bolus followed by a continuous i.v. infusion. To be effective, high serum concentrations are needed and the drug has been reported as causing seizure activity.

Prostaglandin E_2

This is used to maintain the patency of the ductus arteriosus in cyanotic malformations, for example pulmonary atresia, tetralogy of Fallot and tricuspid atresia, until corrective surgery can be performed (Qureshi, 1989).

Caffeine

Full understanding of exactly how caffeine works has not been achieved; it may enhance the contractility of the diaphragm and/or stimulate the respiratory centre. It does increase the heart rate and may cause tachycardia.

In the case of all drugs listed the infant should be on a cardiorater and have regular blood pressure readings as clinically appropriate. Any bradycardia or tachycardia should be reported, and if necessary the drug or drugs not given until medical advice has been sought.

THE PRESENT AND THE FUTURE

Research into cardiac anomalies is ongoing and new treatments are being developed all the time. Prenatal prevention of lesions where possible is desirable, and health promotion to encourage sensible drinking and awareness of the link between some drugs and defects will hopefully reduce the incidence. Ultrasound scans are now used routinely to check the development of the heart *in utero*.

Many young women who have a CHD themselves have survived, thanks to modern medicine, but they need counselling, rigorous antenatal screening and preconception advice. Counselling should also be offered to parents with a family history of cardiac anomalies, or who feel that they are at risk, perhaps from environmental factors such as industrial pollution.

Many infants' abnormalities are picked up and correctly diagnosed in the neonatal period, thereby enhancing their prognosis by the institution of correct management. A blue baby gives a dramatic clue to all observers that something is seriously amiss. In general, if the infant is displaying respiratory distress (gasping, grunting or indrawing), although cardiac pathology cannot be ruled out, he needs respiratory support. If the infant is settled and comfortable but blue, then a cardiac condition should be suspected.

REFERENCES

Adelman, R.D. (1988) The hypertensive neonate. *Clinics in Perinatology* **15**(3), 567–85.

Brunner, L.S. and Suddarth, D.S. (198) *The Lippincott Manual of Paediatric Nursing*, 2nd edn, Harper and Row, New York.

Catzel, P. and Roberts, I. (1984) *A Short Textbook of Paediatrics*, 2nd edn, Hodder and Stoughton, London, pp. 123–50.

Chiswick, M. (1981) Patent ductus arteriosus in premature babies. *British Medical Journal* **283**, 1490–1.

Desai, S. (1992) Interpretation of a normal chest X-ray. *Nursing Standard* **7**(7), 38–9.

Ferguson, A.W. (1979) Recognizing cardiac failure in infancy. *Update*, 519–26.

Fleming, P.J., Spiedel, B.D. and Dunn, P.M. (1986) *A neonatal Vade-Mecum*, Lloyd Luke (Medical Books) Ltd, London.

Grossglauser, L. (1992) Neonatal radiology: assessment of the quality of the neonatal chest X-ray film. *Neonatal Network* **11**(7), 69–72.

Jolly, A. (1991) Taking blood pressure. *Nursing Times* **87**(15), 40–3.

Keeley, S.R. and Bohn, D.J. (1988) The use of inotropic and afterload reducing agents in neonates. *Clinics in Perinatology* **15**(3), 467–84.

Klaus, M. and Fanaroff, A. (1986) *Care of the High Risk Neonate*, Ardmore Medical Books, W.B. Saunders Company, Philadelphia, p. 292.

Levene, M., Tudehope, D. and Thearle, J. (1987) *Essentials of Neonatal Medicine*, Blackwell Scientific Publications, Oxford.

Lum, L.G. and Jones, M.D. (1977) The effect of cuff width on systolic blood pressure measurements in neonates. *Journal of Pediatrics* **91**, 963–6.

Moss, A.J., Duffle, E.R. and Emmanouilides, G. (1963) Blood pressure and vasomotor reflexes in the newborn infant. *Pediatrics* **32**, 175–9.

Marieb, E. (1992) *Human Anatomy and Physiology*, 2nd edn, Benjamin Cummings Publishing Company, California, pp. 604–32.

Qureshi, S. (19897 Signs of neonatal heart disease. *Nursing* **3**(36), 16–19.

Rigby, M.L., Pickering, D. and Wilkinson, A. (1984) Cross-sectional echocardiography in determining persistent patency of the ductus arteriosus in preterm infants. *Archives of Disease in Childhood* **59**, 341–5.

Roberton, N.R.C. (1987) *A Manual of Neonatal Intensive Care*, 2nd edn, Edward Arnold, London.

Roberts, A. (1990) Systems of life: the cardiovascular system. Part Two. *Nursing Times* **86**(50), 53–6.

Silove, E. (1983) Use of E-type prostaglandins in infants with pulmonary atresia and an intact ventricular septum, in *Paediatric Cardiology*, Vol 1, Churchill Livingstone. Edinburgh, pp. 254–62.

Sreeram, N. and Wren, C. (190) Supraventricular tachycardia in infants: response to initial treatment. *Archives of Diseases of Childhood* **65**(1), 127–9.

Stork, E.K., Carlo, W.A., Kleigman R.M. *et al*. (1984) Hypertension redefined for critically ill neonates. *Pediatric Research* **18**, 321A.

Till, J.A. and Shinebourne, E.A. (1991) Supraventricular tachycardia: diagnosis and current acute management. *Archives of Diseases of Childhood* **66**, 647–52.

Turill, S. (1992) Supported positioning in intensive care. *Paediatric Nursing* **4**(4), 24–7.

Wakely, C. (1989) Cardiac catheterisation. *Nursing* **3**(36), 20–3.

10

Infant neurology

Doreen Crawford

The brain and central nervous system (CNS) develop in advance of most of the other organs and systems in the body. They are susceptible to malformation and damage during embryonic and fetal life. Hazards include viral infection, radiation, drugs and other toxins such as excessive alcohol. Insult to the neurotissue can result from hypoxia and malnourishment, from placental insufficiency, from severe maternal illness and deprivation.

There are critical periods of development during which these hazards can exert their influence and cause damage. This may occur before the mother is aware of her pregnancy. The earliest recognizable neurotissue is found approximately 18 days after conception, but there is debate about the accurateness of staging in embryology. The embryogenesis of the brain and central nervous tissue is complex; however, a basic comprehension of normal development allows appreciation of the structure and function of the central nervous system and aids understanding of defective development and neuropathology. It is the aim of this book to give a simple overview; for more detail, the reader is referred to several excellent texts.

ANATOMY OF THE CENTRAL NERVOUS SYSTEM

Neurological development continues throughout gestation and is not complete until the end of the first decade. Embryological development is divided into three stages:

- Neurulation
- Secondary canalization
- Retrogressive differentiation.

Neurulation (very early development)

This stage covers postconceptual age 18–27 days. During this time early neurotissue appears as an area of thickened embryonic neuroectoderm. This becomes known as the neural plate, which will eventually develop into the brain and spinal cord. The neural plate invaginates (forms a groove), flanked by the neural folds; as this groove deepens, the topmost edges of the neural folds begin to fuse at approximately 22–24 days, giving rise to the neural tube. The neural folds do not fuse simultaneously: initially they fuse near the middle, opposite somites 2–7 (O'Rahilly *et al.*, 1977) and continue in both cephalic (towards the top) and caudal (towards the bottom) directions. The neural tube is formed by the 4th week of pregnancy (Marieb, 1992).

Neural tube defects, such as anencephaly and myelomeningocele, are a result of failure of the neural tube to fuse and will be discussed in detail later.

Secondary canalization

This stage covers days 28–51 and is a period of explosive development. With neural tube closure, the cephalic end expands and constrictions appear, dividing this part of the neural tube into three primary brain vesicles called the prosencephalon (the forebrain), the mesencephalon (the midbrain) and the rhombencephalon (the hindbrain). Further subdivision of the forebrain and hindbrain results in five structures called the secondary brain vesicles. The prosencephalon divides and forms the telencephalon (endbrain) and diencephalon (interbrain). The telencephalon, with further development, eventually results in the cerebral hemispheres. The diencephalon is the posterior part of the forebrain. Three swellings occur on each side of the diencephalon and eventually result in the thalamus, epithalamus and hypothalamus. The mesencephalon remains undivided. The rhombencephalon constricts to form both the metencephalon (afterbrain), which becomes the pons and cerebellum, and the myelencephalon (spinal brain), which becomes the medulla oblongata. The midbrain and hindbrain structures, with the exception of the cerebellum, eventually become the brain stem.

Retrogressive differentiation

This occurs between 52 and 80 days. Some of the embryonic landmarks are lost, such as the tail and the structures within it.

During embryogenesis the brain develops its general shape: a framework for the sophisticated nervous system. In the period following embryogenesis there is rapid neuroblast multiplication, when the adult number of cells are laid down. Final maturation of these cells with myelination may not occur until the individual is several years old.

Development of the ventricles

The central cavity of the neural tube remains continuous and becomes enlarged in four areas, resulting in the ventricles. These are lined with ependymal cells and filled with cerebrospinal fluid (CSF). With the convolutions of the brain and spinal cord, owing to the restricted space for development, the lateral ventricles become well defined 'C'-shaped structures by approximately 12 weeks' gestation. Each lateral ventricle communicates with the third ventricle and the third ventricle is continuous with the fourth. Within the fouth ventricle, there are three apertures which connect with the subarachnoid space and bathe the brain in CSF.

Close to the ventricles is the highly vascular subependymal germinal matrix. Between 10 and 20 weeks' gestation this area serves as a main site of cerebral neuroblasts. It is of particular interest to neonatal nurses as it is the most common origin of intraventricular haemorrhage (IVH). Many thin-walled vessels around this area are prone to bleeding, in certain circumstances, if premature delivery has occurred. As the fetus matures, the matrix progressively decreases in size and by 36 weeks it has undergone nearly complete involution (Volpe, 1989). According to Levene, Tudehope and Thearle (1987), it is rare to see such a haemorrhage in term infants. IVH will be discussed later.

Development of the cerebral hemispheres

The cerebral hemispheres arise from the telencephalon. Owing to rapid growth and restricted space, they are forced backwards and sideways (posteriorly and laterally) and shroud the diencephalon and midbrain. At 15 weeks' gestation, the cerebral hemispheres are smooth and have no sulci or gyri. Convolution of the cerebral cortex, which gives the cerebral hemispheres their familiar external pattern, facilitates an increase in cortical size without an increase in cranial volume. The number of sulci and gyri increases until, at birth, the surface of the cerebral cortex covers twice the visible area.

There are many causes of neuropathogenesis: some are related to deviation from normal development. Few conditions have such an impact on the individual and his family as malformation or malfunction of the neurological system. The nurse is in a unique position to support and care for all concerned, whatever the reason for admission.

NEUROLOGICAL CONDITIONS SEEN IN THE NEONATAL UNIT

- Birth asphyxia and trauma
- Seizures
- Structural malformations and hydrocephalus
- Intracranial haemorrhage
- Meningitis
- Neonatal hypotonia: the 'floppy infant'

This list is not exhaustive nor is it in any order of priority; some of the conditions are seen more frequently than others, and some of the most common will be discussed here.

Birth asphyxia

Volpe (1987) suggested that 90% of hypoxic, ischaemic cerebral injuries occurred antepartum or intrapartum. As obstetric screening procedures become more sophisticated the number of severely asphyxiated infants and the number subjected to unnecessary obstetric intervention should decline. Hypoxic insult is no respecter of gestation: although the preterm infant is more at risk, term infants are also affected.

There are various degrees of severity. Infants with mild asphyxia who rapidly respond to minimal resuscitation, who have good APGARS scores and observant mothers, may not even be admitted to the neonatal unit. Others are less fortunate and need a period of observation. Severely asphyxiated infants who have been in terminal apnoea have a variable and not always favourable prognosis. Many of these will require full supportive pulmonary ventilation and some may never be able to self-ventilate.

Following terminal apnoea (Chapter 4), spontaneous respiration cannot occur. Prolonged resuscitation can occasionally revive an infant who is profoundly asphyxiated, but may result in severe neurological sequelae. Initial assessment cannot accurately predict outcome. Levene (1988) concluded that resuscitative measures should be abandoned if an infant has had no cardiac output for 10 min, or has failed to breathe spontaneously 30 min after the establishment of cardiac output.

Complications of severe asphyxia

Infants with severe asphyxia are very sick and may have cardiovascular, renal and gastrointestinal as well as cerebral complications (Perlman, 1989).

The cardiovascular effects of asphyxia may result in instability, with hypotension and poor perfusion. The heart, although more resilient than some other organs, can be damaged by ischaemia, resulting in arrhythmia and cardiac failure. If treatment is to continue, the infant will need skilled medical and nursing care. This may involve the management of several lines, giving infusions of volume expanders such as human albumin to maintain blood pressure and help correct acidosis as well as dopamine to improve vascular tone and raise blood pressure. Such fluid input needs to be balanced with careful monitoring of output, as it is vital not to overload the infant.

These infants are prone to cerebral oedema occurring as a result of intracellular and extracellular accumulation of fluid, for which little can be done except restrict fluids. Mannitol and frusemide may be used, provided that cardiac and renal perfusion is adequate. Cerebral oedema may give rise to signs of raised intracranial pressure, such as increasing blood pressure, decreasing heart rate and irregular respiratory pattern. Regular observation of these vital signs can greatly assist management.

Cerebral oedema and brain injury may result in an irritable and restless infant who can be hyperresponsive to stimulation.

He should be kept warm and comfortable in a quiet environment, and not overstressed by too much handling.

Impaired renal function is common, even in cases of mild asphyxia. Severe asphyxia can result in both tubular and cortical necrosis. These infants need careful monitoring of fluid balance and all urine tested for protein and blood. If the damage is minimal no further intervention is required; others will require resin ion exchange enemas or dialysis.

Gastrointestinal complications such as necrotizing enterocolitis may occur from intestinal tissue hypoxia (Chapter 6).

The prognosis for asphyxiated infants is variable: recovery can occur within hours. If, after a few days, other signs of neurological abnormality occur, the prognosis is bleak. Severe asphyxia may result in profound stupor or convulsions, which may be difficult to control.

Neonatal seizures

Convulsions, fits, seizures, 'blue do's', funny turns, twitching and jitteriness are all terms which are frequently heard and understood in neonatal unit culture. Understanding is easy when there is an infant in front of you displaying the described activity. Brown and Minns (1988) suggested that the term seizure should be used to describe any paroxysmal event which may or may not be a fit. Although there is a classification of seizure types, many do not occur or are difficult to recognize in the neonate. Many seizure activities reported by nurses are generalized motor disturbances which may be accompanied by apnoea.

Management of seizure activity is aimed at the underlying cause as well as control. Prescribed medication by bolus or by continuous infusion may include drugs such as phenobarbitone, phenytoin, benzodiazepines such as diazepam and clonazepam, as well as paraldehyde.

Causes of seizure activity

- Asphyxia
- Metabolic disturbance
- Intracranial haemorrhage

- Malformation
- Genetic
- Infection
- Toxicity

Asphyxia
Asphyxia, resulting in hypoxic ischaemic encephalopathy, is the most common cause of neonatal seizures and these may be difficult to control (Levene, 1987). The full range of anticonvulsants may be tried, singly or in combination, until activity is controlled. As this may result in high serum drug levels in infants who have ischaemic damage to other organs, such drastic polypharmacy may be hazardous (Mizrahi, 1989). Clark (1989) suggested that some seizure activity may be the result of excitatory amino acids in traumatized brains, resulting ultimately in neuronal death. This research suggests that it may ultimately be possible to block the activity of such amino acids with a therapeutic agent.

Metabolic seizures
Hypoglycaemia, hypocalcaemia and hyponatraemia all cause seizure activity which responds to correction of the underlying cause. Rare metabolic disturbances are best left to specialist units to diagnose and manage. Unfortunately, the ability to diagnose exceeds the ability to cure, and for many families genetic advice is necessary to prevent recurrence.

Intracranial haemorrhage
Seizure activity resulting from intracranial haemorrhage occurs because of the presence of blood in the meninges or ventricles, brain tissue damage, compression from extensive blood clot or ischaemia due to interruption of the blood supply.

Malformation
A structurally malformed brain or a rare genetic syndrome may manifest seizure activity, as may cystic areas which are the result of periventricular leucomalacia. Hydrocephalus results in surprisingly few seizures, provided that the intracranial

pressure is not elevated. Management of the infant with a hopelessly abnormal brain may result in ethical dilemmas during which the parents and the family will need all the support that the nurse can give.

Infection

Infants with severe infection and meningitis may display seizure activity, which should be treated by anticonvulsants. The cause of seizure activity from infection varies: it may arise from secondary metabolic disturbance, dehydration or neurotoxins produced by bacteria, as well as meningeal irritation, emboli or thrombosis. Final resolution of this seizure activity depends on the initial cause and the success of antibiotic therapy.

Toxity

Kernicterus is now a rare cause of neonatal seizures. Seizures due to fetal alcohol syndrome and withdrawal from narcotics in the infants of addicted mothers are rare. Seizure caused by toxins produced by infection has already been discussed.

Intraventricular haemorrhage

Levene (1987) described five important types of intracranial haemorrhage (his book is recommended reading, as further explanation is beyond the scope of this chapter). The most common are intraventricular haemorrhages, which occur in premature infants as a result of rupture of delicate blood vessels. Several factors are thought to predispose to this, such as poor condition at birth, respiratory distress syndrome, acidosis and high levels of CO_2. Sudden swings between hypoxia and hyperoxia and infusion of base may also be implicated. Fluctuation of blood pressure may also contribute, as may sudden stressors such as insensitive handling, physiotherapy and endotracheal suction (Perlman and Volpe, 1983).

The sicker and more premature the infant, the likelier is intraventricular haemorrhage. As always, prevention is preferred to cure. Nursing interventions to reduce the risk of IVH include consideration of the infant's position (intracranial pressure was found to be lowest when the head was slightly elevated and in the midline) (Kling, 1989). Obstruction of venous outflow caused by tight strapping to protect infusion sites or secure endotracheal tubes has been implicated. Whenever possible, strapping should not circumvent the head. Other causative factors are beyond medical control and nursing prevention.

Different therapeutic agents have been tried to limit the occurrence and extent of haemorrhage, including vitamin E, fresh frozen plasma and indomethacin. It is difficult to accurately predict the final extent of disability, if any (Andersen, 1989).

Structural malformations and hydrocephalus

The main categories of structural malformation are:

- Anencephaly, where there is developmental failure resulting in the absence of the forebrain. The incidence is about 1 in 1000 (Roberton, 1993) and the defect is incompatible with life. No attempt at resuscitation should be made. Sometimes there are signs of life and the infant may move and occasionally gasp, but the situation remains hopeless and where possible the family should be cared for together, with sensitive support for the parents. There is some risk of recurrence and the families involved need counselling. Increasingly parents are asking about organ donation.
- Encephalocele, which occurs when there is a failure of midline closure. It is comparatively rare and 80% of lesions are occipital (Levene, 1987). The defect can be skin-covered. The prognosis can be poor and depends on how much brain tissue is in the sac. Complications during delivery can result in severe damage and full assessment should be made as soon as possible.
- Spina bifida occulta. This is a defect in the spine, and in many cases the diagnosis is made by X-ray for unrelated problems or by examination and chance; many cases go undetected. The cord and meninges are normal and no disability need be involved.

- Spina bifida cystica, which can be further divided into meningocele and meningomyelocele. Meningocele is a herniation of the meninges and a gathering of cerebrospinal fluid within the defect. It can occur anywhere along the spinal cord and disability need not arise as the cord is structurally normal. Rapid surgical intervention is recommended. In meningomyelocele the defect can be open and much more severe as it can involve the spinal cord. Disabilities resulting from this lesion can be extensive.

These structural malformations are caused by a failure of part of the tube to fuse. This occurs in the first month of pregnancy and many factors have been incriminated, such as genetic, familial, dietetic, toxins and environmental factors; sadly there is a high risk of recurrence. Recent research has suggested that a vitamin deficiency is a major causative factor in the development of neural tube defects (Czeizel, 1993). Extensive media coverage has resulted in maternal feelings of guilt. Improved prenatal diagnosis results in fewer of these infants coming to the neonatal unit (Seller, 1989). Much work has been done since Lorber (1971) initially postulated that 'surgery at all costs' was not always in the best interests of the child. The decision to treat actively or conservatively is not made in isolation but involves the family, physiotherapists, medical and nursing staff. Prior to active treatment, careful assessment is made and surgery performed as soon as possible, provided that there is adequate skin cover, to prevent ascending infection. Tissue expansion is now possible (Moss, 1992), which can provide extra skin, but if the lesion is so vast that early primary closure is not possible the resulting neurological urological and orthopaedic deficits will be unavoidable.

Improved surgical techniques have enhanced the overall prognosis of infants with myelomeningocele (Noetzel, 1989). For infants with hydrocephalus at birth, simultaneous shunt placement is desirable.

Not all neonatal units have facilities for neurosurgery and the infant will need to be transferred. Photographs of the child should still be taken for the parents, whether the child is malformed or not.

Surgeons' preferences and local protocols differ; however, the lesion should be kept covered and moist with a non-adherent sterile dressing. Paxton (1990) continues to recommend saline gauze. In small infants who have difficulty maintaining their temperature, this may not be ideal. A sterile 'U' drape, as used in transporting infants with exomphalos could be used, as could clingfilm or other non-adherent materials. None of these are absolutely ideal or universally recommended.

To try and minimize contamination by soiling and limit any further neurological damage, the infant should be kept prone. This method of management usually means that he is nursed exposed in an incubator to maintain warmth and facilitate observation. Unfortunately, this provides a physical barrier between the parents and their offspring.

There is no reason why the infant cannot be fed milk until approximately 4 hours before surgery, when a dextrose infusion should be started to maintain hydration and blood glucose. Postoperatively, the infusion is continued until the infant is ready to consume milk. The cannula is maintained for antibiotic therapy, if prescribed. He is still nursed prone and his dressing and drainage are monitored for signs of oozing. Frequent observation of the head circumference is vital to detect hydrocephalus. Nursing observation of bowel and bladder function can be useful to establish the extent of associated urinary and bowel problems, and occasionally manual expression of the bladder may be necessary to prevent urinary stasis.

Once the infant has recovered and the lesion healed sufficiently, intensive limb physiotherapy is commenced and the parents can make up for all the cuddles they were perhaps afraid to give preoperatively.

Hydrocephalus is treated by the insertion of a shunt, which prevents intracranial pressure from building up because of dilated fluid-filled ventricles. Surprisingly, the procedure disturbs the infant very little unless complications occur; many return from theatre hungry and ready to feed.

Meningitis

Infection of the meninges (the two delicate membranes that cover the brain) may occur before, during or after birth. Intrauterine infection assumes transplacental crossing of organisms or severe ascending infection following premature rupture of the membranes. Infection during birth and in the neonatal period can come from contamination by hands, instruments, inhalation, ingestion or inoculation. The sicker the infant, the greater the intervention required and therefore the more likely the risk of infection.

The preterm baby has a less than effective immunity system, with reduced levels of immunoglobulin synthesis, few circulating white cells and complement levels which are about half that of an adult (Davies, 1988). Prevention of such infection would be ideal and stringent hygiene regulations apply at all times when caring for such vulnerable infants. Unfortunately neonatal meningitis is common and a major neonatal emergency. The initial signs are often non-specific. In neonatal unit jargon, infants may go 'off their feeds': this means that the infant has not taken his usual amount of feed with the accustomed enthusiasm or has not tolerated the feed and vomited; look 'off colour': this can mean that the infant is pale, mottled, flushed or jaundiced; not 'handle well': this can mean that the infant is irritable and not settling, not welcoming attention, arching and fussing, tense or hypotonic. His temperature may fluctuate and there is often a wide gap between the core and peripheral temperatures owing to poor perfusion. Blood glucose may be elevated as part of a generalized stress reaction, vital signs may deviate from his usual baseline, and seizure activity, tense and bulging fontanelle, posturing such as opisthotonos and increasing head circumference are later signs.

Neonatal nurses are in a prime position to detect these early signs. If their intuition is to prove useful to the infant, resulting in prompt detection and treatment, nurses need to be specific and make accurate descriptions.

Most units perform full infection screens, including lumbar puncture, readily and some may commence intravenous broad-spectrum antibiotic therapy on clinical suspicion, while awaiting the results. Lumbar puncture is not well tolerated by very small, sick infants who tend to become cold and stressed. Owing to the extreme back-bend required to widen intervertebral spaces their respiratory function is compromised. The nurse assisting with the procedure should ensure that emergency equipment is close at hand and that supplementary oxygen is available should the infant's colour change and he become cyanosed. In infants who are bordering on needing ventilatory assistance, it is often preferable to intubate the airway prior to performing the puncture.

Debate exists about the necessity for lumbar puncture. Research has suggested that, in cases of meningitis, there is concurrent septicaemia and positive microbial results would be obtained from blood culture. Such an invasive procedure should not be routine (MacMahon, Jewes and de Louvois, 1990).

Neurological observations are open to wide interpretation but posture, irritability and rousability are good guides to neurological stability; meningeal irritation can result in a high pitched cry. Measurement of head circumference and monitoring of vital signs during the acute stage of the illness should be performed to detect raised intracranial pressure or deteriorating condition. To prevent cerebral oedema, fluid restriction may be prescribed and balanced with accurate measurements of output. Some infants will require anticonvulsants and some will develop neurological sequelae. Infants with mengingitis are often very sick and need full intensive care. The care of the family and siblings is just as important, and is discussed in Chapter 1.

Neonatal hypotonia

The term 'floppy infant' describes the loss of body tension and tone, which results in an abnormal posture when the infant is handled and delayed developmental motor milestones. It can originate centrally as a result of severe asphyxia or from the neurological sequelae of illness and damage. It may also be caused by a genetic defect such as Down's syndrome or a neuromuscular disorder, many of which are very rare. A comprehensive review of causes of neuromuscular disorders can be found in Roland (1989) and is beyond the scope of this book. Some disorders are progressive, such as the muscular dystrophy group, which may not be evident in the newborn. These infants, if admitted for any other reason, should be actively treated as they can live to their late teens or early 20s. Their families require diagnostic assessment and genetic counselling, which should be performed on an outpatient basis, with the support of the families' health visitor.

Infants with spinal muscular atrophy (Werdnig–Hoffman disease) may require admission to the neonatal unit because of respiratory distress, and initially be ventilated. They pose difficult ethical problems owing to their very bleak prognosis. There is no treatment available and arguably the only kind method of management is nursing care. This would ideally be done at home, although it can be difficult to withdraw ventilator support from an infant with breathing difficulties. Many of these conditions result from consanguineous relationships or genetic abnormalities and genetic advice is recommended.

INVESTIGATIONS USED TO AID DIAGNOSIS

A lumbar puncture is performed to obtain a specimen of CSF for examination by culture or chemistry. This is one of the most invasive yet most common investigations to take place on the neonatal unit. A variation on the lumbar puncture, the ventricular tap, may be used to aid the diagnosis of haemorrhage.

Ultrasound scans are not invasive but do require that the infant is handled. The equipment is large and may look fearsome to the parents, so their consent and a brief explanation may reassure them. Other methods of imaging are increasingly being employed, such as computerized tomography (CT) and magnetic resonance scans. Trounce and Levene (1988) and Flodmark (1988) describe these and discuss their advantages and disadvantages.

ETHICAL ISSUES

The care of neonates with neuropathology is an expanding area and also one of the many ethically difficult and grey areas in the specialty, as the outcome is often so variable. A Health Economics Group, in 1993, questioned the concept of care for infants weighing less than 500 g. Other ethical issues concern the donation of organs from infants with anencephaly (Forst, 1989) and the measurement of neonatal brain death (Ashwal, 1989). Ethics are discussed in Chapter 17.

REFERENCES

Anderson, G. (1989) Prediction of outcome in infants born after 24–28 weeks gestation. *Acta Paediatrica Scandinavica* **360**, 56–61.

Ashwal, S. (1989) Brain death in the newborn. *Clinics in Perinatology* **16**(2), 501–18.

Brown, F. and Minns, R. (1988) Seizure disorders, in *Foetal and Neonatal Neurology and Neurosurgery*, (eds M. Levene, M. Bennett and J. Punt), Churchill Livingstone, Edinburgh, pp. 487–513.

Clark, G. (1989) Role of excitatory amino acids in brain injury caused by hypoxic ischaemia, status epilepticus and hypoglycaemia. *Clinics in Perinatology* **16**(2), 459–74.

Czeizel, A. (1993) Prevention of congenital abnormalities by periconceptual multi-vitamin supplementation. *British Medical Journal* **6893**(306) 1645–8.

Davies, P. (1988) Bacterial and fungal infections, in *Foetal and Neonatal Neurology and Neurosurgery* (eds M. Levene, M. Bennett and J. Punt), Churchill Livingstone, Edinburgh, pp. 427–49.

Flodmark, O. (1988) Computed tomography and magnetic resonance imaging of the neonatal nervous system in *Foetal and Neonatal Neurology and Neurosurgery* (eds M. Levene, M. Bennett and J. Punt), Churchill Livingstone, Edinburgh, pp. 122–38.

Frost, N. (1989) Removing organs from anencephalic infants: ethical and legal considerations. *Clinics in Perinatology* **16**(2), 331–7.

Kling, P. (1989) Nursing interventions to decrease the risk of periventricular haemorrhage. *Journal of Obstetrics, Gynaecology and Neonatal Nursing* **18**(6), 457–64.

Levene, M. (1987) *Neonatal Neurology*, Current Reviews in Paediatrics, Churchill Livingstone, Edinburgh.

Levene, M. (1988) Management and outcome of birth asphyxia, in *Foetal and Neonatal Neurology and Neurosurgery* (eds M. Levene, M. Bennett and J. Punt), Churchill Livingstone, Edinburgh, Chapter 34.

Levene, M., Tudehope, D. and Thearle, J. (1987) *Essentials of Neonatal Medicine*, Blackwell Scientific Publications, Oxford.

Lorber, J. (1971) Results of treatment of myelomeningocele: an analysis of 524 unselected cases with special reference to possible selection for treatment. *Developmental Medicine and Child Neurology* **13**, 279–303.

McMahon, P., Jewes, L. and de Louvois, J. (1990) Routine lumbar punctures in the newborn, are they justified? *European Journal of Pediatrics* **149**(11), 797–9.

Marieb, E. (1992) *Human Anatomy and Physiology*, 2nd edn, Benjamin Cummings Publishing Company, California, pp. 378–422.

Mizrahi, E. (1989) Consensus and controversy in the clinical management of neonatal seizures. *Clinics in Perinatology* **16**(2), 485–500.

Moss, A. (1992) Plastic surgeons notebook. The technique of tissue expansion. *Professional Care of Mother and Child* **2**(10), 330.

Noetzel, M. (1989) Myelomeningocele: current concepts of management. *Clinics in Perinatology* **16**(2), 311–29.
O'Rahilly, R. and Gardner, E. (1977) The developmental anatomy and histology of the human central nervous system, in *Handbook of Clinical Neurology: Congenital Malformations of the Brain and Skull* (eds R. Vinken and G. Gruyn), Myrianthopoulos, Amsterdam, pp. 15–40.
Paxton, J. (1990) Transport of the surgical neonate. *Journal of Perinatal and Neonatal Nursing* **3**(3), 43–9.
Perlman, J. (1989) Systemic abnormalities in term infants following perinatal asphyxia: relevance to long term neurologic outcome. *Clinics in Perinatology* **16**(2), 475–84.
Perlman, J. and Volpe, J. (1983) Suctioning in the preterm infant: effects on cerebral blood flow, velocity, intracranial pressure and arterial blood pressure. *Pediatrics* **72**(3), 329–34.
Roberton, N. (1993) *A Manual of Neonatal Intensive Care,* 3rd edn. Edward Arnold, London.
Seller, M. (1989) Perinatal diagnosis of neural tube defects. *Midwife, Health Visitor and Community Nurse* **25**(11), 458–62.
Trounce, F. and Levene, M. (1988) Ultrasound imaging of the neonatal brain, in *Foetal and Neonatal Neurology and Neurosurgery,* (eds M. Levene, M. Bennett and J. Punt), Churchill Livingstone, Edinburgh, pp. 139–48.
Volpe, J. (1987) *Neurology of the Newborn,* W.B. Saunders, Philadelphia.
Volpe, J. (1989) Intraventricular haemorrhage and brain injury in the premature infant. Neuropathology and pathogenesis. *Clinics in Perinatology* **16**(2), 361–86.

FURTHER READING

Roland, E. (1989) Neuromuscular disorders in the newborn. *Clinics in Perinatology* **16**(2), 519–45.
Williams, P. and Warwick, R. (1980) *Gray's Anatomy,* 36th edn, Churchill Livingstone, Edinburgh, pp. 802–1226.

11

Nursing care of a baby in renal failure

Emily Logan

The rapid evolution of renal medicine has meant that babies who in the past were treated conservatively are now being taken on to end-stage renal failure programmes within the first week of life, with optimistic predictions of transplantation. The road to transplantation is long and tortuous and presents a myriad of challenges to nursing management, but when a 7 kg toddler can receive a cadaveric transplant from a 50-year-old donor, what is the limit to renal nursing?

The causes of renal failure in neonates are varied, and can be grouped under the headings of acute, chronic and end-stage renal failure. This chapter does not aim to give a comprehensive review of renal failure in neonates, but addresses the nursing care of the more common complications. These issues, outside the paediatric nephrology environment, may become problems to the less experienced practitioner. The knowledge and understanding of the underlying pathophysiology is an integral part of the provision of safe and appropriate care.

Acute renal failure has a rapid onset that is most often reversible once the cause had been identified. Causes (Arbus and Farine, 1986) are:

- hypovolaemia
- early cord clamping
- sepsis
- congenital heart disease
- hypoxia

- renal vein thrombosis
- renal artery embolization
- obstructive uropathies.

Chronic renal failure has an insidious onset and does not necessitate dialysis, but it usually progresses to end-stage disease. Causes of chronic renal failure (Fine, 1986) are:

- hypoplasia
- dysplasia
- cystic disease
- hereditary diseases.

End-stage renal failure occurs when kidney function is no longer compatible with life and requires replacement therapy, i.e. dialysis.

The regulation of homoeostasis, chemical equilibrium and acid–base balance are well known functions of the kidneys. The kidneys are also important for the regulation of blood pressure, activation of vitamin D and erythopoiesis. Chronic and end-stage renal failure have an effect on all the kidney's functions, whereas acute renal failure does not affect the activation of vitamin D and erythropoiesis.

HOMEOSTASIS AND ASSESSMENT OF FLUID BALANCE

Homeostasis is the condition in which the body's internal environment remains relatively constant, within limits (Tortora and Anagnostakos, 1987). At birth, water constitutes 75–80% of body weight in term infants and a larger proportion in those born prematurely (Nash, 1978). Intracellular fluid accounts for two-thirds of total body fluid, with the remaining one-third being extracellular. This fluid is contained within different compartments in the body and is constantly moving to achieve a state of equilibrium.

Intake and output

It is imperative to record accurate hourly fluid balance. The infant's fluid status needs to be assessed continuously, to determine whether there is a fluid volume excess or deficit, and to elicit in which compartment the fluid lies.

Intake

The fluid regime should be prescribed on a daily basis and sometimes more often if the infant is unstable. With an infant in renal failure who needs fluid restriction, intake is based on the previous day's urinary output plus insensible water losses which, in a term infant, is 20 ml/kg/day for the first week and 40–50 ml/kg/day for a preterm infant (Halliday, McClure and Reid, 1989). Insensible losses are increased under radiant heaters or with a fever, and decreased with ventilated patients.

Output

Ninety-three percent of term infants pass urine within the first 24 hours of life, regardless of gestational age (Clark, 1977). The measurement of urinary output in the infant is extremely important. A term infant should pass 2–5 ml/kg/h. Measuring the volume will help assess what phase of renal failure the infant is in, and this is particularly important in the acutely ill infant.

Oliguria: <0.5 ml/kg/h
Anuria: <1 ml/kg/day
Polyuria: >200 ml/h

(Goetzman-Wennberg, 1991)

All urine specimens should be checked for the presence of protein and blood, with the pH and specific gravity measured using urinary dipsticks. Specimens may need to be sent daily to the laboratory for culture and/or electrolytes. In the neonatal group, the odour of infected urine is noticeable with obstructive uropathies and the assessment of clarity is important as it relates to infected urinary tracts and the degree of haematuria. Urinary pH measurement is important, especially in infants with tubular dysfunction, and specific gravity will determine urine concentration.

Blood and protein testing is important, as an infant with nephritis will have microscopic or macroscopic haematuria and proteinuria, whereas the infant with nephrosis will have proteinuria.

The stream may be abnormal in babies with urinary tract anomalies. To assess the volume of urine passed, nappies should be weighed and, if this does not prove accurate enough, urine bags can be used. Urethral catheters are not a first line of choice for measurement because of the risks of bacteraemia.

It is useful to document on a fluid balance chart when diuretics have been given, to indicate the sequence of events.

If a baby is polyuric the problem may be exacerbated by giving a glucose intravenous solution which will induce an osmotic diuresis.

If the urinary output is low then the bladder should be palpated, because if extended it protrudes into the abdominal space.

Temperature

Peripheral and core temperatures should be measured continually. The shin (toe) and core temperatures should be within 2 °C of each other. A larger temperature gap could be indicative of dehydration.

Blood pressure

As blood pressure helps in estimating the circulating volume, it is imperative that attention be paid to accuracy. In an infant that is acutely ill, blood pressure is often volume-dependent. The nurse must use her knowledge and judgement and discuss with the medical team when administering prescribed drugs. A high blood pressure can be misleading if it is part of a compensatory mechanism associated with dehydration. In this situation it is best to rely on other signs, i.e. temperature gap.

Oedema

This is usually related to lower urinary tract obstruction and congenital nephrotic syndrome. Unlike in infants with cardiac problems, oedema presents itself in the morning, as a peri-orbital phenomenon.

Respiratory rate

Tachypnoea will indicate fluid excess. It is important to alert medical staff to air hunger breathing and the presence of acidosis.

Heart rate

A dehydrated infant will have a tachycardia and an overloaded infant may have a gallop rhythm.

Central venous pressure (CVP)

This is useful when accurate but unfortunately it is difficult to measure in neonates and hence rarely done in a general neonatal unit. A CVP catheter is passed into the subclavian vein and the pressure is measured in the superior vena cava. Ideally, pressure should be kept between 3 and 5 cmH_2O.

Weight

Despite the accuracy of fluid charts, it is best to confirm by checking the infant's weight. Technologically advanced equipment includes a set of bed scales which are placed under the wheels of a cot and sling scales in which the baby can be weighed undisturbed on a hammock-like apparatus.

CHEMICAL EQUILIBRIUM AND ELECTROLYTE DISTURBANCES

Sodium

Sodium represents about 90% of extracellular cations. It is necessary for the transmission of impulses in nervous and muscle tissue and it plays a role in fluid balance. Hypernatraemia is a plasma concentration of sodium greater than 145 mmol/l. The signs and symptoms of hypernatraemia are:

- restlessness
- fits
- coma

- cerebellar haemorrhage
- hypertension
- death.

Other factors to consider include the infant's state of hydration, any sodium supplementation in drugs or intravenous fluids and the urinary sodium loss.

Hyponatraemia is a plasma concentration less than 130 mmol/l. Low sodium levels can cause the following problems:

- cerebral oedema
- vomiting
- restlessness
- disturbed consciousness
- fits
- coma.

Potassium

Potassium is the most abundant cation found in the intracellular fluid. It is present to help maintain fluid volume in cells and influences acid–base balance. Extracellularly, it is essential for the functioning of muscle tissue, including cardiac muscle. With sodium and calcium it regulates neuromuscular excitability and stimulation necessary for the transmission of nerve impulses. Hyperkalaemia is a plasma concentration greater than 5.5 mmol/l. The signs and symptoms of hyperkalaemia are:

- muscle weakness
- abdominal pain
- vomiting
- arrhythmias
- cardiac arrest
- diarrhoea (Watson, 1991)
- ECG changes:
  peaked T waves
  reduced R wave
  increased PR interval
  QRS blends with T waves (Gower, 1983)

If the infant needs a blood transfusion, fresh rather than stored blood (in which the potassium content is higher) should be used.

Hypokalaemia is a plasma concentration less than 3.5 mmol/l. It does not usually occur with renal disease but as a result of treatment prescribed, for example diuretic therapy and dialysis with a low dialysate potassium. Polyuria, as occurs in the diuretic phase of acute renal failure, may cause potassium depletion.

Calcium

Calcium is an extracelluar electrolyte. It has a role in clotting, neurotransmitter release, muscle contraction and the normal heartbeat. Hypercalcaemia is a plasma concentration greater than 2.6 mmol/l, and often the symptoms may not be obvious. Ensure that the infant is not on any drugs that will increase calcium levels, i.e. calcium carbonate in babies with chronic renal failure, or vitamin D therapy.

Hypocalcaemia is a plasma concentration less than 2.2 mmol/l. This occurs as part of chronic renal failure. It can also happen in acute renal failure, particularly in a baby on bicarbonate dialysis, with which calcium cannot be used simultaneously.

ACID–BASE BALANCE

The kidneys are involved in the principal buffer system, the carbonic acid–bicarbonate system, where they play a primary role in the regulation of bicarbonate concentration through tubular secretion. This is achieved by the acidification of urine, which eliminates hydrogen ions and conserves bicarbonate and the elimination of ammonium ions and retention of bicarbonate (Tortora and Anagnostakos, 1987) (Figure 11.1). Acid–base balance is shown in Table 11.1.

An infant with renal disease develops metabolic acidosis through the loss of bicarbonate or the accumulation of acid. Renal losses of bicarbonate are caused by:

- proximal renal tubular acidosis
- Fanconi's syndrome
- chronic renal failure

- accumulation of acid
- distal renal tubular acidosis
- acute renal failure
- chronic renal failure.

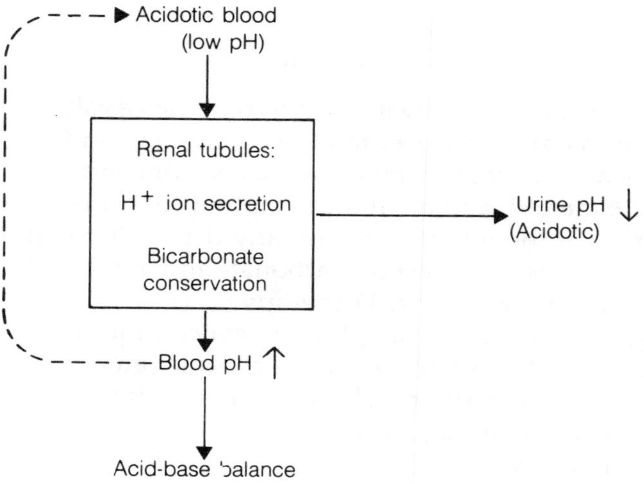

Figure 11.1 Acid–base balance (adapted from Tortora and Anagnostakos, 1987).

Table 11.1 Acid–base

Acid–base status	*Renal function*
Respiratory acidosis	Conservation of bicarbonate ions
Non-renal metabolic acidosis	Excretion of hydrogen ions
Metabolic alkalosis	Excretion of bicarbonate ions

(after Gower 1983)

REGULATION OF BLOOD PRESSURE

Where the loop of Henle re-enters the cortex, the afferent arteriolar cells are thickened. These specialized cells, which are called granular cells, produce renin (Tortora and Anagnostakos, 1987). The renin–angiotensin cascade functions notably in acute renal failure, as is shown in Figure 11.2.

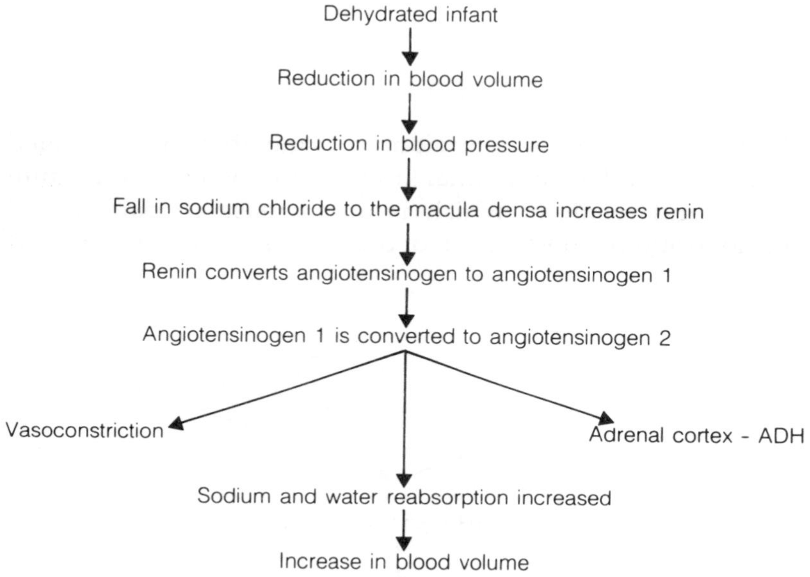

Figure 11.2 The renin–angiotensin cascade (Lote, 1987).

The measurement of blood pressure is often underestimated as a simple skill. Details of how to measure an infant's blood pressure are given in Chapter 9. Consistency in measurement can be ensured by recording which limb was used, the size of the cuff and the method. Measurements taken when the baby is crying or sucking are usually higher than normal. The systolic measurement is more consistent than diastolic, so it is not imperative to measure diastolic pressure with renal failure. Drugs that may affect blood pressure, such as sedatives, have to be taken into consideration. Any infant with suspected hypertension needs to have a four-limb blood pressure taken to exclude non-renal causes such as aortic coarctation. A lower than normal blood pressure may indicate a dehydrated infant.

Arterial blood pressure monitoring may be used in some units. This information is important, as the association between umbilical arterial catheters and renal artery thrombosis is well documented in infants who experience hypovolaemia, leading to long-term sequelae including renal atrophy and hypertension (McGraw, 1986).

VITAMIN D METABOLISM

The role of the kidneys in vitamin D metabolism is detailed in Figure 11.3. Dysfunctional kidneys do not activate vitamin D, the end result of which is an increase in parathyroid hormone and the destruction of bone by osteoclasts in an effort

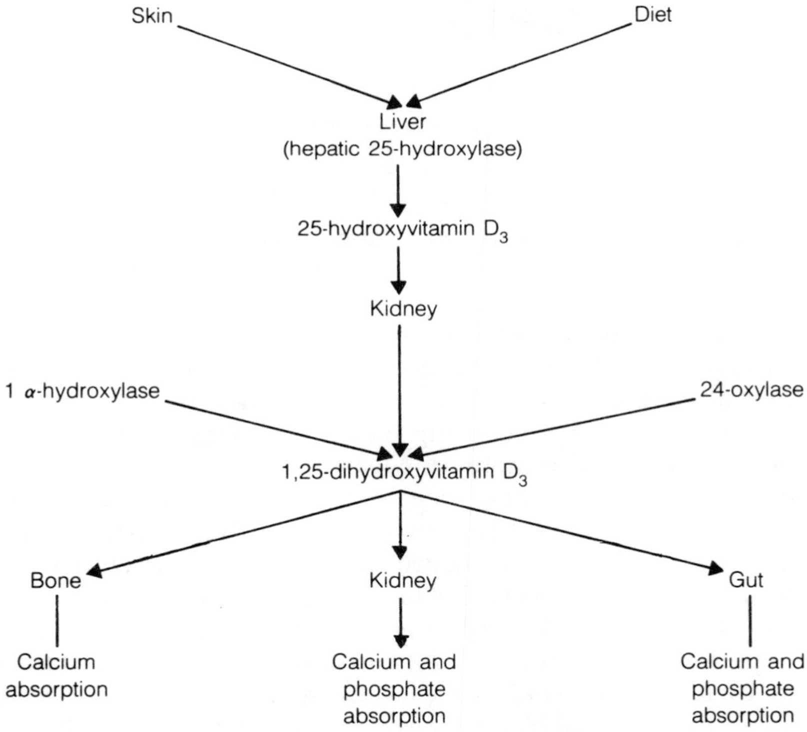

Figure 11.3 Vitamin D metabolism and the kidneys.

to increase blood calcium. The long-term effects of this are hyperparathyroidism and osteomalacia. Infants in chronic and end-state disease are given vitamin D in its active form to avoid this cascade.

ERYTHROPOIESIS

The kidneys produce the erythropoietic factor that converts plasma protein into erythropoietin. Absence of the erythropoietic factor causes chronic anaemia in those with chronic renal disease. Giving a blood transfusion is usually avoided because it may cause fluid overload and will not treat the existing chronic problem. Regular transfusions can cause iron overload and the production of cytotoxic anti-HLA antibodies, which can contribute to rejection of a transplanted kidney. Anaemia is now treated with recombinant human erythropoietin to avoid such complications. The neonatal nurse must explain to parents why blood transfusions are avoided in this situation.

PERITONEAL DIALYSIS

Peritoneal dialysis has always been first choice in the treatment of neonates in acute renal failure as it is safer in a haemodynamically unstable infant. The guidelines for chronic renal failure are similar but less aggressive. Indications for dialysis are:

- hyperkalaemia
- fluid overload
- rapidly rising plasma urea and creatinine in the presence of oliguria
- metabolic acidosis
- to create space for nutrition
- to remove specific poisons
- pulmonary oedema
- end-stage disease.

The peritoneum is chosen because it is a highly vascular semipermeable membrane with a large surface area. The peritoneal catheter is inserted aseptically under sedation unless contraindicated. In most intensive care areas a manual peritoneal dialysis set is used consisting of three dialysate bags, a filling burette, a warming coil, a draining burette and a drainage bag. Nephrology units tend to use automated cyclers which can perform a 50 ml exchange. Each set is changed daily and the effluent sent to the laboratory for microscopy.

Planning the dialysis

A skilled nephrologist will assess a 'dry weight' which is the optimum weight for the infant with a normal blood pressure. This is the target weight for planning the dialysis session. Using the guidelines discussed the infant's fluid status is assessed. Access to the intravascular space is only available in the infant, and if the fluid is in the third space it cannot be removed until that fluid has been shifted by colloid; 20% albumin is used in infants with congenital nephrotic syndrome. Acute renal failure associated with fluid overload may require fluid restriction. Fluid needs on dialysis are based on

- insensible losses at 20 ml/kg/day;
- the amount of ultrafiltrate;
- urinary output.

The infant's blood chemistry, including plasma albumin and haemoglobin, is checked. If both are low or the albumin alone, the removal of fluid will be more difficult because of reduced osmotic pressure in the intravascular space. The infant is weighed to determine how much excess fluid needs to be removed. Cycle volumes are based on the child's weight at 20–30 ml/kg (Donaldson *et al.*, 1983).

Depending on the infant's blood status additives may be needed, for example bicarbonate or potassium. Heparin is added to the dialysate (200–500 units/l), unless contraindicated and the concentration of glucose varies according to volume status. Lignocaine can be given to alleviate pain.

If fluid is sitting in the interstitial space with a low plasma albumin it is dangerous to increase the concentration of glucose, as this leads to hypovolaemia.

The acidotic infant on bicarbonate dialysis is at risk of becoming hypocalcaemic, as there is no calcium in the dialysate.

Potassium removal is very efficient, especially in the first couple of hours, when the gradient between serum potassium levels and the dialysate is greatest.

Ensure that all blood results are scrutinized to avoid unnecessary interruption of the circuit: in a chronic dialysis patient the peritoneum is their lifeline.

Starting dialysis

Always drain first, as the peritoneum is filled with fluid during insertion of the catheter. If the fluid is bloodstained, fill and drain the peritoneum without a dwell (waiting time), followed by frequent exchanges to avoid clotting of the catheter. The prescription sheet should indicate clearly the parameters of safety with regard to fluid excess or deficit.

Cycles

Times may vary from 30 min to 2 h, depending on the infant's needs.

Fill time: 10 min	hourly cycles
Dwell: 30 min	
Drain: 20 min	

Fill and drain times should be as little as possible as dialysis only takes place during a dwell. Smaller volumes are used at the beginning, building up to 30 ml/kg. Gentle clearance of urea is important, particularly in the presence of uraemia, as this can lead to imbalance, with resulting signs of cerebral oedema and raised intracranial pressure.

Mechanical troubleshooting

Problems with draining can be associated with a badly positioned infant or catheter. He may reabsorb fluid if he is dehydrated and hypoalbuminaemia may cause problems as the albumin level may be too low to pull off fluid. It may take a couple of cycles before ultrafiltration begins; wait and see what happens in the next cycle before intervening. Peritonitis also reduces the permeability of the peritoneum (Wu and Oreopoulos, 1988).

Problems with filling are usually catheter-related. There may be omentum adherent to the catheter which would indicate the need for a new catheter. A kinked line will prevent access.

Complications

Fluid balance

Fluid overload usually results from inefficient dialysis and is best overcome by increasing the frequency of cycles. Glucose may need to be added to the dialysate. Dehydration may occur if the infant's fluid status has been inaccurately assessed, or may result from aggressive dialysis.

Individuals respond differently to dialysis: some lose fluid very quickly and some do not, so it is best to start with a weak glucose solution until it is known how the infant is going to respond. If the ultrafiltrate is in excess of the desired amount but the baby needs dialysis, it is best to get intravenous fluids prescribed and continue dialysis. If the infant has a temperature gap do not be tempted to increase the glucose concentration to compensate for the dehydration as the glucose is not accessible to the body.

Respiratory

Dyspnoea may result from fluid overload or splinting of the diaphragm, especially in ventilated patients. The former is resolved by increasing the number of cycles and the latter by reducing the cycle volume. Sitting the infant upright or tilting the bed is also beneficial.

Hyperglycaemia

Sugar is absorbed from the dialysate into the blood most commonly in the infant who is dry, and is best avoided by gentle removal of fluid. The blood sugar levels need to be checked 4–6-hourly.

Hypotension

This is best avoided by watching closely the amount of fluid being removed, as blood pressure drops with hypovolaemia.

Electrolyte disturbances

Low levels of electrolytes means over enthusiasm (i.e. more salts were dialysed out than was necessary) and increased levels mean inefficient dialysis. Blood chemistry needs to be checked 6-hourly in the acute phase. Increasing the cycle volume will improve solute clearance.

Potassium and calcium are the two electrolytes that cause most problems, potassium because it dialyses so efficiently and calcium in an acidotic infant as it cannot be added to the dialysate with bicarbonate, in which case it is given intravenously.

Peritonitis

Good precise technique is the key to the avoidance of peritonitis. Rates of peritonitis are increased in patients who have a greater number of connections made (Leehey, Gandi and Daugirdas, 1988). *Staphylococcus epidermidis* accounts for a majority of peritonitis (Michael *et al.*, 1987).Fungal peritonitis is uncommon but is the most serious type, which carries with it a morbidity and mortality (Forwell, 1987). Be alert to infants with fungal infections elsewhere, i.e. suprapubic catheters and central lines, especially if fluid is leaking. Catheter removal is necessary with fungal infection which, for a chronic dialysis infant, is a disaster.

The nurse must observe for signs of peritonitis, which include a cloudy fluid, pyrexia, abdominal pain and irritability.

Leakage of fluid around catheter

In acute access, the catheter is best secured with gauze and adhesive tape and left untouched until removal. However, if there is a fluid leak or pyrexia the dressing should be changed and watched closely, as glucose dialysate provides a fine growth medium for bacteria. If leaking persists, the catheter is best removed and replaced in a different site and dialysis recommenced using smaller volumes.

Blocked catheter

This usually occurs because the catheter has been misplaced, there is omentum adherent, or it is blocked by fibrin. Heparin can be added to the dialysate or the line can be flushed with 10 ml of saline and heparin 1000 units. Urokinase can be placed in the catheter and left for a few hours.

A good technique is the key to successful peritoneal dialysis. All bags should be attached and the system left closed until disposal the next day. If the infant is very unstable and needs frequent prescription changes, additives should be added to one bag only to avoid breaking the system.

The effluent should be observed and sent for culture if necessary, and gloves should be worn when disposing of drainage fluid.

NUTRITION IN RENAL FAILURE

Diet in renal failure is part of the process aimed at impeding the progression to end-stage disease. In the neonatal period, dietary problems are experienced in the management of infants in acute renal failure and less so in those with chronic renal failure. Dietetic advice is imperative, as early as possible, to avoid unnecessary dialysis because of poor dietary control. If an infant sucks it is best to feed orally; if not, enteral or parenteral feeding may be started.

Guidelines to nutritional requirements in the first 6 months

Age	*Energy*	*Protein*
	Conservative management	
0–6 months	120–150 kg/day	1.8 g/kg/day
Peritoneal dialysis		
0–6 months	120–150 kg/day	2.2–3.0 g/kg/day

(Coleman and Watson, 1992)

An infant in acute renal failure will be in a hypercatabolic state and needs an increased amount of energy to meet the demands of this state. Adequate nutrition will alleviate the symptoms produced by raised plasma urea and expedite recovery (Haycock, 1991). As urea is a protein metabolite, the undesirable symptoms produced by a raised plasma urea require protein to be restricted. Infants who are on peritoneal dialysis need extra protein to compensate for the loss during dialysis. In the acute phase, expressed breast milk can be fortified by the dietitian and the infant may be put to the breast when he is polyuric and fluid restriction is no longer necessary. Mature human milk contains 0.7 mmol/100 ml of sodium and 1.5 mmol/100 ml of potassium. Maternal diet alters the composition of fatty acids in human milk but does not affect potassium or sodium, therefore in a baby who is hyperkalaemic there is no reason to alter a mother's diet (DHSS, 1988).

DRUGS IN RENAL FAILURE

Nephrogenesis is complete at 36 weeks (Fleming, Speidel and Dunn, 1986). Glomerular filtration rate in full-term infants at birth is approximately 25 ml/min/per 1.73 m^2; that of a 31-week gestational age infant is 10–20 ml/min/per 1.73 m^2, and remains low for the first 2–3 weeks of life (Chevalier, 1986). It is important to remember that renal excretion is not as efficient in the first few weeks of life, and therefore dosages of drugs must be prescribed accordingly. Blood levels may need to be checked after a first dose, particularly with aminoglycosides. The frequency of administration relates to the infant's renal function, i.e. a baby in end-stage renal failure may only need a dose of vancomycin every 48 h to maintain therapeutic levels.

PSYCHOSOCIAL ASPECTS

'But he looks so normal' is a term heard over and over again from parents with newly diagnosed infants in renal failure. The concept of renal failure does not seem tangible to parents and can sometimes take years before the symptoms make sense to the anxious eye. When there has been an antenatal diagnosis parents are anxious but ready to take information on board.

Those diagnosed postnatally are often bewildered and need information reinforced.

Babies no longer die of renal failure alone, and it is important to assure parents of the many treatments available to support an infant in renal failure. Management of these infants cannot be achieved without all members of the relevant multidisciplinary team, including social worker, psychologist, counsellor, dietitian, nurse, doctor, consultant and any person relevant to provision of this care on a unit. Regular meetings of the team increase awareness of the many parental worries and help alleviate unnecessary anxieties. Each problem experienced in the dialysis may be a separate entity for that carer, but the cumulative result is a living nightmare for the parent.

CONCLUSION

The kidneys, although encapsulated as a separate organ, have the potential to cause a host of problems. Management of renal failure is primarily supportive until the infant reaches a suitable weight for transplantation. The outcome for acute renal failure is good and, if well managed, the baby will recover fully. Chronic renal failure is progressive and, if well managed, dialysis can be delayed.

An understanding of the pathophysiology will enable the nurse to anticipate and prevent potential complications and provide good nursing care. Renal failure certainly tests the clinical acumen of any nurse, but its challenge can be met if knowledge and expertise is increased.

REFERENCES

Adelman, R.D. (1978) Neonatal hypertension. *Paediatric Clinics of North America* **25**, 99–100.

Arbus, G.S. and Farine, M. (1986) Acute renal failure, in *Clinical Paediatric Nephrology*, (ed R.J. Postlethwaite), Wright, Bristol, pp. 197–217.

Chevalier, R.L. (1986) Renal diseases in neonates, in *Clinical Paediatric Nephrology* (ed R.J. Postlethwaite), Wright, Bristol, pp. 329–50.

Clark, D.A. (1977) Times of first void and first stool in 500 newborns. *Journal of Paediatrics* **60**, 457–9.

Coleman, J.E. and Watson, A.R. (1992) Nutritional support for the child with acute renal failure. *Journal of Human Nutrition and Dietetics* **5**, 99–105.

DHSS (1988) *Report on Health and Social Subjects 32, Present Day Practice in Infant Feeding: Third Report,* HMSO, London.

Donaldson, M.D.C., Spurgeon, P., Haycock, G.B. *et al.* (1983) Peritoneal dialysis in infants. *British Medical Journal* **286**, 759–60.

Fine, R. (1986) Conservative management of children with chronic renal faiure, in *Clinical Paediatric Nephrology* (ed R.J. Postlethwaite), Wright, Bristol, pp. 217–26.

Fleming, P.J., Speidel, B.D. and Dunn, P.M. (1986) *A Neonatal Vade-Mecum,* Lloyd-Luke (Medical Books) Ltd, London.

Forwell (1987) Control Nephrology, pp. 110–113.

Goetzman-Wennberg, (1991) *Neonatal intensive care handbook.*

Gower, P.E. (1983) *Nephrology,* Grant McIntyre, London.

Halliday, H., McClure, G. and Reid, M. (1989) *Handbook of Neonatal Intensive Care,* 2nd edn, Baillière Tindall, London.

Haycock, G.B. (1991) Renal disease, in *Textbook of Paediatric Nutrition,* pp. 240–2.

Leehey, Gandhi and Dougirdas (1989) Peritonitis, in *Handbook of Dialysis.*

Lote, C.J. (1988) *Principles of Renal Physiology,* 2nd edn, Croom Helm, London.

McGraw, M.E. (1986) Large kidneys, in *Clinical Paediatric Nephrology* (ed R.J. Postlethwaite), Wright, Bristol, pp. 70–82.

Michael, Adu, Gruer and McIntyre (1987) Bacteriological spectrum of CAPD peritonitis. *Contributions to Nephrology* **57**, 41–4.

Nash, M. (1978) in *Paediatric Kidney Disease,* Vol. 1.

Tortora, G.J. and Anagnostakos, N.P. (1987) *Principles of Anatomy and Physiology,* 5th edn, Harper and Row, New York.

Watson, A.R. (1991) The management of acute renal failure. *Current Paediatrics* **1**, 103–7.

Wu and Oreopoulos (1988) Diminished peritoneal ultrafiltration and solute permeability, in *Handbook of dialysis.*

12

Neonatal infection

Ann and Daniel Dooley

The newborn baby in a special care neonatal unit is in a uniquely vulnerable situation with regard to infection. Several factors contribute to the high incidence of infection, including:

- poor immune response in preterm babies;
- artificially warm enclosed environment in incubators;
- use of invasive procedures such as ventilation, cannulation and drains.

The rates for neonatal septicaemia give an indication of the increased risk of infection, with preterm babies experiencing a 5–8 times higher incidence than term babies (Driscoll *et al.*, 1982). Some neonatal infections can be attributed to the baby already being infected at time of admission to the neonatal unit, but nursing staff must be aware that nosocomial (hospital-acquired) infection rates in neonatal units can be as high as 25% (Donowitz, 1989). Infection control measures must therefore be carefully devised and implemented to protect the neonate from further risk of infection.

The newborn baby is unable to communicate verbally the distress caused by infection, and will often lack the classic signs which would be found in more mature infants and adults. Careful monitoring, coupled with appropriate use of infection screening procedures, is vital if any infection is to be diagnosed in its early stages. An understanding of the above points will give nursing staff a greater awareness of the needs of the newborn baby and help optimize the nursing care provided.

IMMUNE RESPONSE TO INFECTION

The newborn baby's immune system will offer some degree of protection against infection by certain microorganisms, but the extent of this protection will vary greatly according to the gestational age at delivery. At term, the baby will have high levels of maternal immunoglobulin G (IgG) (the only immunoglobulin to cross the placenta), which will offer protection against the range of pathogens to which the mother has been exposed, i.e. streptococci, pneumococci and meningococci. However, in premature babies this level of maternal IgG will be reduced, making them particularly vulnerable to infection by these pathogens.

Immunoglobulin M (IgM) is the immunoglobulin class responsible for combating Gram-negative infections but, due to its large molecular size, it does not cross the placenta. Since IgM levels in premature babies are reduced, and even in term babies are only found at 20% of adult levels, this predisposes them to Gram-negative infections by organisms such as *Escherichia coli*, and this accounts for the high pathogenicity of these organisms at this stage in life.

The other major class of immunoglobulin is immunoglobulin A (IgA) which, again, does not cross the placenta but can be of great significance in the newborn baby's response to infection, because it is present in very high concentrations in colostrum and breast milk. Also present in breast milk is a protein called lactoferrin, which has a synergistic role with IgA in preventing gastroenteritis caused by pathogenic strains of *E. coli*. These enteropathogenic *E. coli* have a high metabolic requirement for iron, to allow replication and growth; however, lactoferrin has a high affinity for free iron, thereby depriving the *E. coli* of this essential metabolic component and making them susceptible to attack by IgA.

SPECIFIC RISK FACTORS FOR INFECTION

Preterm neonates born as a result of a labour complicated by prolonged rupture of membranes (PROM) are at a greater risk of infection than those born in non-PROM labours (Levine, 1991). This risk is increased twofold if the duration of PROM was more than 48 hours. Subsequent delivery by caesarean section is also a risk factor. These neonates may therefore require closer observation for any sign of early-onset infection and, according to local policy, consideration for active antimicrobial prophylaxis.

Other researchers have shown that low birth weight and prematurity are, in themselves, specific risk factors, as are abnormal vaginal presentation and antepartum fetal tachycardia (Spaans *et al.*, 1990). Following delivery, other factors associated with increased likelihood of infection have been identified, such as the presence of intravenous cannulae (Bryant, 1990; Roberts and Gollow, 1990; Hruszkewycz *et al.*, 1991) and assisted ventilation (Slagle *et al.*, 1989).

DETECTION AND DIAGNOSIS OF INFECTION

Specimen taking

Compliance with laboratory requirements when taking specimens for the detection/diagnosis of neonatal infection is an aspect of nursing care which is often overlooked. This is not generally as a result of failure to follow guidelines but, rather due to ignorance and lack of communication between laboratory and nursing staff. For example, the type of specimen container and the type of swab used will determine the acceptable delay allowed before processing the specimen in the laboratory. Examples of this are the use of sterile universal containers for urine instead of urine containers with boric acid, and the use of normal transport swabs instead of charcoal swabs when attempting to culture *Neisseria gonorrhoeae* from suspected ophthalmia neonatorum.

In general, swabs, secretions, endotracheal tube tips and intravenous line tips should arrive at the laboratory within 4 h of being taken. If this is not possible, certain specimens may be placed in a refrigerator overnight, without significant detriment to the culture results. Notable exceptions to this are specimens taken when looking for delicate organisms such as *Chlamydia trachomatis* isolation. In these cases the transport of the specimen direct to the laboratory specimen reception should be arranged and, if outside normal working hours, consideration must be given to contacting the laboratory to arrange for urgent processing or appropriate storage upon receipt.

Microbiology/virology request forms

The details provided by medical and nursing staff on microbiology/virology request forms are of great importance in determining the extent of investigations undertaken and the significance placed on any findings. Date of onset of symptoms, duration of illness, other predisposing medical conditions, all recent and current antimicrobial therapy, and a full description of specimen site and patient's details will all influence the final laboratory report and should therefore be included wherever possible.

The Gram stain

The Gram stain is a laboratory technique which allows visualization of certain microorganisms and human cells. When performed directly in specimens, this stain can give an indication of the cellular response to infection (i.e. presence of leucocytes) as well as the type of bacteria/fungi present. The Gram stain also has a use in the preliminary identification of bacteria according to their Gram reaction. Examples of Gram stain reactions for commonly encountered pathogens are given in Table 12.1 (these are also included under the sections dealing with the specific pathogen). The morphology of bacteria is also included in a Gram stain result to aid any presumptive diagnosis of infection.

Table 12.1 Gram stain reaction and bacterial morphology of certain bacterial pathogens encountered in neonatal infections

Gram reaction and morphology	*Common neonatal pathogens*
Gram-positive cocci	*Staphylococcus aureus* β-haemolytic streptococci
Gram-positive bacilli	*Listeria monocytogenes* *Clostridium* species
Gram-negative bacilli	*Escherichia coli* *Pseudomonas aeruginosa*
Gram-negative cocci	*Neisseria gonorrhoeae*
Gram-negative coccobacilli	*Haemophilus influenzae*

Non-microbiological tests

As well as the bacterial and virology specimens that will be taken when infection is suspected, other tests will be carried out to aid the diagnosis. These may include:

- haematology requests, such as full blood counts;
- chemical analysis, such as blood gases and electrolyte levels;
- radiography if respiratory or necrotizing enterocolitis is suspected.

BACTERIAL AND FUNGAL INFECTION

β-haemolytic streptococci (BHS)

β-haemolytic streptococci are a group of Gram-positive cocci which produce a wide range of toxic factors responsible for the pathogenicity. These include haemolysins, which can be tested for in the laboratory, and are responsible for their name. BHS are grouped serologically (Lancefield groups) with groups A, B, C, D and G being of most significance in neonatal infection.

Group B streptococci are at present the major cause of neonatal meningitis (Fleigner and Garland, 1990). The infection is usually perinatally acquired following prolonged rupture of membranes or during traumatic delivery. Following perinatal exposure, group B streptococci are often isolated from eye, ear and gastric aspirate cultures, hence the value of full infection screens in babies following a long labour or trauma birth.

Group A streptococci are the classic pyogenic streptococci responsible for scarlet fever, glomerular nephritis and wound infections. They are often responsible, along with groups C and G streptococci for infected umbilical stumps, as well as eye, ear and respiratory infections.

Group D streptococci (Faecal Streptococci/*Enterococcus faecalis*), are less pathogenic members of this group but are occasionally found in urinary tract infections and septicaemia.

Coliform bacilli

The coliform bacilli are a group of Gram-negative bacilli commonly associated with a faecal/intestinal origin but also found in the general environment. Included in this group is *Escherichia coli*. Colonization of the intestinal tract occurs in the first week of life and superficial skin contamination soon thereafter. Unlike healthy babies, newborns, hospitalized in neonatal units, are initially colonized with Gram-negative bacterial flora found in the neonatal unit, and not from bacteria acquired from the mother perinatally. This may have serious consequences if the unit contains endemic strains of virulent or multiple drug-resistant coliforms, since these newly colonized babies represent a reservoir for continued infection within the neonatal unit. Examples of this effect have been documented with particular strains of *Serratia marcescens* causing infection over a long period of time (Wake, Lees and Cull, 1986).

Coliform bacilli do not produce the wide range of toxins found in other pathogens, and therefore physical damage to infected areas are less severe. However, prompt treatment of any infected site is essential to reduce the risk of infection spreading, since coliform bacilli are a major cause of neonatal meningitis and septicaemia.

Candida albicans (Thrush)

Candida albicans is a commensal of the vaginal tract found in low numbers in 10–30% of healthy women. During vaginal delivery the baby is exposed to this opportunistic pathogen and may be at risk from infection. The main sites of candidal infection are the mouth and groin. In the case of oral candidiasis, the mucous membranes develop white spots or a coating which resists gentle scraping. The condition responds rapidly to regular mouth care with nystatin drops. Candidiasis of moist skin folds, particularly the groin region, is recognizable by the characteristic reddening of the affected area, often with satellite lesions occurring in close proximity. In cases of candidiasis affecting the groin region, there is a risk of subsequent urinary tract infection, therefore if there is any suspicion of this a specimen of urine should be submitted for culture, specifically requesting Candida culture.

Listeria monocytogenes

Listeria monocytogenes is a Gram-positive bacillus responsible for meningitis and septicaemia in immunocompromised individuals, pregnant women and newborn babies. The main source of maternal infection is the consumption of contaminated foods, although dietary advice, which is now widely available, appears to be reducing the incidence of adult infections. Maternal infection results in abortion in 90% of cases, whereas an infection at the time of delivery places the baby at high risk of developing neonatal meningitis.

Neisseria gonorrhoeae

Neisseria gonorrhoeae (Gonococcus) is a Gram-negative diplococcus responsible for the sexually transmitted disease gonorrhoea. Its main significance in neonates is as the cause of the purulent neonatal conjunctivitis (ophthalmia neonatorum) although disseminated infection involving sites such as the vagina and rectum can occur if the maternal infection is acute at the time of delivery. Ophthalmia neonatorum usually presents following undiagnosed gonococcal infection in the mother, resulting in perinatal infection during vaginal delivery, with the characteristic purulent conjunctivitis appearing within 48 h of birth. In cases of purulent conjunctivitis, treatment must be started immediately following the taking of swabs for culture, and not delayed until the results are available. Any swabs taken for suspected ophthalmia neonatorum must be taken to the microbiology laboratory without delay if *Neisseria gonorrhoeae* is to be cultured successfully, since these bacteria are very fragile and die off quickly in transport swabs.

Haemophilus influenzae

Haemophilus influenzae is a Gram-negative coccobacillus which is predominantly a pathogen of the respiratory tract, eyes and ears in neonates. Contrary to common misconception, *Haemophilus influenzae* is not responsible for influenza ('flu'), which is caused by the influenza viruses. In neonates, *Haemophilus influenzae* is a rare cause of meningitis and septicaemia but it should be noted that this organism becomes of increasing importance in older infants and children, being one of the major causes of paediatric meningitis.

Myobacterium tuberculosis

Myobacterium tuberculosis is a bacterium which does not respond to the Gram stain reaction and therefore requires specialized stains for its identification. The most common stain is the Zeihl–Nielsen stain (ZN stain) which involves treatment with acid and alcohol, giving rise to the terminology acid alcohol-fast bacilli (AFB or AAFB). In recent years the incidence of neonatal tuberculosis infection in Europe has been very low. However, due to a combination of factors, including the emergence of drug-resistant strains and increased infection on AIDS patients, the overall incidence of tuberculosis is increasing worldwide, with an accompanying increase in the risk of neonatal tuberculosis as a result. Intrauterine tuberculosis is rare and inevitably results in abortion or stillbirth, with perinatal infection from the mother being the main source of infection. If neonatal infection is suspected, as well as investigating the infant, examination of the mother for tuberculosis must be made, since the demonstration of tubercle bacilli in infected neonates is unreliable. Treatment consisting of long-term multiple antibiotic therapy is started in the absence of proven neonatal tuberculosis, due to the devastating consequences of this disease.

Infected infants and mothers should be nursed in isolation if 'open' tuberculosis is diagnosed. Staff should be screened for tuberculosis when starting work, because of the high infectivity of the disease in neonates and because, in its early stages, tuberculosis may be asymptomatic yet infectious.

Pseudomonas aeruginosa

Pseudomonas aeruginosa is a Gram-negative bacillus. Its main pathogenesis in neonates is in conjunctivitis, skin infections and complications as a result of heavy colonization of endotracheal tubes. The latter occurs due to the very favourable conditions for the growth of *Ps. aeruginosa* in the warm humidified environment, and results in greatly increased secretions in heavily colonized infants.

One characteristic of *Ps. aeruginosa* is the production of green pigments which, when visible in infected secretions and discharge and accompanied by the typical rancid smell of pseudomonal infection, may assist diagnosis before laboratory reports are available.

Staphylococcus aureus

Staphylococcus aureus is a Gram-positive coccus, responsible for a wide range of infections in neonates. Since the organism is ubiquitously distributed in the hospital environment, colonization of the infant's nose and skin occurs within 5 days in up to 90% of cases. The commonest manifestations of staphylococcal infection are conjunctivitis, omphalitis and skin infections, although abscesses, septicaemia, osteomyelitis and respiratory tract infections also occur. Infections usually respond to flucloxacillin, although certain strains of methicillin-resistant *Staphylococcus aureus* (MRSA) are not responsive and must be treated alternatively.

Other species of staphylococci, such as *Staphylococcus epidermidis* (also called *Staphylococcus albus* and coagulase-negative *Staphylococcus* also cause infections in neonates, usually bacteraemia. A high risk factor in this case is the presence of central lines and umbilical catheters, which tend to be colonized from the skin, thereby giving rise to infection.

Syphilis

Syphilis is caused by the spirochaete *Treponema pallidum*. Congenital syphilis has been largely eradicated in developed countries due to antenatal screening programmes. Non-attendance for full antenatal care, primary infection late in the third trimester and failure of treatment in diagnosed cases currently account for approximately 5–10 cases annually in the UK. Intrauterine infection results in very poor prognosis, with intrauterine growth retardation, hydrops fetalis and preterm labour common, if abortion does not occur. Approximately 60% of cases of congenital syphilis have no clinical symptoms apparent at birth, but go on to develop long-term sequelae of ocular and aural impairment, bone lesions and neurological involvement. Of the clinically symptomatic infants, the main feature is a macropapular rash, particularly on the back, thighs, palms and soles. Treatment of congenital syphilis is by penicillin, with long-term serological and developmental follow-up.

Chlamydia trachomatis

Chlamydia trachomatis is taxonomically linked to bacteria but the diagnosis is made by virological laboratory techniques, because of its failure to grow outside human cells. In neonates the main clinical manifestations of infection with *Chlamydia trachomatis* are conjunctivitis and pneumonia. The increase of sexually transmitted infection in adults during the last decade, with over 1600 reported cases in women in 1989, is making this organism a pathogen of increasing importance in neonates, with perinatal infection occurring in around 60–70% of cases of maternal infection. Treatment is by erythromycin, either orally or intravenously, since topical treatment of chlamydial conjunctivitis will not prevent any subsequent chlamydial pneumonia.

SITES OF INFECTION

Conjunctivitis

The most common causes of neonatal conjunctivitis are staphylococci and Gram-negative organisms such as *E. coli* and *Ps. aeruginosa*. These generally present as non-purulent conjunctivitis with inflammation of the conjunctiva and eyelids. In more severe cases of purulent conjunctivitis, infection with *Neisseria gonorrhoeae* must be considered and aggressive antimicrobial treatment commenced immediately (following the taking of a swab for microbiological confirmation). Another cause of purulent conjunctivitis is perinatal infection with *Chlamydia trachomatis*, so chlamydial cultures should be taken to exclude this.

Meningitis

Neonatal meningitis is one of the most serious bacterial infections encountered in the newborn. Mortality is high, even with early antibiotic treatment, and long-term sequelae are common in survivors (Wald *et al.*, 1986). The classic symptom of headache, neck stiffness and photophobia cannot be communicated by the infant to his carers, and irritability and poor feeding are often the only visible signs of meningitis. The main causes of neonatal meningitis are Group B streptococci and coliforms, although other organisms are occasionally implicated.

In suspected neonatal meningitis a full infection screen should be performed, including lumbar puncture. The cerebrospinal fluid of a neonate differs in two respects from that of an adult: it contains a higher number of white blood cells (mainly polymorphs) and has a higher protein content. Since both these factors play a role in the diagnosis of meningitis, these differences make the preliminary laboratory results less useful than in adults, due to the overlap with normal ranges found in children and adults. Conclusive evidence of bacterial infection will only be available after 18–24 h, when cultures have grown, since Gram staining of the CSF will not always show bacteria, if present in low numbers. Progressively more sensitive tests to confirm the presence of pathogens in CSF are being developed, such as latex agglutination tests. These are enabling earlier presumptive diagnosis of the causative agents of meningitis to be made, although antibiotic sensitivities must still wait for culture results to be available.

Umbilical stump infection (omphalitis)

The umbilical stump is colonized by bacteria at birth and, although the bacterial load may be reduced by cleansing and topical administration of antiseptics, it is still a site which is prone to infection. The administration of antiseptics has also been shown to delay the drying and separation of the cord and, since all bacteria cannot be eradicated from the stump site, this may increase the duration of vulnerability to umbilical stump infection. It is normal to find some redness at the edge of the skin as the cord separates, but any greater sign of infection, such as discharge of pus, requires attention. The main causes of infection are *Staphylococcus aureus*, coliform bacilli and β-haemolytic streptococci. As well as damage to the umbilical site there is further risk of systemic spread of infection, so this condition should always be given close attention.

The use of umbilical arterial catheters has been documented to correspond to an increased risk of systemic infection in preterm neonates, therefore when these are in place scrupulous attention to cord care must be given.

Gastrointestinal infections

Gastroenteritis is now a relatively uncommon occurrence in neonatal units in the developed world. The main infectious causes are of viral aetiology, since improved infection control measures and general hygiene have reduced the chance for spread of bacterial gastroenteritis. Occasional outbreaks due to bacterial pathogens do still occur, with enteropathogenic *E. coli* and *Salmonella* sp. being implicated. In all cases of gastroenteritis isolation of the infected baby is required, with careful assessment of fluid balance to prevent dehydration and electrolyte imbalance. Oral rehydration therapy is of limited efficacy in neonates, so intravenous fluids may be required.

Necrotizing enterocolitis (NEC) is a condition of uncertain aetiology with many predisposing factors, such as congenital heart defects, exchange transfusions and early enteral feeding. The current explanation for its cause is that, rather than being a primary infection caused by specific pathogens, the initial event leading to NEC is an episode of intestinal ischaemia (Gall, 1986). This then allows invasion of the intestinal mucosa with normal gas-producing bowel flora such as *E. coli* and *Clostridium* sp. giving rise to the formation of the characteristic gas pockets.

Urinary tract infections

Urinary tract infections (UTI) occur in neonates either as a result of ascending infection or as a secondary infection during bacteraemia. In cases of repeated infection, there is a strong correlation with obstructive abnormalities of the urinary tract, and therefore subsequent follow-up may be required to exclude this. The overall incidence of neonatal UTI ranges from 0.1% to 1% of all babies, with males experiencing between three and eight times the infection rate found in females (Ginsburg and McCracken, 1982). In preterm babies under 2500 g birth weight, UTI rates of 3–10% have been reported (Klein, 1990).

The diagnosis of neonatal UTI is made difficult due to problems associated with obtaining clean-catch urine specimens for analysis. Both bag urine specimens and free-flowing specimens can be suitable but are prone to contamination. If these produce inconclusive results then suprapubic aspiration may be performed. Also of importance is the type of specimen container used, since often only very small volumes of urine can be collected. The standard urine specimen containers will contain boric acid powder, which acts as a preservative and prevents subsequent multiplication of bacteria during transit to the laboratory, and this allows accurate estimations to be made of the bacterial number at the time of sampling. However, if the urine specimen container cannot be filled to the recommended level, the concentration of boric acid can reach bactericidal levels, resulting in a decrease in bacterial count. This can be overcome by using sterile universal containers, the specimen must then be transported to the laboratory without delay to prevent any bacteria multiplying and giving inaccurate culture results.

NON-BACTERIAL INFECTIONS

Toxoplasma gondii

Toxoplasma gondii is a protozoan parasite whose natural host is members of the cat family, with the domestic cat being the primary host in Europe. Human infection is as a result of either direct contact with cat faeces or indirect contact with contaminated foods. This may be by ingestion of unwashed vegetables contaminated with infective sporocysts, or by ingestion of undercooked meat from secondary hosts who have been infected and developed infective tissue cysts. Severe infection occurs in 10–20% of infected neonates, with clinical features of hydrocephalus, retinochoroiditis, cerebral calcification, hepatitis, pneumonia, myocarditis and myositis. Antimicrobial therapy is available for confirmed cases of congenital toxoplasmosis and consists of a combination of antiparasitic drugs, normally taken for a duration of 12 months.

Rubella

Congenital rubella infection is a rare occurrence in the UK, with only approximately 20 cases being reported annually; however, public awareness is very high due to vaccination programmes which have been in place since 1970. The most well known clinical manifestations of congenital rubella infection are cataracts and heart defects. Other common manifestations are bone lesions, cryptorchidism, diabetes mellitus, hepatomegaly, splenomegaly, meningoencephalitis, microcephaly, patent ductus arteriosus, pulmonary stenosis and retinopathy.

As well as the actual nursing care delivered to the infected neonate, attention must be given to the fact that these neonates are highly infective and excrete large amounts of the rubella virus. Studies have shown that by 3 months approximately 60% are still active excreters, but by 1 year continued excretion is very rare. Therefore the infected neonate should be isolated and cared for only by staff who are known to have antibodies to rubella. Since occasional cases of reinfection have been documented, it is advisable to exclude any members of staff who may be pregnant, even if antibodies to rubella have previously been detected. Advice should also be given to the mother not to expose the baby to women who may be pregnant, following discharge from hospital, until the risk of excretion has diminished.

Herpes simplex virus (HSV)

Two types of HSV are major pathogens to man: HSV-1, which causes cold sores, generally around the mouth and nose, and HSV-2, which is the major cause of genital herpes (although cross-infection may occur with both HSV-1 and HSV-2). In adults, infection with both HSV-1 and HSV-2 occurs first as a primary infection, following which the lesion heals and the virus remains latent in the cells of the central nervous system. The latent virus may then be reactivated to produce lesions at the site of original infection. In contrast to the other infections covered in the TORCH syndrome (toxoplasma, rubella, cytomegalovirus and herpes simplex virus), HSV only rarely causes intrauterine infection. Infection normally occurs during delivery, since active maternal genital herpes results in the shedding of virus by the mucous membranes of the cervix and vagina.

Perinatally acquired HSV infection presents in three forms: localized mucocutaneous infection (20%); localized neurological infection (30%); and disseminated infection (50%). When only the mucous membranes are involved the lesions will appear in 9–11 days and there is only a small chance of long-term sequelae. The more serious neurological infections present later, at 15–17 days, and result in mortality in 20% of untreated cases, with 60% of survivors suffering long-term sequelae. In cases of disseminated HSV infection, the clinical manifestations appear in 9–11 days and include brain, liver and skin involvement, with 80% mortality in untreated cases. With appropriate antiviral treatment (acyclovir for at least 10 days), this mortality is reduced to 20%, with 50% of survivors suffering long-term sequelae.

Neonates with HSV infection should be isolated to prevent the spread of infection until antiviral treatment is complete. Since HSV-1 infection in adults is very common and transmission, under non-mucosal contact situations, rare, staff with cold sores need not be excluded from work as long as standard infection control procedures are practised.

Cytomegalovirus (CMV)

CMV is the most common cause of congenital infection, resulting in approximately 120–180 symptomatic cases annually in England and Wales. CMV is one of the herpes viruses and therefore the neonatal congenital infection can be as a result either of primary maternal infection during pregnancy or reactivation of latent infection occurring during pregnancy. Almost all of these neonates who exhibit symptoms at birth will suffer long-term sequelae. The clinical manifestations of congenital CMV infection include hepatomegaly, splenomegaly, cerebral calcification, microcephaly, prolonged jaundice, petechiae, thrombocytopenia and pneumonitis. In addition to these symptomatic neonates, an equal or slightly greater number who are infected yet asymptomatic at birth can be expected to develop long-term sequelae later in life, of which the main symptom is deafness.

Perinatal infection also occurs at the time of delivery, if active maternal infection is present. In neonates who are not infected at birth, studies have shown that breastfeeding and close contact with their seropositive mothers is a major source of infection in early life. Neonates with CMV infection excrete large amounts of virus and are potentially infective to health care staff. However, standard infection control procedures have been shown to be effective in preventing transmission to staff and other babies, so isolation is not required.

Respiratory syncytial virus (RSV)

RSV infection in neonates is one of the few exclusively nosocomial viral infections in neonates. There have been no proven cases of intrauterine infection, as transmission occurs either from aerosol inhalation or contact with infected material in the neonatal unit, or by contact with infected visitors or members of staff, who are often asymptomatic. Infants with suspected or proven RSV infection should be nursed in isolation, and any members of staff or visitors with signs of infection (in adults, often only a mild cold) be excluded from the unit.

In mild infections, the main symptoms are rhinorrhoea and coughing, but in severe infection bronchiolitis is seen. Neonates with predisposing factors such as congenital heart defects and bronchopulmonary dysplasia are more prone to develop these severe infections. Another consequence of RSV infection is viral otitis media, which presents in up to 20% of cases.

Human immunodeficiency virus (HIV)

Congenital infection with HIV can occur as a result of intrauterine, perinatal or neonatal infection through breastfeeding. Of these possible modes of infection only the first will normally be apparent to staff in neonatal units, because of the dysmorphic features which may be found in infants infected early in pregnancy. Most clinical manifestations of congenital HIV infection only become apparent at around 6 months of age, and therefore neonatal unit staff will not come into frequent contact with them, since most babies will probably have been discharged by this time. If extended treatment in the neonatal unit is required, then staff must be aware of the increased susceptibility to infection of these babies and provide care accordingly. Immunization against common childhood infections has been shown to be beneficial and should be encouraged. As in the case of hepatitis B infection risk, all specimens sent for pathology examination should indicate the high-risk status of the specimen.

Hepatitis B virus (HBV)

Congenital HBV infection is predominantly perinatal, since intrauterine infection accounts for less than 5% of cases. The main clinical significances of congenital HBV infection are the long-term sequelae of cirrhosis and hepatocellular carcinoma, with acute neonatal hepatitis occurring very rarely. The risk of neonatal transmission is related to the time of maternal infection, as well as the serological markers present at the time of delivery, with infection in the third trimester and presence of HBsAG giving the highest correlation with neonatal infection. Most neonates who are congenitally infected will develop HBsAG antibodies at around 2–3 months of age, and will progress to the chronic carrier state.

In an attempt to prevent perinatal infection from HBV-positive mothers, active immunization with HBV vaccine will be given, as will passive immunization with anti-HBV immunoglobulin, according to the infectivity of the mother at delivery. Studies have shown that breastfeeding does not increase the risk of neonatal transmission in HBsAG-positive mothers and should not, therefore, be discouraged.

Measures to reduce the risk of infection to health care staff must be implemented where neonates are born to HBV-infected mothers; these will depend on local infection control policy and also on the serological status of the mother. To reduce the risk to pathology staff dealing with specimens from these babies, the risk of HBV infection should always be marked clearly on any request forms.

CONCLUSION

The diagnosis, treatment and care of neonates with infection is a complex subject which has been given an overview here, which should not be considered exhaustive. In cases of infection caused by pathogens which are not detailed here, and where further knowledge is desired, the titles recommended in the Bibliography provide information in greater depth. Drawing on these resources will allow nursing staff to deliver care in a more informed way not only to the neonate but also to the family, who will need reassurance if their baby is ill due to infection.

REFERENCES

Bryant, B.G. (1990) Drug, fluid and blood products administered through the umbilical artery catheter: complication experiences from one NICU. *Neonatal Network* **9**(1), 43–6.

Donowitz, I.G. (1989) Nosocomial infection in neonatal intensive care units. *American Journal of Infection Control* **17**(5), 250–7.

Driscoll, J.M., Driscoll, Y.T., Stier, M.E. *et al*. (1982) Mortality and morbidity in infants less than 1000 grams birthweight. *Pediatrics* **69**, 21–6.

Fliegner, J.R. and Garland, S.M. (1990) Perinatal mortality in Victoria, Australia: role of group B streptococcus. *American Journal of Obstetrics and Gynaecology* **163**(1), 1609–11.

Gall, L.S. (1986) The role of intestinal flora in gas formation. *Annals of the New York Academy of Sciences* **150**, 27–30.

Ginsburg, C.M. and McCracken, G.H. (1982) Urinary tract infection in young infants. *Pediatrics* **69**, 409–12.

Hruszkewycz, V., Holtrop, P.C., Batton, D.G. *et al*. (1991) Complications associated with central venous catheters inserted in critically ill neonates. *Infection Control and Hospital Infection* **12**(9), 544–8.

Klein, J.O. (1990) Bacterial infections of the urinary tact, in *Infectious Diseases of the Fetus and Newborn Infant*, 3rd edn, (eds J.S. Remmington and J.O. Klein), W.B. Saunders, Philadelphia, pp. 690–9.

Levine, C.D. (1991) Premature rupture of membranes and sepsis in preterm neonates *Nursing Research* **40**(1), 36–41.

Roberts, J.P. and Gollow, I.J. (1990) Central venous catheters in surgical neonates. *Journal of Paediatric Surgery* **25**(6), 632–4.

Slagle, T.A., Bifano, E.M., Wolf, J.W. and Gross, S.J. (1989) Routine endotracheal cultures for the prediction of neonatal sepsis in ventilated babies. *Archives of Disease in Childhood* **64**(1), 34–8.

Spaans, W.A., Knox, A.J., Koya, H.B. and Mantell, C.D. (1990) Risk factors for neonatal infection. *Australian and New Zealand Journal of Obstetrics and Gynaecology* **30**(4), 327–30.

Wake, C., Lees, H. and Cull, A.B. (1986) The emergence of *Serratia marcescens* as a pathogen in a newborn unit. *Australian Paediatric Journal* **22**(4), 323–6.

Wald, E.R., Bergman, I., Taylor, H.G. *et al*. (1986) Long term outcome of group B streptococcal meningitis. *Pediatrics* 77(2), 217–21.

FURTHER READING

Greenough, A., Oxborne, J. and Sutherland, S. (eds) (1991) *Congenital,Perinatal and Neonatal Infections,* Churchill Livingstone, Edinburgh.

Isaacs, D. and Moxon, E.R. (1991) *Neonatal Infections,* Butterworth Heinemann, Oxford.

13

Nursing care of a baby with jaundice

Doreen Crawford

Jaundice can be described as a yellow discoloration of the skin and mucous membranes. Biochemically, jaundice is a state of hyperbilirubinaemia in excess of 25 μmol/l and is not usually evident until levels of 85–100 μmol/l are reached. Experienced neonatal nurses and midwives notice most cases of jaundice, although subjective measurement can be influenced by green or yellow clothing or the nursery decoration, as well as poor lighting. Jaundice affects 80% of the premature and as many as 50% of term infants. It is a symptom not a disorder, and there are many possible causes.

PHYSIOLOGY OF THE BILIRUBIN METABOLISM

Bilirubin is the catabolized product of haem, the red protein of the erythrocyte, and is processed in the liver and spleen and in tissue macrophages as a result of microsomal activity. For further details of the degradation of haem refer to Rodgers and Stevenson (1990). In newborn infants the circulating level of bilirubin is increased owing to the shorter lifespan of fetal erythrocytes, the greater proportion of red cells to body weight and the immaturity of the liver.

Bilirubin is conjugated in the liver by converting insoluble unconjugated bilirubin to water-soluble bilirubin. Each molecule of unconjugated bilirubin is conjugated with two molecules of glucuronic acid and is then catalysed by the enzyme glucuronyl transferase. Conjugated bilirubin is excreted into the bile and then into the duodenum and small intestine. In older children the process ends here, with the conjugated bilirubin further reduced to stercobilinogen by bacteria in the bowel. However, in the newborn infant a second pathway exists due to the 'sterile' uncolonized bowel and the slow clearance of bowel contents because of poor peristalsis. Conjugated bilirubin is hydrolysed by glucuronidase back to unconjugated bilirubin, which is reabsorbed and transferred via the enterohepatic circulation for further hepatic metabolism.

The fetal liver is a fairly inactive organ as the maternal liver processes the bilirubin from spent erythrocytes. If haemolysis is excessive, the cord and the amniotic fluid may be stained yellow by the excess pigment. Haemopoiesis may fail to keep pace with the demand for erythrocytes and secondary anaemia can result.

Neonatal jaundice is important because of the risk of kernicterus, which occurs when bilirubin crosses the blood–brain barrier (Bratlid, 1990). The term comes from the discovery that the brains of dead and severely jaundiced infants were yellow (Schmorl, 1903). Although very rare, kernicterus is fatal in 75% of cases. Infants who do survive suffer fits, mental retardation and postural and behavioural disability (Swanwick, 1989).

Hyperbilirubinaemia has been incriminated in hearing impairment (Vohr *et al.*, 1989). There is no exact level at which unconjugated bilirubin will become pathological as this varies with the maturity, weight and health of the infant. Large, term infants can tolerate greater levels than small, sick, premature infants (Newman and Maizels, 1990).

With so many possible causes of jaundice the infant could be subjected to a battery of unnecessary investigations. A fortunate aid to diagnosis is the time and pattern in which the jaundice appears (Table 13.1).

Table 13.1 Jaundice 'timetable'

Early jaundice	Jaundice apparent at birth or appearing within 24 hours. This requires urgent investigation
Prolonged jaundice	Jaundice which appears by days 2–3 of life but fails to clear after 10 days
Recurring jaundice	Jaundice which has cleared returning
Profound jaundice or jaundice with a greenish tinge should always be investigated immediately regardless of time of onset	

INVESTIGATIONS

The investigations performed will reflect the manner in which the jaundice occurred and the severity of the condition: the rarer the cause the more profound the investigation.

Bilirubin measurement

Bilirubin measurement is the first and the most obvious investigation. Non-invasive transcutaneous bilirubinometry methods exist (Schumacher, 1990) which are very useful but cannot replace serum estimation. Most neonatal units have a bilirubinometer to measure bilirubin from the serum of a centrifuged sample of blood. More sophisticated tests which split the levels of conjugated and unconjugated bilirubin require laboratory testing. If phototherapy is in progress at the time of blood harvest, the light should be temporarily switched off.

Coombs test

This detects the presence of antibodies coating the erythrocytes, by using a reagent which causes the cells to agglutinate, resulting in a positive test.

Full infection screen

A full infection screen will vary from unit to unit and may include a chest x-ray, blood samples for TORCH (toxoplasmosis, others (e.g. syphilis), rubella, cytomegalovirus, hepatitis) culture, lumbar puncture, urine for culture, gastric aspiration and endotracheal aspiration, and suspicious-looking sites would be swabbed.

Blood and urine tests

- The ethnic group and the family history will indicate whether blood tests for specific investigation of sickle-cell disease or G-6PD are appropriate. Other tests are:
- blood and urine for specific investigation of metabolic disorders e.g. galactosaemia;

- urine for conjugated bilirubin;
- infant's blood group;
- mother's blood group;
- haemoglobin, blood film and reticulocytes.

Other tests

- Thyroid function tests
- Liver function tests
- Liver ultrasound
- Cholangiogram
- Liver biopsy
- Exploratory laparotomy

TREATMENT FOR JAUNDICE

Treatment to reduce unconjugated bilirubin levels will be either phototherapy or exchange transfusion. The method used will depend on the actual level of bilirubin and how rapidly this level of bilirubin rose, as well as the clinical condition and the weight of the infant. Exchange transfusion gives rapid results, whereas phototherapy takes longer.

Pharmacological methods of reducing bilirubin levels are possible (Valaes *et al.*, 1990) as many chemicals bind to bilirubin. Phenobarbital has been therapeutically used but is not popular. A breakthrough may come with the clinical success of haem oxygenase inhibition.

Phototherapy

Phototherapy, initially used in the late 1950s (Cremer *et al.*, 1958), is the first-line method of management. The equipment consists of a number of fluorescent light tubes which emit light in the blue-green band of the visible spectrum (420–470 nm) (Ennever, 1990). Phototherapy works by converting unconjugated bilirubin by photodegration to a biliverdin-like pigment, which is water-soluble and harmless. Phototherapy is never given for raised conjugated bilirubin levels as it results in bronze infant syndrome, owing to the different photodegration products produced. There are a few complications, which are discussed below; however, it is non-invasive and is very effective, usually within a couple of days.

Potential risk of eye damage

Radiation from this light band has been shown to cause retinal damage in animal models, and consequently infants having this therapy must have eye protection with a tinted screen or eye shields, but exposed infants are extremely mobile and can wriggle out from under a tinted screen. If eye shields are used then the eyes should be checked for corneal abrasion. This sort of damage is rare but should be avoided.

Potential risk of hypo/hyperthermia

Light at this wavelength does not emit much heat and the exposed infant can get cold. Incubators should be set in the correct thermoneutral range and the individual's temperature monitored constantly, as some need more help to maintain their temperature than others.

Potential risk of dehydration

Phototherapy may decrease the bowel transit time and result in diarrhoea, probably as a result of bowel wall irritation caused by the presence of photoisomers of bilirubin. Jaundiced infants are commonly drowsy and may not wake for feeds. Some units recommend a 25% increase in fluids.

Potential risk of skin irritation and damage

Deposits of bile salts in the skin can cause irritation and itching: strong term infants can scratch and traumatize themselves. Redness and inflammation can occur from a photosensitive reaction resulting in the release of histamine from mast cells. This condition is exacerbated if lotions are used or if the nappy area is not thoroughly cleansed of urine and excreta prior to commencing therapy. Skin care using warm water should be performed 4–6 hourly, to maintain skin integrity.

Information for parents

The greatest disadvantage of phototherapy is the impact that the treatment can have on the parents. New mothers, especially at about the 3rd day, are in a vulnerable position; having a very jaundiced infant means extra blood tests, which may result in a distressed infant and increased maternal anxiety. With today's flexibility in care the baby need not be admitted to the neonatal unit solely for phototherapy: he can be managed adequately on the postnatal ward, where the mother can remain the primary caregiver and have continuous contact with him. A detailed explanation given to both parents and perhaps backed up with a written supplement, can reduce anxiety.

Exchange transfusion

Exchange transfusion, first used in 1951, is the second line of management and is not undertaken lightly as it has several potentially hazardous complications. This is commonly used in conjunction with phototherapy. It is effective in that it not only removes excess bilirubin but also, in the case of rhesus disease, removes antibodies and corrects anaemia. The amount of blood to be exchanged will depend on the infant's condition, but commonly about 90–95% of blood volume is replaced.

Transfusion can be performed by continous removal of the infant's blood from the umbilical vein, balanced by continuous transfusion of donor blood into another limb. This has the advantage of ensuring that there is no serial fluctuation in the circulating volume. Flow rates can be difficult to manage, and if catheter complications in one line occur the procedure should stop immediately so as not to lose track of the fluid balance.

An alternative is serial withdrawal and replacement of aliquots of 5, 10, 20 ml of blood, preferably using the umbilical vein. The volume removed and replaced with each cycle depends on the condition, weight and tolerance of the infant. It is very time-consuming as it is performed slowly. It is often difficult to maintain concentration during such a repetitious procedure, so various types of chart have been designed to ensure the correctness of the fluid balance.

Both methods are equally efficient and both have the potential for serious haemodynamic, metabolic and mechanical complications. Whenever the umbilical vein is used, the position of the cannula is always checked by X-ray.

Haemodynamic alterations

The infant's vital signs should be continuously monitored to detect changes from the baseline or progressive subtle alterations. Too-rapid removal or replacement of blood can result in disastrous haemodynamic complications. All emergency equipment and drugs should be checked and available.

Metabolic alterations of exchange transfusion

In the past walking donors were used but, owing to the difficulties involved in screening these donors, fresh banked blood is now used. Hyperkalaemia and arrhythmia can occur in infants who have received blood more than 2 days old. The way blood is stored means that the citrate present in banked blood to prevent it clotting can cause hypocalcaemia in small infants who have had comprehensive exchanges. Frequent blood gas, glucose and electrolyte levels should be taken to ensure tight control of the metabolic status.

Mechanical complications of exchange transfusion

As with any invasive procedure there is a risk of introducing infection, so an exchange transfusion should be performed under aseptic conditions. Close observation of the lines going to the infant should be made to prevent air emboli.

Other medical complications

Thrombosis of the aorta and of the portal vein has been reported and exchange transfusion, via the umbilical vein, has been incriminated in necrotizing enterocolitis.

Risk of hypothermia

An infant undergoing exchange transfusion needs continuous monitoring of his temperature. If the incubator doors are likely to be open for a long period, he is best nursed under a radiant heat source. This ensures maximum visibility and optimal control of his temperature. If unstable and already in an incubator, the desirability of a radiant warmer needs to be balanced with the undesirable effect of extra handling. A heat shield (which restricts access) or bubble wrap (which restricts visibility) may need to be considered.

Infusion of cold blood would result in chilling, so blood should be given through a specialized blood warmer; blood should never be left out to warm up.

CAUSES OF JAUNDICE

Table 13.2 lists the categories into which the causes of jaundice in the neonatal period can fit.

Table 13.2 Categories into which the causes of jaundice in the neonatal period can fit

Haemolytic jaundice	Occurs when excess haemolysis of red cells results in a level of bilirubin which overloads clearance mechanisms
Hepatocellular jaundice	Occurs when the infant's liver cells are unable to fulfil the normal functions
Obstructive jaundice	Occurs when the biliary tree is blocked and drainage of bilirubin cannot occur

Causes of jaundice at birth or occurring within 24 h

Haemolytic causes of jaundice often appear in the first 24 h of life, and always need investigating. These include:

- rhesus haemolytic disease;
- ABO incompatibility;
- congenital infection;
- severe overwhelming acquired infection;
- abnormality in shape or composition of the red cell, such as hereditary spherocytosis, α-thalassaemia, G-6PD and sickle-cell anaemia.

Erythroblastosis fetalis

This is a severe antibody-mediated haemolytic destruction of erythrocytes resulting in profound anaemia, causing cardiac failure and generalized oedema. It occurs when the mother has been sensitised to an antigen present on the fetus's erythrocyte and subsequently produces antibodies to this antigen. A Rh – mother carrying an Rh + infant is the most common case, but other antibodies can be involved. This sensitivity can result from the birth of a previous infant, a spontaneous miscarriage, termination of pregnancy and small antepartum haemorrhages. A detailed history may alert the obstetric and neonatal team to an infant at risk. Other risks are obstetric procedures such as chorionic villus sampling or amniocentesis.

The rhesus status of every pregnant woman is obtained. Rh – women should be given injections of anti-D with every risk incident. Antenatally, serial antibody measurements are taken and if these rise, intervention may be necessary. In a severely affected fetus the risk of early delivery versus the risk of a hostile uterine environment needs to be balanced. Occasionally the dramatic step of giving an intrauterine transfusion is made.

These infants demand a high level of care and expertise. Initial management of a severely affected infant includes:

- resuscitation
- correction of acidosis
- drainage of effusions
- immediate exchange transfusion
- administration of diuretics
- sensitive handling of the family.

Successful resuscitation means that intensive care and support of the family will be required, as will the management of repeated exchange transfusions and small top-ups to relieve anaemia.

Congenital infection

Congenital infections, as causes of jaundice, include cytomegalovirus (CMV), rubella, herpes, toxoplasmosis and syphilis etc. Transplacental transmission of the virus, parasite or spirochaete has important and long-term ramifications for the infant. Maternal infection with herpes may influence the mode and timing of delivery to avoid vaginal contact. CMV, rubella and herpes are potentially infectious so, as well as treatment and management of the presenting condition and the jaundice, universal precautions will need to be applied. The jaundice may be a mixed haemolytic and hepatocellular type.

Haemolysis due to shape and structure of the red cell

Glucose-6-phosphate dehydrogenase deficiency (G-6PD) is an inherited enzyme defect rendering the erythrocyte prone to haemolysis when exposed to environmentally determined trigger factors such as infection, drugs and some foods. α-Thalassaemia is a genetically transmitted cause of an abnormal red-cell protein structure, causing serious haemolytic disease. Hereditary spherocytosis and sickle-cell disease are abnormalities in the shape and structure of the red cell; if severe haemolytic disease is present in the neonatal period jaundice will occur.

Jaundice occurring from days 2–5

- Physiological jaundice
- Infection
- Excessive bruising
- Drugs
- Metabolic diseases such as galactosaemia
- A few rare genetic syndromes such as Gilbert's or Crigler–Najjar

Physiological jaundice

Physiological jaundice is an accepted deviation from normal. The 'pathology' results from the imbalance between bilirubin production and excretion. Physiological jaundice may be exacerbated by dehydration and poor feeding. It arises on day 3 and is resolved by day 10, causing no damage and requiring no active treatment. Parental anxiety can be encountered, so sympathetic explanation and reassurance may be appreciated. The jaundice resulting from excessive bruising is similar in origin as it occurs from the haemolysis of extravascular blood loss caused by severe trauma, e.g. a difficult breech extraction, which can be compounded if the infant is premature. Some of these infants need phototherapy.

Infection

Infected infants are always actively treated and many will need phototherapy. Bacterial infection causes erythrocyte destruction, liberating bilirubin. Infection causes the infant to be severely ill and shut down, subsequently impairing the ability of the liver to handle this extra load.

Drugs

Drugs such as oxytocin, used during labour, compete with bilirubin for bonding sites. As a consequence the free bilirubin level is raised, sometimes sufficiently to warrant phototherapy.

Metabolic disorders

These are numerically very rare and not all cause a rise in unconjugated bilirubin; phototherapy may not be indicated. These disorders may occur in the same period as physiological jaundice, but may be initially mild then gradually deepen and fail to resolve, resulting in a need for investigation.

Prolonged jaundice

- Breast milk jaundice
- Endocrine disorders, hypothyroidism and hypopituitarism
- Neonatal hepatitis
- Biliary atresia
- Other obstructive causes

Breast milk jaundice

The cause of breast milk jaundice is unknown (Poland and Ostrea, 1986): it is a diagnosis almost by default, once other causes are ruled out. Usually the levels, although unconjugated, are not high enough to warrant treatment and it is regarded as harmless except for the trauma to the mother's esteem. Sadly, many of these mothers tend to give up breastfeeding, which is unnecessary but effective in clearing up the jaundice.

Hypothyroidism

Although this can result in prolonged jaundice owing to sluggish metabolism, there are usually sufficient clues to aid diagnosis. Treatment is with thyroxine and, if diagnosed quickly, the prognosis is good.

Hypopituitarism

This is very rare. If suspected, management is best in a specialist unit.

Neonatal hepatitis

This results in severe, prolonged, conjugated jaundice. Other indications are often non-specific and diagnosis may be delayed. Phototherapy is unnecessary and management is best in a specialist unit, as over half of these infants will go on to develop cirrhosis or chronic liver failure.

Biliary atresia

This causes obstructive jaundice owing to the absence of the bile ducts; bile produced cannot drain away. It is a rare condition and may not present in the neonatal period; however, it is a diagnosis which should not be missed. Clinic nurses and health visitors are well placed to alert the family to an intractable problem and direct the infant to medical attention. Stools are pale owing to the absence of stercobilin, and the jaundice has a greenish tinge. Prognosis depends on how quickly repair can be attempted. The aim of repair is to establish bile drainage into the small intestine. With no intervention, diminished bile flow results in biliary cirrhosis, portal vein hypertension, varices, ascites and chronic liver failure (Kedzierski, 1991). With uncorrectable disease transplantation becomes necessary, usually during the 2nd year of life. Recent advances in liver reduction have made the outlook better but problems in tissue typing and insufficient organ donors remain.

Other causes of obstructive jaundice exist and include inspissated bile, cystic fibrosis, rare tumours and cystic lesions.

REFERENCES

Bratlid, D. (1990) How bilirubin gets into the brain. *Clinics in Perinatology* **17**(2), 449–81.

Cremer, R., Perryman, P., Richards, D. *et al*. (1958) Influence of light on the hyperbilirubinaemia of infants. *Lancet* **1**, 1094–7.

Ennever, J. (1990) Blue light, green light, white light, more light, treatment of neonatal jaundice. *Clinics in Perinatology* **17**(2), 467–81.

Kedzierski, M. (1991) Liver disease in babies and children. *Nursing Standard* **5**(43), 30–3.

Newman, T. and Maisels, M. (1990) Does hyperbilirubinaemia damage the brain of healthy full term infants? *Clinics in Perinatology* **17**(2), 331–58.

Poland, R. and Ostrea, E. (1986) Neonatal hyperbilirubinaemia, in *Care of the High Risk Neonate*, 3rd edn, (eds M. Klaus and A. Fanaroff), Ardmore Medical Books, W.B. Saunders Company, Philadelphia, pp. 239–261.

Rodgers, P. and Stevenson, D. (1990) Developmental biology of heme oxygenase. *Clinics in Perinatology* **17**(2), 275–91.

Schmorl, G. (1903) Zur Kenntniss des Ikterus Neonatorum, insbesondere der dabei auftretenden Gehirnveranderungen. *Verhandlung Deutsche Pathology Gesellschaft* **6**, 109.

Schumacher, R. (1990) Noninvasive measurement of bilirubin in the newborn. *Clinics in Perinatology* **17**(2), 417–35.

Swanwick, T. (1989) The causes of neonatal jaundice. *Nursing* **3**(39), 3–5.

Valaes, T. and Harvey-Wilkes, T. (1990) Pharmacologic approaches to the prevention and treatment of neonatal hyperbilirubinaemia. *Clinics in Perinatology* **17**(2), 245–73.

Vohr, B., Lester, B., Rapisardi, G. *et al*. (1989) Abnormal brain stem function and acoustic cry features in term infants with hyperbilirubinaemia. *Journal of Pediatrics* **115**, 303–8.

FURTHER READING

Levene, M., Tudehope, D. and Thearle, J. (1987) *Essentials of Neonatal Medicine*, Blackwell Scientific Publications, Oxford.

Marieb, E. (1992) *Human Anatomy and Physiology*, 2nd edn, Benjamin Cummings Publishing Company, USA.

Roberton, N. (1986) *A Manual of Neonatal Intensive Care*, 2nd edn, Edward Arnold. London.

14

Nursing care of a baby in pain and discomfort

Margaret Sparshott

EFFECT OF PAIN AND DISCOMFORT ON THE NEWBORN BABY

It is the duty of a nurse to act as the patient's advocate, especially so for the neonatal nurse, whose charges cannot speak of their sufferings and cannot protect themselves by either flight or fight. This inability to 'speak for themselves' has led many people to doubt that newborn babies can feel pain at all. If you are obliged to inflict pain for the good of others, the task is made easier if you can pretend they do not feel it. This absolves you of all guilt and allows you to proceed without worrying about the distress you may be causing. But research has shown that babies given analgesia during heart surgery tend to be less stressed, both during and after the operation, than those who have had to do without (Anand and Hickey, 1987).

The elements involved in the pain pathway are in place from an early gestational age, and babies are neurologically capable of feeling pain from 30 weeks' gestation and probably before. Fetal development can be affected by life events stress in the mother and, since this is a time of rapid increase in cortical brain cell structure, adverse experience may affect the balance of neurological development of the cerebral cortex (Connolly and Cullen, 1983). The question of pain and its effects on the newborn is therefore of vital importance when future quality of life is considered.

The newborn baby has no subjective experience of pain. He has, as yet, no knowledge of his environment; he is absorbing this from day to day. The infant develops and grows through his relationship with the encompassing world and the people it contains, and it is mainly through this relationship that personality comes into being. For this development, a gradual awareness of pain and discomfort is essential, as the stimulation of discomfort as well as an awakening interest in his surroundings will aid the infant to pass from complete dependence to independence. Both positive and negative experience are necessary for the growth of the individual, but this must come about gradually. It is what Winnicott (1965) referred to as the 'graduated failure', meaning that no mother is perfect, and this is one of the things every baby must learn.

It is potentially harmful, however, if the environment impinges too soon, too sharply or too persistently; the infant will not be able to cope with the adaptation necessary to withstand it. He will be forced into a knowledge that is totally inappropriate at this stage, and to defend himself he will regress and withdraw (Huteau, 1988). This regression can be beneficial if it is only temporary and, once the cause is removed, can be reversed. Early prolonged traumatic experience in infancy, however, has been diagnosed by psychoanalysts in adults suffering from feelings of persecution (Balint, 1968), and a syndrome of 'needing' pain has been identified in some small children who have undergone traumatic experiences in infancy (Herzog, 1983).

The environment of a neonatal unit, in which the fragile baby must be maintained, is inappropriate at best and frequently appears to offer nothing but discomfort. To keep such a baby alive, it is necessary to inflict many traumatic procedures upon him, and to do this knowingly can only add to the stresses of the caregiver. This is the dilemma which faces all those caring for the sick newborn and will be examined in this chapter.

INFANT RESPONSES TO PAIN AND DISCOMFORT

In order to improve the lot of sick and preterm babies in hospital, the neonatal nurse must first understand how these babies communicate their feelings, since they are unable to speak. The response that each infant makes will depend on his gestational age, his physical condition and his state of consciousness at that time.

The 'states of consciousness' or 'sleeping/waking states' are a cycle of states in which a healthy newborn baby passes his daily life. He progresses from deep sleep to light sleep (or rapid eye movement sleep), then through drowsiness to a quietly awake and alert state, and from wakefulness with considerable motor activity and some fussy crying, to crying as he becomes hungry. Once hunger is satisfied, he retreats into deep sleep and the cycle begins again (Brazelton, 1984).

The internal 'state' of a baby will affect his ability to receive stimuli from and respond to the environment; it is at the time of quiet wakefulness that the baby is most attentive to what is going on around him and this is the time he needs stimulation from his caregivers. His attention span is short, however, and a well term baby is able to retreat into a state of sleep, shutting off unwanted external stimuli (Wolff, 1966). On the other hand, a sick or preterm baby may be incapable of this response and will consequently be at the mercy of environmental pressure. It is important that the baby exhibiting 'shut out' signs should be handled as little as possible (Als *et al.*, 1986).

Babies 'speak' through their actions and reactions and are incapable of telling a lie. If a baby shows signs of stress, something is wrong; he may be complaining of the onset of pain, or simply of a soiled nappy. It is the degree of behavioural and physiological expression, combined with the neonatal nurse's own knowledge and understanding of the baby himself, which must guide her in uncovering the root of the problem.

The three types of pain and their symptomatology experienced by a newborn baby should be distinguished from each other. These are acute, extreme, and chronic or long-lasting pain.

Acute pain

This is usually highly localized, sharp and transitory. It is experienced by the infant during the performance of traumatic procedures, when handled postoperatively or spontaneously in conditions such as colic.

Extreme pain

Extreme pain may be experienced in illness such as necrotizing enterocolitis, meningitis or glaucoma.

Chronic or long-lasting pain

This type of pain is intractable and persists over a period of time. It is usually associated with illnesses such as cancer, but the symptoms may also be seen in infants who, due to their precarious state, are repeatedly subjected to traumatic procedures (Sparshott, 1989).

Behavioural responses to acute pain

Vocalization

The baby indicates that he is distressed by the way he cries. Interpretation of sound spectrography of infants' crying suggests that cries differ not so much in their origin (hunger, pain etc.) as in their intensity, pitch and duration (Michelsson, Jarvenpaa and Rinne, 1983), but hunger is probably not distinguishable from pain to the baby and the fussy crying of the hungry baby will eventually lead, if he is not satisfied, to the cry of pain. This 'pain cry' has been described as 'a sudden long and strong initial cry ... followed by a long period of absolute silence, due to apnoea; ultimately this gives way and short gasping inhalations alternate with expiratory coughs' (Bowlby, 1969). If there is no response to this cry, it will develop into the loud, braying cry of anger or tantrum, which is very difficult to appease.

Sound spectrography also shows that sick, light for gestational age, preterm babies, or babies suffering from birth trauma, have a particularly high-pitched shrill penetrating cry, which is hard to ignore and demands a response (Michelsson, Jarvenpaa and Rinne, 1983). Very low birth weight babies undergoing ventilation may be seen to gape round the endotracheal tube (Figure 14.1). This is known as the 'silent cry' (Wolke, 1987).

Facial expression

A neonatal facial coding system was adapted by Grunau and Craig in 1987, using adult facial coding systems and the

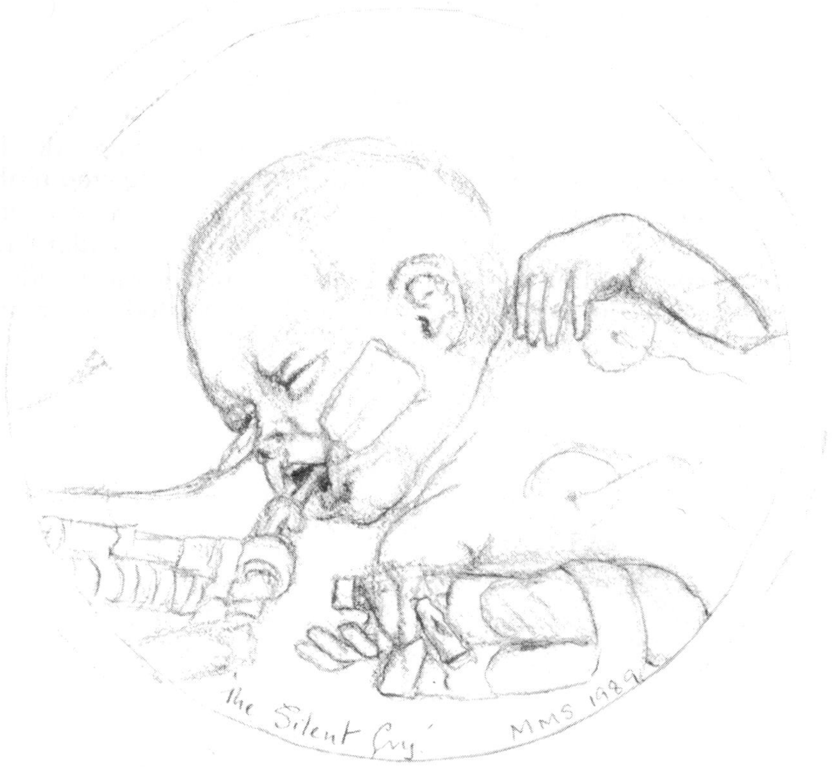

Figure 14.1 The 'silent cry'.

baby's response to a painful stimulus (heel-prick blood sampling). These specific facial changes – eye squeeze, brow contraction, nasolabial furrow, taut/cupped tongue and open mouth (Figure 14.2) were quite different from facial responses to other stimuli, such as rubbing the heel. For practical purposes, this pattern of reaction may be termed a 'pain expression'.

Grunau and Craig discovered that healthy term babies disturbed for heel prick during deep sleep would, provided they were not overhandled, react less violently than babies disturbed during the quiet alert state (Figure 14.3). Babies also react differently to different technicians, suggesting that it is to the baby's advantage if he is handled by someone who has a good technique (Grunau and Craig, 1987).

Body movements

There is frequently a violent thrashing or extension of all extremities and sometimes a withdrawal of the affected limb from the site of the injury. A well term baby may even sideswipe with the unaffected limb, showing considerable motor coordination at this stage (Dale, 1986). The Moro reflex may be present, but it is less specifically associated with pain and its origin may rather be a fear of falling.

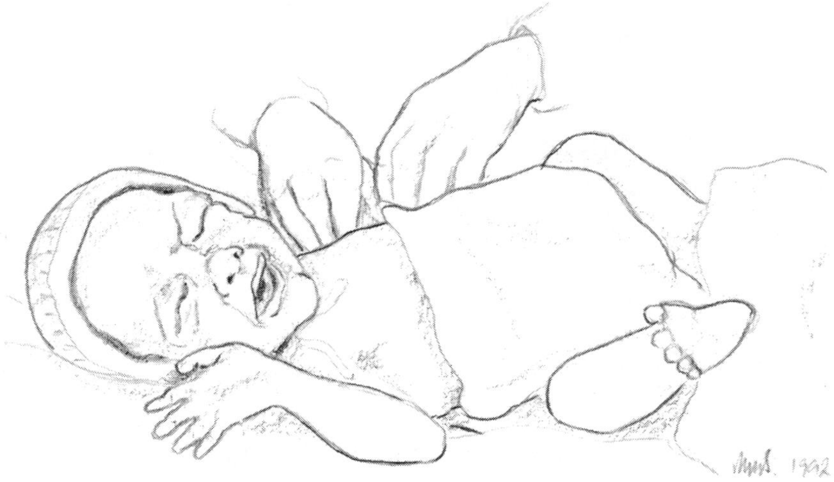

Figure 14.2 Pain expression.

Physiological changes in acute pain

Cardiovascular

Increases as well as decreases in heart rate have been observed during procedures in healthy full-term babies, but bradycardia is more frequent in fragile infants (Williamson and Williamson,

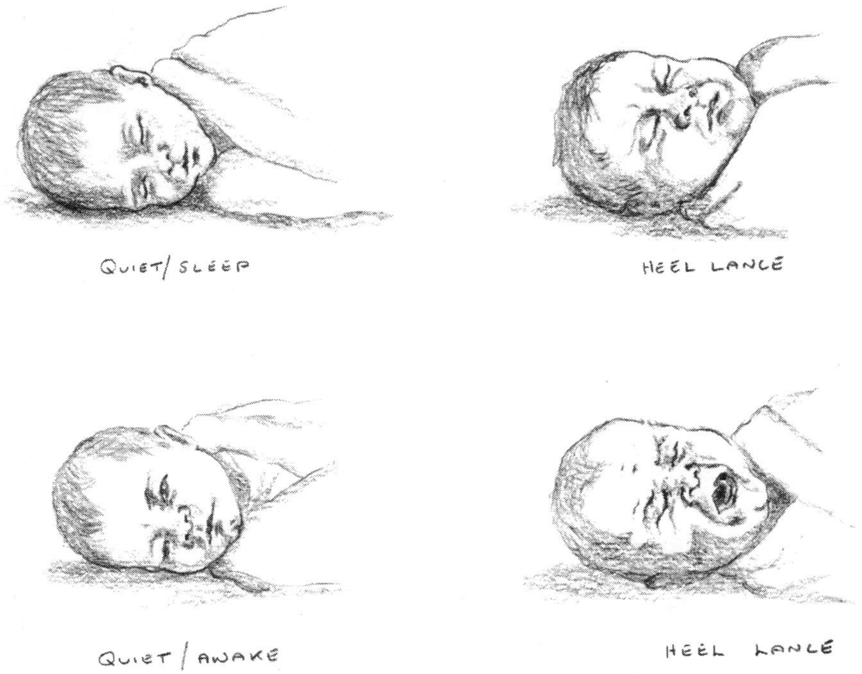

Figure 14.3 Facial behaviour of the newborn. Upper row depicts an infant prior to the heel-rub during quiet sleep, and the reaction to heel-lance. The bottom row depicts the reactions to the same procedures during the quiet awake phase. (Based on Grunau and Craig (1987).)

1983; Anand and Hickey, 1987; Brown, 1987). Increase in blood pressure has been noted during traumatic procedures. Increase in cerebral blood flow and increase in intracranial pressure can occur during endotracheal suctioning (Perlman and Volpe, 1983; Brown, 1987).

Respiratory

Hyperventilation can follow prolonged crying in term infants, but decrease in respiratory rate and apnoea are more likely to occur in fragile infants (Brown, 1987; Wolke, 1987). Increase in $TcPo_2$ may occur, owing to crying, but a decrease will be more common (Williamson and Williamson, 1983; Brown, 1987; Wolke, 1987). Overhandling and suctioning can cause $TcPo_2$ to fall (Long, Philip and Lucey, 1980). Oxygen saturation will be affected in the same way.

Temperature regulation

A deficit between core and peripheral temperatures is also an indication of stress in a baby.

Palmar sweating

Palmar sweating increases during painful procedures in babies from at least 37 weeks' gestation (Harpin and Rutter, 1982).

Endocrine

Changes in the endocrine system have been observed following ventilation, chest physiotherapy, endotracheal suctioning and circumcision with minimal anaesthetic, a response which has measurably decreased in sedated infants (Anand and Hickey, 1987). Overhandling can also lead to a release of plasma catecholamines, hormones whose raised levels are associated with stress (Lagercrantz *et al.*, 1986).

Pain assessment

The last two physiological changes, palmar sweating and endocrine response, are of no practical value to the nurse assessing a baby in her care, but all the others mentioned are alarm signals and, when observed, every possible source of stress should be investigated. In fact, physiological changes are the only means open to the very preterm infant to indicate stress from whatever cause, since he is too immature to coordinate behavioural responses. A tool for assessing pain using facial expression, cry, breathing patterns, movement of limbs, and state of arousal has been developed by Lawrence *et al*. (1993). This is called the Neonatal Infant Pain Scale (NIPS).

Other factors besides pain may underlie a stress reaction, but obviously, if the baby is undergoing traumatic procedures, pain must be considered as a possible cause.

Responses to extreme pain

Since crying cannot indicate the intensity of pain felt, it is sometimes difficult to assess when an infant is in extreme pain. There are certain abnormal positions of the limbs, an axial stiffness with head extension and an antalgic position of the body at rest, which may indicate intense suffering (Figure 14.4). The antalgic position is a defensive attitude adopted by the body against pain (Gauvain-Piquard, 1986). The infant in extreme pain may stop crying for a short while when picked up and cuddled but, since the pain persists, he will begin again as soon as he is returned to his cot.

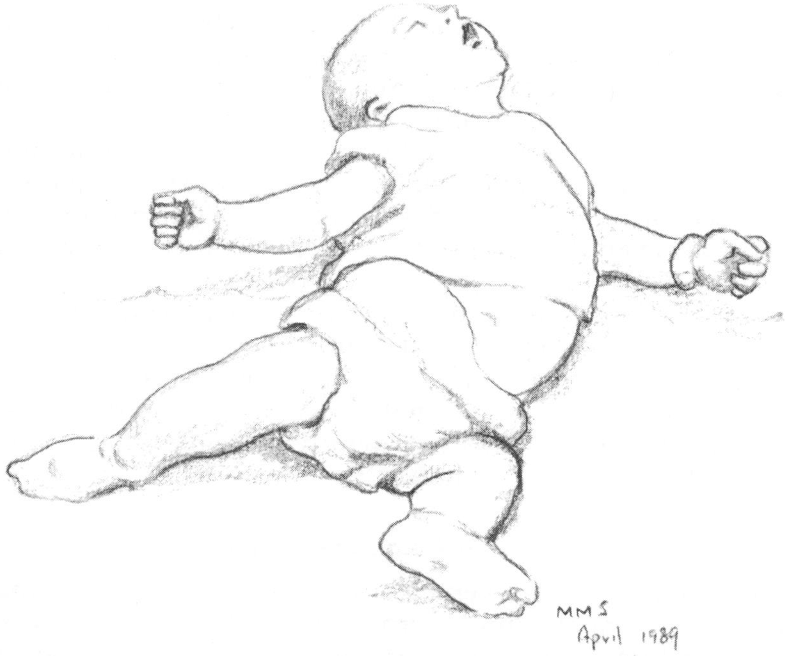

Figure 14.4 Abnormal position of an infant in extreme pain. (from Gauvain-Picquard, A. (1987) Le douleur d'un enfant. *Revue de l'Infirmière* **15** with permission.)

Responses to chronic or long-lasting pain

Lasting pain has a very different symptomatology. It may endure for several hours, days or weeks, and is not easy to diagnose as the symptoms are more discrete. If an infant suffers for a long time without relief, he will cease to struggle or cry since this wastes valuable energy (Gauvain-Piquard, 1986). He will withdraw into himself (as already described) and, the younger the infant and the greater the intensity of the pain, the more quickly he will cease to make responses. It is hard to recognize that this infant is suffering. The signs are negative: no crying, reduced motor activity, diminished communication with the outside world, diminished alertness and sometimes even an expression of hostility. The infant appears apathetic, listless and unresponsive to the caregiver (Gauvain-Piquard, 1986).

CATEGORIES OF ENVIRONMENTAL DISTURBANCE

Once the nurse has interpreted the baby's messages and believes him to be in pain, what action should she take? This will depend on the type of pain suffered and the individual baby's responses to treatment. A chart showing the main sources of pain, discomfort and disturbance likely to be encountered in the neonatal unit, balanced by the corresponding ways in which they may be treated, should help the nurse to identify the problem and choose the most acceptable way of providing comfort (Table 14.1). Since the baby has as yet no subjective experience, the items of these categories are interchangeable; for example, heel prick may be hardly disturbing to the term baby in deep sleep but will be painful to the fragile infant who is unable to 'shut off' unwanted experience. It is for the nurse, knowing the baby, to discover which method of consolation will suit him best (Sparshott, 1991a).

Disturbance and cherishment

Disturbance can be prevented by attention to light and sound levels. Permanent lighting, providing no difference between night and day, may contribute to the absence of circadian rhythm which is present in intrauterine life. Dimmer switches can be used in the special care nurseries. In intensive care individual lamps reduce the light intensity, as does partly covering the incubators with a cloth, allowing observation but protection from direct light.

Sound levels in excess of 60 dB(A) are potentially harmful to the newborn baby and British and American safety standards

Table 14.1 Categories of environmental disturbance and their treatment

Pain	*Discomfort*	*Disturbance*
Intubation	Monitoring	Light
Chest drain insertion	Physical examination	Noise
Venepuncture	Extubation	Cold
Heel prick	Range finding, due to insecurity	Heat
Suctioning	Chest physiotherapy	Nappy change
i.m. injection	Electrode removal	Position change
Wound cleansing	Rectal temperature	Nakedness
CPAP	Passage of NG or OP tube	Weighing
Lumbar puncture	i.v. medication	Overhandling
Arterial or suprapubic stab	Splinting	Feeding by NG or OP tube
Surgery	Physical restraint	Bottle feeding when too weak
Illness, e.g.	Phototherapy	Isolation
meningitis,	Urine bag removal	Separation
necrotizing enterocolitis	Adhesive tape removal	Lack of stimulation if well
	Hunger	Noxious taste/odour

Therapy	*Consolation*	*Cherishment*
Prevent pain by:	Music and sound	Day and night lighting
	Provision of boundaries	Noise reduction
Technique	Containment	Minimal handling or stimulation
Preparation beforehand	Stroking and massage	Clothing and coverings
Choice of equipment	Swaddling	Parental presence
Abstention	Rocking	Soft toys
Grouping care	Non-nutritive sucking	Musical toys and cassettes
	Breastfeeding	Pictures
Treat pain by:	Encouragement of self-consolation (hand to mouth movement)	Mirrors
Analgesia	Encasement	Mobiles
Local anaesthetic	Correct positioning	Baby carriers
Anaesthetic cream		Baby chairs
Treat intractable pain by:		Skin-to-skin contact
		Pleasant taste/odour
Relief of symptoms		
Containment		
Narcotic analgesia		

require that this level should not be exceeded within an incubator (Wolke, 1987). Noise can be reduced by avoiding the slamming of incubator doors or the placing of solid objects on the top of incubators, and by being aware of the disturbance caused by such extraneous sounds as the radio, loud voices and laughter. It is the behaviour of caregivers that is responsible for most of the raised sound levels. Babies do respond well to the sound of the gentle human voice and parents should be helped to understand that speaking lovingly to their baby can contribute to his wellbeing.

Strict observance of 'minimal handling' will allow periods of rest for the fragile infant. Ways to accomplish this are for caregivers to group care, using one sample of blood for several tests or by helping parents to see for themselves when it is best not to disturb their baby. Suitable stimulation should be offered, particularly by parents, to the well baby in the quiet alert state, who is waking up to the world (Chapter 15). A booklet designed for the parents of a preterm baby explaining how he is likely to behave and what actions they can take to maintain him in a state of wellbeing, will help them to feel involved (Sparshott, 1990).

Discomfort and consolation

The integrity of the skin as the surface of the body is of vital importance to a newborn baby, both physiologically and psychologically (Sparshott, 1991b,c). Attention should be paid to the siting of electrodes and the use of adhesives. If strapping is used in splinting it should be backed, to allow the minimum of adhesion to the skin, and if possible material should be used which is easy to detach. The positioning of the splint is also important, to ensure that the splinted limb is maintained in as natural a position as possible.

Babies do not like to be exposed and will waste energy 'range finding'. Suitable clothing, swaddling and the provision of barriers against which they can rest will promote a sense of security.

Following a traumatic procedure, the caregiver should console the baby in the way that suits him best (Table 14.1). This will be discovered over a period of time by trial and error, and parents should be encouraged to play the role of comforter.

The isolation of the newborn baby in an incubator is one of the most unnatural features of neonatal intensive care, and parents should be encouraged to participate in the care of their baby as soon as they feel confident to do so. The majority of parents, constantly watching their baby, soon become sensitive to his needs and learn just what form of stroking and caressing will suit him best.

For the fragile baby for whom even the gentle stimulation of stroking is too much, the technique of 'containment' or 'encasement' may be beneficial (Als, 1986). The caregiver places one hand very gently over the top of the baby's head and the other hand very gently over the trunk, thus containing his body in the warmth of human contact without demanding any response in return.

Pain and therapy

Unfortunately, many of the traumatic experiences that a baby undergoes in the neonatal unit are unavoidable if he is to survive with a good quality of life. It is the task of the caregiver to alleviate this suffering as much as possible.

Pain can be prevented by attention to such details as choice of equipment, preparation of the baby beforehand and grouping of care. For example, the use of mechanical lancets for the taking of blood samples has been shown to cause the least damage, whereas over-zealous squeezing of the heel adds to the trauma (Harpin and Rutter, 1983). Studies of infants undergoing circumcision without local anaesthetic showed that as much distress was caused by immobilizing the babies on a cold slab and drenching then with cold antiseptic solution, as by the incision itself (Williamson and Williamson, 1983). Doctors and nurses arranging their care of the baby to coincide will allow longer periods for rest and sleep.

The practice of a good technique is also essential to avoid inflicting unnecessary suffering. Nurses and doctors are more likely to become skilled at such procedures as heel-prick blood sampling and the siting of intravenous infusions with experience, and this is enhanced by the establishment of a permanent qualified staff in neonatal units.

Intractable pain can be alleviated by as far as possible relieving the symptoms, and by the use of narcotic analgesia.

Consolation techniques are unlikely to benefit the baby in extreme or long-lasting pain.

Morphine is the opioid analgesic most commonly used in the treatment of both acute and chronic pain. It is usually administered intravenously, either by bolus or by continuous infusion. Close monitoring and strict observation are necessary in view of the possible side effect of depression of respiration, and facilities for ventilation should be at hand (Koren *et al.*, 1985).

Of the non-opioid analgesics paracetamol is the most widely used, particularly in the treatment of peripheral pain. Its preparation for infants is in the form of an elixir or rectal suppository.

Lignocaine is the most widely used nerve block and is effective as a local skin anaesthetic, as it works rapidly; for example, it can be used in the elective insertion of a chest drain. Its disadvantages are that it is not suitable for use in an emergency and that, since it is administered by subcutaneous injection, it is itself painful. EMLA cream is a local anaesthetic used topically to anaesthetize the skin, but it needs to be applied at least 1 h before the performance of a traumatic procedure. EMLA cream has not, to date, been recommended by the manufacturers for use with newborn babies, since the effects of absorption through the skin of the newborn are as yet unknown.

PAIN MANAGEMENT

Believing that babies are not capable of feeling pain is a protective mechanism against the stress of being obliged to inflict pain on a being who is helpless and can neither fly nor fight. To see an infant in pain is very shocking; to be forced to inflict pain, even in the baby's interests, makes it even less supportable. But pain does exist and denying it will not make it go away.

The nurse, acting as the baby's advocate, should be able to demonstrate the baby's reactions to painful stimuli. Verbally accusing the doctor of hurting a baby will only rouse antagonism, since traumatic procedures must be performed for the baby's eventual wellbeing. However, if the nurse can show that the baby is suffering or is maybe even compromised

Table 14.2 Management of pain in the special care baby unit: plan of care

Problem	*Goal*	*Nursing intervention*	*Nursing evaluation*
Pain from:			
Traumatic procedures	Prevention of unnecessary suffering Maintenance of a safe environment Restoration to a state of equilibrium	1 Observe: State of consciousness Physiological signs prior to procedure 2 Perform or assist with procedure: Causing as little disturbance to baby as possible Maintaining safe environment by keeping baby warm and in most comfortable position Suggesting administration of local anaesthetic if appropriate 3 Note time taken over procedure 4 Note immediate behavioural and physiological response 5 Comfort and console baby until calm once procedure is completed 6 Suggest administration of analgesia if necessary 7 Observe state of baby and physiological changes 8 Note time taken and methods used to restore baby to a state of equilibrium	Goal is achieved when baby is restored to state of equilibrium; the shorter the time the greater the success of the nursing intervention
Post surgery	As above	1 Anticipate that pain will be experienced 2 Ensure that appropriate analgesia has been prescribed 3 Observe for signs of pain 4 Take appropriate action by: Alleviating symptoms Administration of analgesia 5 Observe state of baby and physiological changes 6 Note time taken and methods used to restore baby to equilibrium	As above
Illness (extreme and lasting pain)	As above	As in post surgery	As above

Note: Observations of state, maintenance of safe environment and attempts to comfort and console should be made in all cases

Table 14.3 Chart to show an individual baby's reaction to pain

Date & Time			
STATE (before procedure)			
Asleep			
Awake			
Crying			
Heart rate*			
Respiration			
Blood Pressure*			
TcPo_2 (or O_2 sat)*			
PROCEDURE time taken (minutes)			
REACTION			
NURSING ACTION			
Voice			
Stroking			
Massage			
Cuddle			
Rocking			
Swaddle			
Non-nutritive sucking			
Breast/bottle feed			
Analgesia			
RESULT			
Asleep			
Awake			
Crying			
Heart rate*			
Respiration			
Blood pressure			
TcPo_2 (or O_2 sat)*			
ACHIEVED			
1–3 minutes			
3–5 minutes			
5–10 minutes			
CODE			

by the pain felt, the doctor is more likely to avoid inflicting pain, by use of analgesia or other means.

The most reliable way to maintain adequate sedation for the newborn is for the medical staff to establish a 'pain protocol', such as that proposed by Andrews and Wills (1992). For neonatal nurses, a care plan for the pain management of a newborn baby (Table 14.2) can be used in combination with a chart (Table 14.3) showing the individual baby's reactions to the traumatic procedure, and which method of consolation or analgesia proved to be the most effective (Sparshott, 1989).

SUMMARY

An understanding of infant behaviour is of vital importance to the neonatal nurse. Not only will this enable her to identify signs of pain and discomfort in her patient, it will also allow her to see when he is comfortable and at rest. Each individual baby has his own needs and what pleases one will not always satisfy another. It is by means of behavioural responses and physiological changes that he communicates pain and pleasure. Once these are understood, all the actions listed in Table 14.1 (and many more) are available for the nurse to try and, if she fails, to choose an alternative. The baby will soon let her know when she has made the right choice for him.

REFERENCES

Als, H. (1986) A synactive model of neonatal behavioural organisation: framework for the assessment of neurobehavioural development in the premature infant and for the support of infants and parents in the neonatal intensive care environment, in *The High Risk Neonate*, (ed J. Sweeney), Haworth Press, London, pp. 3–53.

Anand, K.J.S. and Hickey, P.R. (1987) Pain and its effects in the newborn neonate and fetus. *New England Journal of Medicine* **317**(21), 1321–9.

Andrews, K. and Wills, B. (1992) A systematic approach can reduce side effects. *Professional Nurse* **7**(8), 528–32.

Balint, M. (1968) *The Basic Fault*, Tavistock Press, London.

Bowlby, J. (1969) *Attachment*, The Hogarth Press and the Institute of Psycho-Analysis, London.

Brazelton, T.B. (1984) *Neonatal Behavioural Assessment Scale*, 2nd edn, Blackwell Scientific Publications, Oxford.

Brown, L. (1987) Physiological responses to cutaneous pain in neonates. *Neonatal Network* **6**, 18–22.

Connolly, J.A. and Cullen, J.H. (1983) Maternal stress and the origins of health status, in *Frontiers of Infant Psychiatry*, (eds. J.D. Call, E. Galenson and R.L. Tyson) Basic Books Inc., New York.

Dale, J.C. (1986) A multidimensional study of infants' responses to painful stimuli. *Pediatric Nursing* **12**(1), 27–31.

Gauvain-Piquard, A. (1986) *The Infant Experiencing Pain: His Modes of Defence and Relationship With His Environment*, Third World Congress of Infant Psychiatry and Allied Disciplines, Stockholm, August 7.

Grunau, R. and Craig, K. (1987) Pain expression in neonates: facial action and cry. *Pain* **28**, 395–410.

Harpin, V.A.H. and Rutter, N. (1982) Development of emotional sweating in the newborn infant. *Archives of Disease in Childhood* **57**, 691–5.

Harpin, V.A.H. and Rutter, N. (1983) Making heel pricks less painful. *Archives of Disease in Childhood* **58**(3), 226–8.

Herzog, J. (1983) A neonatal intensive care syndrome: a pain complex involving neuroplasticity and psychic trauma, in *Frontiers of Infant Psychiatry*, (eds. J.D. Call, E. Galenson and R.L. Tyson), Basic Books, New York.

Huteau, M. (1988) Travail de recherche sur les sons et les prématures. *Soins Gynecologie-Obstetrique-Puericulture-Pediatrie* **84**, 11–20.

Koren, G., Butt, W., Chinyanga, H. *et al.* (1985) Post-operative morphine infusion in newborn infants: assessment of deposition characteristics and safety. *Journal of Pediatrics* **107**(6), 963–7.

Lawrence, J., Alcock, D., McGrath, P., *et al.* (1993) The development of a tool to Access Neonatal Pain. *Neonatal Network* **12**(6), 59–65.

Lagercrantz, H., Nilsson, E., Redham, I. and Hjemdahl, P. (1986) Plasma catecholamines following nursing procedures in a neonatal ward. *Early Human Development* **14**, 61–5.

Long, J.G., Philip, A.G.S. and Lucey, J.F. (1980) Excessive handling as a cause of hypoxemia. *Paediatrics* **65**, 203–7.

Michelsson, A-L., Jarvenpaa, A-L. and Rinne, A. (1983) Sound spectrographic analysis of pain cry in preterm infants. *Early Human Development* **8**, 141–9.

Perlman, J.M. and Volpe, J.J. (1983) Suctioning in the preterm infant: effects on cerebral blood flow velocity, intracranial pressure, and arterial blood pressure. *Pediatrics* **72**, 329–34.

Sparshott, M.M. (1989) Pain and the special care baby unit. *Nursing Times* **85**(41), 61–4.

Sparshott, M.M. (1990) *This is Your Baby*. Booklet for parents obtainable from NICU/Derriford Hospital, Plymouth PL6 8HD.

Sparshott, M.M. (1991a) Creating a home for babies in hospital. *Paediatric Nursing* **3**(8), 20–2.

Sparshott, M.M. (1991b) Maintaining skin integrity. *Paediatric Nursing* **3**(2), 12–13.

Sparshott, M.M. (1991c) Psychological function of the skin. *Paediatric Nursing* **3**(3), 22–3.

Williamson, P.S. and Williamson, M.L. (1983) Physiological stress reduction by a local anaesthetic during newborn circumcision. *Paediatrics* **71**(1), 360–400.

Winnicott, D. (1965) The theory of parent–infant relationship, in *The Maturational Processes and the Facilitating Environment*, Hogarth Press, London.

Wolff, P.H. (1966) *The Causes, Controls and Organisation of Behaviour in the Neonate*, International University Press, New York.

Wolke, D. (1987) Environmental and developmental neonatology. *Journal of Reproductive and Infant Psychiatry* **5**, 17–42.

15

Enhancing development in the neonatal unit

Maryke Morris

Advances in neonatology have contributed to the survival of increasingly premature, sick or small babies. However, the intensive nature of the medical and nursing intervention required to maintain life can also mean that early stimulation for these infants is far from normal. Some surviving neonates will exhibit neurological impairments due to complications of prematurity or life-saving treatment (e.g. retinopathy of prematurity due to oxygen therapy). Over the last 15 years, there has been a reduction in major impairments in babies weighing less than 1 kg at birth and a relative decrease in neurological impairments (cerebral palsy, neurosensory hearing loss, blindness, development or intelligence quotient <70) in the number of babies surviving weighing less than 1.5 kg at birth (Wolke, 1991).

Wolke (1991) has concluded that the outcome for low birth weight infants can best be improved by the provision of early developmental support through stimulation and play. Such a programme should be based on theory, dynamic in nature and respect the infant's individual behavioural organization, mother–child interaction and parenting needs.

NEONATAL INFANT DEVELOPMENT

The sensory systems mature in an orderly progression, with that of oral cutaneous responsiveness developing first. Other senses then develop in the following sequence: vestibular (balance), olfaction (smell), gustatory (taste), auditory (hearing) and, lastly, vision (Gottlieb, 1971). It has also been found that a sensory system begins functioning before maturation is complete (Gottlieb, 1971, 1986), implying that experience is necessary for the facilitation, induction, development and maintenance of early neural maturation (Gottlieb, 1976).

Kuo (1967) discovered that changes in the prenatal environment (such as preterm birth) can affect the probability of developing normal behavioural responses. This possibly explains the fact that the preterm infant can easily become disorganized with handling, compared to his full-term contemporary (Korner, 1990). Deviations in the developmental process can occur, depending on the experiences that the infant is exposed to and the type of responses that he receives (Swanwick, 1990) as well as the stress of being in hospital (Wilson and Broome, 1989). In the preterm infant, the neonatal nurse has to facilitate development of the behavioural potentials (Kuo, 1967) to the best of her own and the infant's ability. Being born too soon puts an unexpected load on the immature central nervous system, demanding responses that may not be appropriate to the stage of sensory development that the infant has reached (Horowitz, 1990).

The preterm infant

The preterm infant is caught in a dilemma in that he is missing out on the normal home environment a newborn baby experiences at the same time as being deprived of the unique stimulation that is encompassed in the last few weeks of pregnancy (Korner, 1990). The environment that the newborn preterm infant is exposed to must respond to loss of the supportive womb, indicating a need for containment and supported positioning (Turrill, 1992).

The older preterm baby is deprived of close interaction with a few special people, as well as the play and stimulation a loving home presents, indicating the need for auditory, visual and social stimulation.

Neonatal unit graduates

Studies reporting on the long-term growth and development of infants who required admission to neonatal units came to the conclusion that it was not the size of the baby at birth that indicated future motor, cognitive and behavioural development, but the severity and chronicity of the neonatal illness. Subtle developmental deficits may exist in previously low birth weight, neurologically intact infants, including intelligence quotients at the lower limits of normal (Aylward *et al.*, 1989), delays in the acquisition of language (Vohr, Garcia Coll and Oh, 1988) and motor problems, leading to clumsy children (Marlow, Roberts and Cooke, 1989).

Effects of hospitalization

Hospitalization is disruptive and stressful at any age, and immediately after birth the separation caused can affect nurturing and attachment, altering the pattern of stimulation (Goldberger, 1990). In hospital, the infant is in contact not only with his family and friends but also with the nursing and medical staff and ancillary workers. The disorganized sensory stimuli from the many caregivers and the environment prevents the infant developing a routine and thus beginning to organize his behaviour and the maturing central nervous system. The baby in the neonatal unit requires developmental care as well as medical and nursing care (Gorski, 1991).

SENSORY STIMULATION AND THE NEONATAL UNIT

As has already been discussed (Chapters 1 and 14), the infant in a neonatal unit receives a constant bombardment of stimuli, most of it not suitable or appropriate for his needs. Wolke (1991) defined it as a mismatch between the infant's developmental status and the intensity, type and pattern of stimulation to which he is exposed. The baby in an incubator might be sensorily deprived (Korner, 1990) but is subject to the unit environment. He might have some resilience (Macedo, 1981), but probably not enough to cope all day and every day.

The sick newborn is also deprived of the normal mother–child interaction which, as well as promoting attachment and psychological wellbeing, has an important role in the organizational abilities and behavioural state of the newborn. The caregiver selects a repertoire of appropriate caregiving functions and responses which helps the infant to organize himself (Linn and Horowitz, 1983). When the infant is cared for by many people, he is not subjected to either a limited or a constant repertoire of actions, and this can have far-reaching consequences.

This evidence would lead a considerate neonatal nurse to plan and provide care that meets not only the infant's sickness needs but also his developmental needs. The type and timing of play and stimulation is important for the wellbeing of the preterm baby, and consideration has to be given to his postconceptual age and the stage of sensory development reached (Korner, 1990).

ROLE AND IMPORTANCE OF PLAY

Play is not just recreational for an infant, nor is it always active, organized and supervised. It is one way that an infant can work through and explore feelings, thereby increasing understanding, and is essential for promoting normal development. Within the neonatal unit play adds normality to life in an abnormal environment, which is important both to the infant and his family.

The sick preterm baby is already disadvantaged from his early birth and is at risk for developmental delays. These are compounded when life begins in hospital, in a critically ill state and separated from parents. Play and an appropriate stimulation can compensate for the interruption of uterine life and promote development as would occur *in utero*, following the normal maturational sequence so as to enhance the functioning of the present sense and the development of the following system (Korner, 1990).

Every infant has a right to have some emotional and developmental input during his stay in hospital (Royle, unpub.), through play, stimulation and manipulation of the environment. Infants prescribed and receiving care adjusted to their abilities and behavioural state have been shown to gain weight more quickly (Korner, 1990), require less respiratory assistance and graduate more quickly to full feeds than a matched control group (Als, Hawthorn and Brown, 1986). These infants also exhibited long-term benefits of higher mental development and better social interactions when older (Als, Hawthorn and Brown, 1986).

PLAY AND THE INFANT IN THE NEONATAL UNIT

Play programmes are necessary to help the long-term patient to meet specific developmental goals, and are written respecting the infant's ability to cope with the external environment and sensitive to his medical condition and behavioural state. The sick neonate should have his play scheduled to respect his ability to regulate his cardiac, respiratory and thermoregulatory systems.

Play programmes

Grunwald and Becker (1991) wrote a set of standards which were research-based and form a foundation to begin planning a programme. They include:

- organizing care to suit the infant's behavioural state;
- reducing stress due to invasive procedures;
- promoting motor development by appropriate positions;
- adjusting the visual and auditory environment for the infant;
- parental participation.

The rationale behind play and stimulation is to help maintain homeostasis and provide sufficient appropriate stimulation for the developing neurological systems (Schultz, 1992). Stimulation programmes, as planned for the preterm infant, focus on the senses, notably visual, auditory, tactile and vestibular–kinaesthetic (Gorski, 1991). Touch is the most important sense, which should be accommodated for in the plan.

The 'geriatric' neonate requires directed play for normal growth, physically, intellectually, emotionally and socially. Physically, play helps the infant gain body control, confidence and independence, along with helping coordination and relieving energy, frustration and boredom. The practising of new skills and exposure to new experiences promotes intellectual development, which in turn results in the development of thought, language and vocalization. Emotional needs are met as the infant derives comfort from the involvement of family and carers during routine activities, helping the infant to develop socially. Play is planned to meet these requirements and to stimulate curiosity.

Implementation

It is difficult to ascertain what type of intervention is necessary to promote the best outcome (Korner, 1990). Outcome is affected by the type of stimulation and the regimen, for example to soothe an infant, slow, gentle continuous stimulation is given, and conversely, to rouse him, vigorous, fast intermittent stimulation is necessary (Korner, 1990).

A play programme does not have an easily taught or prescribed aim, and the implementation needs to suit the infant both in how he responds (Korner, 1990) and in his needs. Extra stimulation may not be appropriate in the very sick infant who is struggling to keep a hold on life (Korner, 1990), and an older preterm baby's response can depend on the presence of any cardiopulmonary or neurological complications or insults (Korner, 1990).

An example of a play programme

This play programme was written for a 4-month-old infant born at 30 weeks' gestation who was nursed most of the time in a continuous negative-pressure box. Some activities were implemented inside the box.

Physical

To encourage good posture
  Allow Joshua to lie on sides in good position, with shoulders and hips well over.

To encourage hands together in the midline
  Lay Joshua on side or supine gently bring hands together prompted by elbows.

To encourage head control
  Lay Joshua lengthways down own trunk. Talk to him, encouraging head lifting.

Intellectual

To encourage sucking own fingers
  When bringing hands together, guide from the elbow to mouth.
  Allow Joshua to explore own fingers in mouth.

To allow Joshua to watch own hands
Bring both hands together in line of vision. Hold for a brief time.

To encourage eye contact with Joshua.
Lay Joshua supine. Gain eye contact by talking, singing or an interesting object.

Emotional
To continue input from family
Involve family in all aspects of Joshua's care.

To alleviate any distress caused to Joshua
Comfort Joshua, reassure him and talk to him during painful intervention.

Social
To encourage enjoyment of routine cares
Chats and songs during nappy change. Playful tickling etc.

To encourage smiles and interaction with others
Lots of talking to after gaining eye contact.

Evaluation
Joshua can play with own hands in the midline.
Joshua can watch his own hands and fingers.
Joshua gives beaming smiles to those he knows well, especially Mum and Dad.
Joshua looks at you when you speak to him.

(Play programme reproduced by kind permission of Joshua's parents and Karen Alleyne, Play Specialist).

The role of the nurse

The baby's nurse has a role in ensuring that his days have some sort of resemblance, with care following a predictable routine which is planned in coordination with the parents and play specialist (if available), reflecting his individual needs. Limiting the number of nurses assigned to the infant promotes familiarity and the baby's routine.

It is within the right of the nurse and parents, as the infant's advocates, to delay non-urgent intervention and organize the timing and coordination of invasive procedures (Chapter 14).

Table 15.1 Sleep wake states

Quiet (non-REM)	Eyes shut, breathing regular, no limb movement, no response to sudden noise
Active (REM)	Eyes shut, eyes moving beneath eyelids, breathing irregular, limb movement, startle and blink to sudden noise
Quiet	Eyes open in the midline, no limb movement, startle and blink to sudden noise
Active	Eyes open in the midline, no crying, alternating limb movement, startle and blink to sudden noise
Crying	Eyes open or shut, voicing an opinion, alternating, jittery limb movements, response to sudden noise

In order to assess the infant's developmental needs, a theoretical and practical knowledge base of normal and abnormal responses, newborn reflexes, signs of stress (Chapter 14) and arousal (Table 15.1) is needed, along with an understanding of normal age-related development and behaviour. It is beyond the scope of this chapter to give all the details of infant development and an appropriate textbook on play is recommended reading.

The role of the family

The participation of the family in play is essential to both the infant and the parents. Parents are the constant carers whom the baby recognizes from an early age, generating smiles and responses of familiarity. Play is a normal part of infant care which every parent is capable of, although occasionally a little assistance is needed in realizing their potential, by helping the family develop their parenting skills and by showing them how to play with their baby.

Siblings are a vital source of stimulation, both in playing with the baby and in providing play materials, for example colourful mobiles that can be hung near the baby's head. Any child provides a happy chatter, with lots of kisses and cuddles and exploring fingers to enable the baby to be surrounded by touch.

If the baby is very sick, the family will need reassurance that their loving presence, gentle caresses and soft talking is just as important as the more dramatic actions of the nursing team. Very rarely is the infant so sick and unstable that he cannot tolerate any interaction from his parents, but a cuddle may have to be modified to a gentle touch inside the incubator.

PLAY AND THE SICK PRETERM NEONATE

The preterm baby should not be viewed as an undeveloped full-term baby, nor as a fetus, but as a new human being (Adamson-Macedo, 1990). Appropriate stimulation in the very sick preterm baby helps the infant organize himself, i.e. how he responds to handling, his behavioural status and thus the development of appropriate behaviour along with the maturation of the central nervous system (Horowitz, 1990).

Long periods of rest with minimal stimulation (Collins and Kuck, 1991) are important for these infants. This may mean the placing of a notice requesting that the baby be left alone unless a life-promoting action needs to be taken, grouping handling together, preplanning medical and nursing interventions and shielding the baby from harsh lighting.

Tactile stimulation

With the knowledge that touch is the first sense to mature and be developmentally relevant, it is the most appropriate form of play for the preterm baby. There is debate about what this tactile stimulus consists of, but it seems that any loving touch has a beneficial effect and equates to play just as much as a rattle does in an older infant.

Adamson-Macedo (1990) developed a sequence of stroking, the so-called 'Tick Tac' method, which aimed at delivering a silent, 'gentle and soothing message' that was opposite to the more usual invasive, rough and painful handling the infant received. Stroking the infant, using gentle rhythmic and repetitive actions can be performed using the fingers or palm, so that every part of the body is touched in sequence from head to toe (Macedo, 1984; Rice, 1977; Sparshott, 1991). Any lifting or turning of these small babies should be slow and controlled, with the head and extremities being simultaneously supported (Collin and Kuck, 1991).

An infant too ill to tolerate handling may appreciate being encased by the carer's hands to give comfort (Sparshott, 1989). To do this, one hand is gently placed around the head and the other encloses his buttocks and legs, so that the infant is not disturbed from his position but at the same time can be provided with warmth and security (Sparshott, 1989).

Nesting the baby in a cocoon made from rolled-up sheets and blankets and laying him on a sheepskin or against a cuddly toy all produce pleasing tactile stimulation to the sick baby (Turrill, 1992). Containment not only reduces the stress associated with bad positioning but promotes motor development (Grunwald and Becker, 1991).

Promoting normal infant development

To help compensate for the missed flexed position that occurs after 36 weeks' gestation and which is thought to be responsible for developing active muscle tone (Downs *et al.*, 1991), the infant should be nursed in a supported flexed position (Turrill, 1992). From birth, the infant is exposed to gravity which, in the hypotonic preterm neonate, causes pronounced extension and an artificially held posture, inhibiting normal motor development processes (Fay, 1988). The flexed position can be promoted by the use of bedding rolls and strategically placed toys to provide a barrier in the baby's environment which will not only promote muscular development but will also reduce his energy expenditure, as he has easily defined parameters which enhance the feelings of security and stability (Turrill, 1992).

A soft surface that will distribute the pressure of the heavy brain helps prevent craniofacial deformation. Soft or padded mattresses, beanbags, sheepskins and waterbeds (partially filled i.v. fluid bags) for the paralysed infant allow the skull to grow sideways and not flattened against the relatively hard incubator mattress.

Promoting the development of hearing and seeing

Hearing

To promote the development of hearing, anyone talking to a preterm infant should aim at using a soft, high-pitched voice (Weibley, 1978) and use rhythmic sounds to enhance security and comfort similar to those that the infant was exposed to in the uterus (Salk, 1973). Tapes of womb 'music' have been commercially produced and could be used. The risk of hearing loss can be reduced by minimizing the noisy environment (Chapter 14) and using the quietest equipment available and responding promptly to alarm signals.

Some illnesses and drugs have an effect or consequence on hearing and the neonatal nurse can limit their detrimental effects. Careful monitoring of ototoxic drugs, e.g. vancomycin, gentamicin and frusemide, is necessary and medical advice sought for high blood levels. Uncontrolled hypoglycaemia and high bilirubin levels, along with loud noises, can affect hearing. Absent responses indicating impaired hearing are: no Moro reflex in response to loud noise, no babbling by 4 months of age and the lack of localizing to sound by 6–7 months (Shultz, 1992).

Sight

The preterm infant is able to see patterns and geometric shapes, including the human face, from 36 weeks' gestation (Shultz, 1992). Placing pictures or bright objects 8–12 in from his face and for as long as he can tolerate them will provide visual stimulation (Anderson, 1986). The infant approaching term is able to track objects and should be positioned so as to see the carer's face during feeding and procedures. When not involved in direct interaction, stimulation can be provided from the environment. Imposing a day/night environment has many positive effects on development (Sheldon and Bell, 1987).

Infants at risk of visual impairment include those who have received indomethacin, a blood transfusion or prolonged oxygen. Having a very low birth weight, septicaemia and being one of twins have also been identified as risk factors for visual loss (Shultz, 1992). Indicators of impaired sight include the use of non-visual senses, the absence of blinking and the lack of eye movement in line with rotation of the body (Shultz, 1992).

PLAY AND THE GERIATRIC NEONATE

It is not unusual nowadays to have infants on a neonatal unit for several months, going well beyond their due date into the early months of postconceptual infancy. In some cases, these babies celebrate major developmental milestones and first birthdays, hence the term 'geriatric neonate'. Lack of attention to the emotional and developmental needs of the hospitalized infant, as young as 6 months, has been shown to cause disturbances with a lasting effect (Douglas, 1975), let alone the preterm survivor who has spent all his life in hospital. Unless play is catered for and directed, the infant may be confronted with the same environment and toys, day after day, that are used neither imaginatively nor constructively by the nurse and evoke no stimulation in the baby.

Encouraging play

Organising the baby's day to allow the important inclusion of planned and directed play should be given the same priority in the older neonate as his nursing and medical problems receive. Scheduled play times, in a quiet familiar room, are most appreciated by the wide awake and recently fed infant. In the comfort and security of these surroundings, the baby can respond most positively to the person who is devoting his/her time and attention to him. In the general nursery, there are the constant comings and goings of staff and multiple interactions, leading to continual disruptions in the infant's concentration on other matters.

The infant can assess his priority of needs and will not play if too tired or too hungry. Active play and learning new skills involves the use of energy, which may be more than some babies can spare, e.g. those with bronchopulmonary dysplasia (Goldberger, 1990). As play does not only occur at specified times, there must be the necessary stimulants for play within range all the time and the infant positioned appropriately to make use of his toys. Incorrect positioning, care procedures and medical intervention, along with the lack of rest and sleep, by day and night can all inhibit play.

Suitable environment

The brightly lit, noisy world of the neonatal unit is often very baby-unfriendly. Decor should be planned and inviting to the baby at his eye level and within his line of vision, but friezes and mobiles strategically placed for the benefit of the baby, for example on the ceilings and at the head end of the cot may not always be the most practical. Dimly lit or even dark, quiet rooms are necessary at night, along with the avoidance of interruptions, including specimen taking, as far as possible; nor should midnight become playtime.

Promoting normal infant experiences

The varied involvement of parents and different caregivers may mean that the baby's needs of hunger, discomfort or loneliness may not be treated the same way each time. Nursing care plans need to emphasize the parenting approach specific to each infant and his likes and dislikes, in order to promote some consistency into his day.

The older infant should not spend all his waking hours laid flat in a cot. Some play periods can be spent on a play mat surrounded by various toys that are light and small enough for the baby to grasp, brightly coloured to attract his attention and simple enough for some reaction to be obtained, for example a rattle. Sitting in a baby seat or reclining buggy not only provides a change of position but also allows him to have another view of the world, his play mates and himself. Provided that he is safely strapped in and the chair is stable, mobiles and other toys can be hung within sight and touch so that he can satisfy his own play needs. One advantage of being able to use a buggy, pushchair or pram is that the child can safely be moved from room to room and the parents can take walks about the unit (and perhaps outside). This not only increases their independence but stimulates the infant's interest in his surroundings.

Depending on the baby's stage of development time can be given for self-amusement, but often these graduates of intensive care need assistance in realizing that they have arms and legs which belong to them. Playing with parts of the body, such as guiding the infant's hand to his mouth, and line of vision as well as singing the usual nursery rhymes that facilitate body actions, for example 'pat a cake, pat a cake' is important to the long-term hospitalized infant. Involving parents in these play sessions increases their fulfilment by bringing enjoyment to the infant, who has suffered so much pain and heartache during his short life, and rewards them with beaming smiles and happy babbling. Families where childcare is not at its optimum for such reasons as lack of parentcraft teaching, lower socioeconomic status (Goldberger, 1990) and problems with bonding because of admission to the unit, benefit from involvement in play programmes and the teaching of parenting skills.

Infant development

With the older infant or geriatric neonate the theories of infant development can be considered as a basis for planning and enhancing play. Theories and their application is too vast a subject to be discussed here. For example, Piaget (1963) classed the first 18 months of life as being the sensorimotor period of cognitive development. The young infant has a small repertoire of reflexes and, through repetition and the resulting experiences from these movements, he begins to learn to use his senses to communicate with the environment. Randomized movements, such as sucking everything that touches the lips and reflex grasping on to anything, develop into coordinated actions as do feeling appropriately placed toys and turning to look at objects and in response to familiar voices (Barba, King and Walker, 1992). The infant can be encouraged to make pleasant associations by exploration.

Allowances have to be made in the application of these theories for the baby whose development may be inhibited by his medical management, e.g. babies on long-term continuous positive airway pressure or in a negative pressure box.

Promoting hearing and recognition

Hearing and the recognition of familiar voices can be utilized and encouraged by playing baby or nursery rhyme tapes which can either be bought from a shop or home-made (this gives the advantage that the child can be entertained by familiar voices). Personal stereos can be placed inside an incubator or on a bedside locker. However, tapes and the radio should not be played indiscriminately as there is a time and a place for music, just as there is for eating and sleeping.

Comfort

Much of the nurse's time with these older babies should be spent in pleasant and enjoyable play, which is as important as performing nursing procedures. When a painful procedure has to be performed, thought and attention always needs to be given to the amount of distress that the action will cause and how the infant will best be comforted. This, along with the parents' and baby's preferences, can be written in the nursing documentation.

THE PLAY SPECIALIST

No infant plays naturally in hospital; he needs someone to initiate play (Hogg, 1990). Play does not occur in a timetabled format and should be continuous with the infant's desires. In saying this, neonatal nurses often have heavy workloads and direct most of their time and energy to saving the lives of their critically ill patients, and they omit the play aspect either because of wanting to promote rest and save energy or because of lack of time, knowledge and resources. Play therapy for the convalescent infant may be given a low priority. The importance of play is often realized but not adequately catered for, so a play therapist/specialist can assist in bridging the gap to meet the infant's play requirements.

The play specialist can be a NNEB-trained nursery nurse with an understanding of the neonate, or a qualified neonatal nurse who focuses on the play needs, assisting the infant to achieve his full potential by supporting and advising nurses and parents in play, as well as planning and conducting individual play programmes (Royle, unpub). The play specialist is a valued member of the unit team (Royle, unpub.) who can either work on a referral system, for example when the infant is 1 month postconceptual age or has special needs, or can be involved with every infant on the unit.

REFERENCES

Adamson-Macedo, E.N. (1990) The effects of touch on preterm and fullterm neonates and young children. *Journal of Reproductive and Infant Psychology* **8**, 267–73.

Als, H., Lawhorn, G. and Brown, E. (1986) Individualised behavioural and environmental care for the very low birth weight preterm infant at high risk for bronchopulmonary dysplasia: neonatal intensive care unit and developmental outcome. *Pediatrics* **78**, 1123–32.

Anderson, J. (1986) Sensory intervention with the preterm infant in the neonatal intensive care unit. *American Journal of Occupational Therapy* **40** (1), 19–25.

Aylward, G.P., Pfeiffer, S.I., Wright, A. and Verhurst, S.J. (1989) Outcomes studies of low birth weight infants published in the last decade: a meta analysis. *Journal of Pediatrics* **11**, 515–20.

Barba, L.A., King, D.J. and Walker, C.L. (1992) Infant definitive care unit: developmental care for the hospitalised NICU graduate. *Neonatal Network* **11**(7), 35–41.

Collins, S.K. and Kuck, K. (1991) Music therapy in the neonatal intensive care unit. *Neonatal Intensive Care* **4**(5), 19–24.

Douglas, J.W.B. (1975) Early hospital admissions and later disturbances of behaviour and learning. *Developmental, Medical and Child Neurology* **17**, 456–80.

Downs, J.A., Edwards, A.D., McCormick, D.C. *et al.* (1991) Effect of intervention on development of hip posture in very preterm babies. *Archives of Disease in Childhood* **66**, 797–801.

Fay, M. (1988) The positive effects of positioning. *Neonatal Network* **6**, 5.

Goldberger, J. (1990) Lengthy or repeated hospitalisation in infancy. *Clinics in Perinatology* **17** (1), 197–206.

Gorski, P.A. (1991) Developmental intervention during neonatal hospitalisation. *Pediatric Clinics of North America* **38**(6), 1469–79.

Gottlieb, G. (1971) Ontogenesis of sensory function in birds and mammals, in *The Biopsychology of Development* (eds E. Toach, L.R. Aronson and E. Shaw), Academic Press, New York, pp. 67–128.

Gottlieb, G. (1976) Conceptions of prenatal development: behavioural embryology. *Psychology Review* **83**, 215–34.

Gottlieb, G. (1986) *Discussion*. Winter Conference on Current Issues in Developmental Psychology, Hawk's Cay, Florida.

Grunwald, P.C. and Becker, P.T. (1991) Developmental enhancement: implementing a program for the NICU. *Neonatal Network* **9**(6), 29–45.

Hogg, C. (1990) Standards for play. *Pediatric Nursing* **2**(8), 6.

Horowitz, F.D. (1990) Targeting infant stimulation efforts. *Clinics in Perinatology* **17**(1), 185–95.

Korner, A.F. (1990) Infant stimulation. *Clinics in Perinatology* **17**(1), 173–84.

Kuo, Z.Y. (1967) *The Dynamics of Behavioural Development*, Random House, New York.

Linn, P.L. and Horowitz, F.D. (1983) The relationship between infant individual differences and mother–infant interaction during the neonatal period. *Infant Behavioral Development* **6**, 414–27.

Macedo, E.N. (1981) *Effects of Tactile Stimulation on Preterm Infants*, Paper, Annual Conference of BPS Postgraduate Psychology, Durham.

Macedo, E.N. (1984) *Effects of Very Early Tactile Stimulation on Very Low Birth Weight Infants – a 2 Year Follow Up Study*. Unpublished doctoral dissertation, University of London.

Marlow, N., Roberts, B.L. and Cooke, R.W.I. (1989) Motor skills in extremely low birth weight children at age 6 years. *Archives of Disease in Childhood* **64** 839–47.

Piaget, J. (1963) *The Origins of Intelligence in Children*, 2nd edn, Norton, New York.

Rice, R.D. (1977) Neurophysiological development in premature infants following stimulation. *Developmental Psychology* **13**, 69–76.

Royle, C. (unpublished) *Is There a Need for a Play Specialist on the Neonatal Unit*? HPS Special Study, North Warwickshire College of Technology and Art.

Salk, L. (1973) The role of the heartbeat in the relations between mother and infant. *Scientific American* **228**, 24–9.

Sheldon, S.J. and Bell, E. (1987) Light, sleep and development. *Pediatrics* **79** (6), 1053–4.

Shultz, C.M. (1992) Nursing roles: optimizing premature infant outcomes. *Neonatal Network* **11**(3), 9–13.

Sparshott, M.M. (1989) Minimising discomfort of sick newborns. *Nursing Times* **85**(4), 39–42.

Sparshott, M.M. (1991) Psychological function of the skin. *Paediatric Nursing* **3**(3), 22–3.

Swanwick, M. (1990) Development and chronic illness. *Nursing* **4**(16), 24–7.

Turill, S. (1992) Supported positioning in intensive care. *Paediatric Nursing* **4**(4), 24–7.

Vohr, B.R., Garcia Coll, C. and Oh, W. (1988) Language development of low birth weight infants at 2 years. *Developmental Medicine and Child Neurology* **30**, 608–15.

Weibley, T.T. (1989) Inside the incubator. *Maternal Child Nursing* **14**, 96–100.

Wilson, T. and Broome, M.E. (1989) Promoting the young child's development in the intensive care unit. *Heart and Lung* **18**(3), 274–81.

Wolke, D. (1991) Annotation: supporting the development of low birth weight infants. *Journal of Child Psychology and Psychiatry* **32**(5), 723–41.

16

Neonatal pharmacology

Ian Costello

A large and increasing range of drugs are administered to neonates to treat the cardiovascular, gastrointestinal, neurological and infectious complications often encountered due to prematurity. Rational, safe and effective drug therapy depends on an understanding of the physiological and pharmacological differences that exist between adults, term and premature infants. These differences can account for alterations in drug response and pharmacokinetics (absorption, distribution, metabolism and excretion) and can be helpful in minimizing adverse effects to drug administration.

DRUG ABSORPTION

Absorption is the movement of a drug from its site of administration into the blood circulation. Absorption characteristics differ between oral, intramuscular, rectal and topical (skin) routes of administration.

Oral absorption

The absorption of oral medication is dependent on a number of factors. In the drug itself these are:

- ionization at gastric and duodenal pH
- molecular weight
- degree of lipid solubility.

In the patient they are:
- gastric and duodenal pH
- gastric emptying time

- intestinal motility
- biliary function
- bacterial flora in the intestinal tract
- underlying disease states.

For a drug to be absorbed from the gastrointestinal tract it must be mainly in a lipid-soluble unionized form. As pH affects drug ionization and hence solubility: an acidic (low) pH favours the absorption of acidic drugs, and a basic pH the absorption of basic drugs. Gastric acid secretion is the main determinant of gastric and duodenal pH, and appears to be variable at birth though rarely present in neonates of less than 32 weeks' gestation. Acid secretion patterns in the neonatal period are generally reduced, and may be related to the presence or absence of enteral feeding (Hyman *et al.*, 1983).

The unpredictability of gastric acid secretion and thus gastric and duodenal pH leads to variability in oral drug absorption. The relatively higher, more alkaline pH enables basic drugs such as penicillins to be more rapidly and completely absorbed than acidic drugs such as phenobarbitone or phenytoin, when compared with adults.

Peristalsis and gastric motility are decreased in the neonatal period but remain variable and unpredictable, affecting the absorption of drugs and their concentrations in body fluids. Most orally administered drugs are absorbed in the small intestine. If the rate of gastric emptying of the stomach contents is reduced then the rate of intestinal drug absorption will be reduced, lowering the peak concentration of drug in the plasma. If peristalsis is reduced, then the drug may be in contact with its site of absorption for a longer period, resulting in more complete absorption into the body.

Many other factors affect gastric acid secretion, gastrointestinal motility and drug absorption. Biliary function is reduced, lowering the absorption of lipid-soluble drugs and vitamins. The bacterial flora present in the gastrointestinal tract differ in neonates and affect drug absorption, as certain bacteria are able to metabolize drugs (Table 16.1).

Intestinal motility may be impaired in cardiovascular, metabolic or neurological disease states. Bowel surgery delays motility and may increase acid secretion, and massive bowel resection may reduce the total surface area available for drug absorption.

Table 16.1 Factors affecting gastrointestinal drug absorption

Factors	*Symptoms*
Acid secretion	Small bowel resection
Reduced gastric emptying	Gastro-oesophageal reflux Respiratory distress syndrome Congestive cardiac disease
Gastric motility	Thyroid disease Diarrhoea
Bile salt excretion	Cholestatic liver disease Biliary obstruction

In summary, although oral administration can be a safe and effective route for drug delivery, the unpredictable and erratic absorption of drugs must be taken into consideration. This is important when consistent predictable plasma drug concentrations or complete absorption are required.

Rectal absorption

Rectal administration of drugs may be useful if the oral and intravenous routes are unavailable or impracticable. Drug absorption from the rectum occurs in a similar manner to that in the gastrointestinal tract, and is influenced by similar factors. Since the pH of the rectal area is slightly alkaline, the drugs most suitable for rectal administration are those that will be mainly unionized at this pH and are sufficiently lipid-soluble to cross cell membranes. Drugs may be formulated for rectal use in solution or as a solid suppository. Absorption is more rapid from solution as the initial delay while the suppository dissolves is removed. Clinically effective rectal use of diazepam (Kundsen, 1977) and Aminophylline (Lyon and McIntosh, 1985) has been demonstrated in infants and neonates. This route of administration holds promise for the future, although further controlled studies are needed.

Topical absorption

The epidermis of neonates is thin and immature and, particularly in premature neonates, acts as a poor barrier to the absorption of agents applied to its surface (Harpin and Rutter, 1983). The ratio of skin surface area to body weight is much larger than that of an adult, and can result in relatively greater amounts of a topically applied drug being absorbed. In addition, any trauma to the skin (burns, denudation, inflammation) will increase absorption into the bloodstream. Toxic effects from the topical administration of hydrocortisone, hexachlorophene and phenol have been reported (Tyrala *et al.*, 1977).

Extreme caution is needed when applying any topical agent to neonatal skin, especially if premature, and careful thought should be given to the possible toxic effects if absorption occurs. Although the skin represents a potentially useful route of drug administration, further research is needed and few drugs have been studied.

Intramuscular absorption

Drug absorption following intramuscular administration depends on a number of factors. The drug must be lipid-soluble enough to cross from the muscle tissue into the blood, but must also be stable at muscle pH.

Blood flow to and from the muscle is also important in drug absorption from the site of administration. This is often compromised in infants with poor peripheral blood flow in conditions such as respiratory distress syndrome, hypotension or cardiac failure. 'Drug pooling' can occur, when an apparently ineffective intramuscular dose administered during a period of reduced peripheral perfusion is absorbed when blood flow improves, thereby causing adverse effects or toxicity.

Owing to the variable absorption of drugs, the intramuscular route is generally reserved for occasions when intravenous access is not possible. However, the major limiting factor to the use of multiple intramuscular injections in premature infants is their small muscle mass.

Oral, rectal and intramuscular drug administration is generally limited to non-seriously ill haemodynamically stable infants. For the majority of drugs in the neonatal unit, the intravenous route of administration is used to avoid variable or incomplete absorption.

DISTRIBUTION

The distribution of a drug in the body after administration is affected by a number of factors:

- Route of administration
- Body composition
- Plasma protein drug binding
- Tissue binding
- Vascular perfusion.

The route of administration is important in drug distribution. A drug administered orally passes through the liver before entering the systemic circulation, and if extensive liver metabolism occurs very little may be available for systemic action. Intravenous administration results in direct distribution to the heart and lungs, which may cause adverse effects.

Total body water is increased in the neonate, mainly due to the larger extracellular fluid volume and lower fat content (Figure 16.1). This becomes more exaggerated the more premature the neonate, and results in a lower serum level for

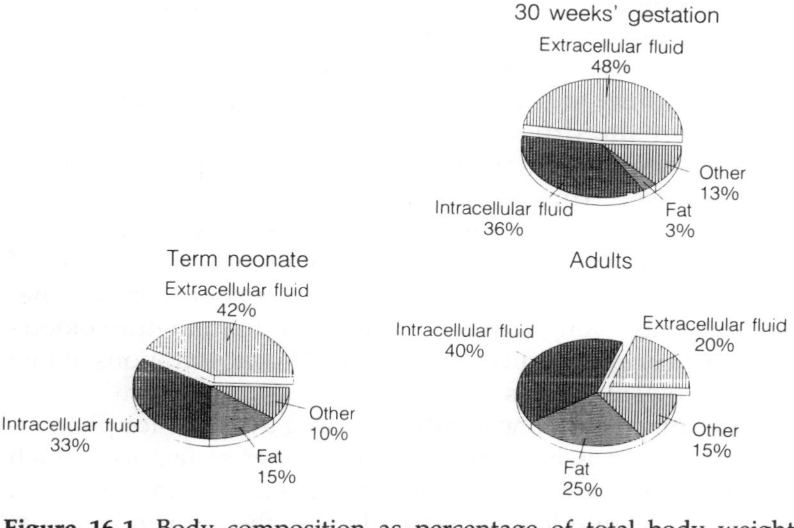

Figure 16.1. Body composition as percentage of total body weight. (Adapted from Besunder *et al.*, 1988).

drugs which distribute mainly into the extracellular fluid when administered in an equal dose based on mg/kg of body weight compared with adults or older children. Drugs affected include penicillins, aminoglycosides (gentamicin, tobramycin) and non-depolarizing neuromuscular blocks such as pancuronium and vecuronium). Similarly, less drug is distributed in fat and muscle tissue.

A proportion of a drug present in plasma is bound to plasma proteins and thus unavailable for systemic action, as only free drug can bind to the target site. Neonates have reduced levels of most plasma proteins and this results in greater amounts of free drug in the plasma. This may lead to an exaggerated pharmacological or toxic response, and may account for the lower therapeutic dose of theophylline required in neonates (6–12 mg/kg) compared to adults (10–20 mg/kg). An increase in free drug available for distribution to liver, kidney and tissues may result in little change in overall plasma concentration, as more drug is removed from the circulation.

Drugs bound to plasma proteins can be displaced from their binding sites by agents such as other drugs or body compounds. Bilirubin is one such agent. The increased production and delayed excretion of bilirubin which occurs in the first few days of life can lead to higher free drug levels. More importantly, decreased bilirubin binding to plasma proteins in the presence of drugs may lead to higher levels of free bilirubin and hence central nervous system toxicity.

Drug binding to plasma proteins varies depending on the structure of the drug. Plasma protein-binding effects only become clinically significant if a drug is highly protein bound, e.g. phenytoin, frusemide and diazepam.

Tissue binding and uptake of drugs is also altered in neonates compared to adults. The increased penetration of many drugs into the central nervous system (morphine, fentanyl, diazepam) may be explained by an immature blood–brain barrier, and results in greater CNS concentrations at low doses or plasma levels.

In summary, the concentration of drug available for pharmacological action is influenced by a number of factors, which can result in a larger dose being required on a mg/kg basis. However, despite lower plasma levels, the concentration at the site of action may be greater, leading to an enhanced pharmacological action. Thus doses of drugs in neonates must be carefully chosen and preferably based on controlled studies and pharmacokinetic information. Extrapolation from paediatric or adult doses is unsatisfactory.

METABOLISM

Many drugs undergo metabolism before excretion from the body. Many organs and tissues are capable of metabolizing drugs, including the lungs, gastrointestinal tract, kidneys and blood. However, the liver is the major organ responsible for drug metabolism. The neonatal hepatic enzyme systems responsible for metabolism are not fully developed. This can result in decreased drug metabolism and prolonged plasma half-lives for many drugs, e.g. theophylline, morphine and diazepam.

The lack of certain liver enzyme systems may result in a drug being metabolized by a different set of enzymes in neonates from that in adults. This leads to the formation of different metabolites, which may be pharmacologically active or toxic. These alternative enzyme systems may be very effective in metabolizing drugs so that little difference is seen between adults and neonates, e.g. paracetamol. Following birth, liver function and enzyme systems mature at varying rates. Blood flow and liver size are relatively greater in infants than in adults and, as liver enzymes mature, a period of increased drug metabolism can occur compared to adults.

Liver function is altered by a number of disease states (RDS, hypoxaemia, septicaemia) and can change rapidly during the neonatal period. Careful monitoring of drug plasma levels and therapeutic response may lead to regular adjustments in dosage. In general, drug metabolism by the liver is decreased in the neonate and this is more marked in premature infants.

EXCRETION

Most drugs or their metabolites are excreted from the body by the kidneys. Renal function develops late in gestation (at approximately 34 weeks) and is thus markedly reduced in premature compared to term neonates. Following birth, renal function improves at a rate that depends on gestation, postconceptional age and concurrent disease state. In term infants an improvement occurs over the first 3–4 days following birth. In premature infants of less than 34 weeks' gestation, renal function is impaired for much longer.

Cardiovascular disease and hypoxia can delay the development of renal function. Drug excretion by the kidneys is thus reduced to varying degrees in neonates and improves as renal function increases, but remains variable.

Drug therapy can affect renal function by reducing renal blood flow (indomethacin) or by toxic effects on the renal tissue (aminoglycosides). Other drugs may increase renal blood flow (dopamine, epoprostenol) and improve renal excretion. Careful monitoring and adjustment of dosage intervals is required for those drugs excreted mainly unchanged by the kidney (aminoglycosides, penicillin, pancuronium, frusemide) in order to avoid drug accumulation and toxicity, and to ensure adequate therapeutic effects.

DRUG RECEPTORS

The action of most drugs is dependent on binding to specific receptors, either extracellularly on individual cell membranes or intracellularly. This initiates a drug-induced response. Neonates may differ in the relative number of receptors and the cellular response to drug binding. Some receptors appear more sensitive to drug binding and an increased drug response occurs at lower doses than expected, e.g. pancuronium and morphine. These receptor differences may explain the toxic effects of certain drugs at low serum levels.

THERAPEUTIC DRUG MONITORING

Therapeutic drug monitoring is the measurement of drug levels in a body fluid to determine whether the drug is within certain concentration limits known to be safe and effective. Normally, serum is the body fluid chosen as it is easily obtainable in a suitable volume for measurement.

Drugs that require close monitoring of serum levels and dosage adjustment are generally those that show only a small difference between therapeutically effective and toxic doses. These are:

- aminoglycosides, e.g. gentamicin, vancomycin
- theophylline
- phenobarbitone
- phenytoin
- digoxin.

Due to the variations in drug distribution, metabolism and excretion already described, therapeutic or toxic serum concentrations for drugs may be different between adults and neonates. Any plasma measurements require careful evaluation and correlation with therapeutic response.

A number of factors can affect the result of serum level measurements and may lead to inappropriate adjustments in dosage thereby increasing the risk of toxicity or ineffective concentrations. Most important is the timing of the serum sample taken for measurement in relation to the dose. This should be sufficient to allow the drug to be fully distributed throughout the body so that the serum measurement will reflect the true concentration of the drug. Sampling times vary between drugs, and are generally standardized and based on adult experience and studies.

The time and rate of drug administration are important in determining the accuracy of serum level measurement. For those drugs that require therapeutic monitoring, standard protocols should be adhered to. If this is not possible, the method of administration and timing of the dose should be documented.

Adverse effects

The incidence of adverse reactions to drugs and their administration is greater in neonates than in infants, children or adults. Incidences of 10–30% (Bonati *et al.*, 1990) have been reported, with 55% of these classified as major adverse effects resulting in clinical deterioration (Aranda *et al.*, 1982). Known adverse effects of drugs often used in the neonatal unit are summarized below. However, many adverse effects are unexpected or difficult to attribute to specific drug therapy, and careful monitoring may improve recognition of these. Specialist advice should be sought from pharmacists or clinical pharmacologists if an adverse effect is suspected.

Drug	*Adverse effect*
Ampicillin	skin rash
Amphotericin	fever
	vomiting
	renal failure
	blood disorders
Digoxin	cardiac arrhythmias
	electrolyte disturbance
Dopamine	cardiac arrhythmias
	hypertension
	peripheral ischaemia
Heparin	haemorrhage
	thrombocytopenia
Indomethacin	renal failure
	hyponatraemia
	intraventricular haemorrhage
	necrotizing enterocolitis
	gastrointestinal bleeding
Morphine	seizures
	respiratory depression
	hypotension

DRUG ADMINISTRATION

Intravenous

The intravenous route is the main route of drug administration to neonates and presents a number of problems. Drug delivery via a syringe pump is the method of choice when precise rates of delivery are required or large volumes used, as this allows complete control over the time and rate of administration. A second method is the antegrade infusion method, in which the drug is injected in the direction of flow via a 'Y' site or burette attached to a primary infusion fluid. Large variations in predicted drug delivery times have been found at the low infusion rates commonly seen in neonates.

The characteristics of the syringe pump or infusion pump may be important. Fluctuations in blood pressure during a dopamine infusion to a premature neonate have been reported

(Schulse *et al.*, 1983). Low-pressure infusion pumps have reduced these problems but careful consideration is still required.

The intraluminal diameter of intravenous tubing is important in determining the characteristics of drug infusion. Tubing with a smaller diameter causes an increase in the speed of flow of the infusion fluid, which reduces the time required for drug delivery, reduces the flush volume and prevents delays in delivery.

The material from which the intravenous tubing is made should also be considered. Some drugs, such as insulin, paraldehyde and glyceryl trinitrate, are absorbed on to certain plastics, causing variations in drug delivery. Leaching of substances from various disposable intravenous administration products is also a problem with paraldehyde and chlormethiazole infusions. Specialist advice from the pharmacy department should be sought to determine the infusion tubing available for administration of these products; polyethylene-lined administration sets are generally recommended.

The use of bacterial and particulate inline filtration devices is now common. Intravenous solutions contain varying quantities of particulate matter, which may produce phlebitis or even pulmonary granulomas. Certain drugs may bind to such filters (insulin) while others may not pass through (amphotericin, lipid). Again, specialist pharmacy advice should be sought.

Inadequate mixing of drug additions to intravenous bags or between a drug solution and the primary infusion fluid can result in inaccurate and dangerous administration of large drug doses. Squeezing of intravenous infusion bags is not an effective method of mixing additives, and the bag should be rapidly inverted several times to ensure even dispersal of the drug. This is particularly important when potassium is added to large-volume intravenous bags. Suitable dilutions of drug solutions should be used to prevent differences in specific gravity resulting in the drug settling out or floating in the primary infusion fluid. This is a particular problem when low infusion rates are used, and can be reduced by using narrow tubing.

Many drugs are administered by 'i.v. push'. This term is ambiguous and should be discouraged. All drugs administered intravenously to neonates should be given slowly over a minimum of 5 min to allow adequate mixing with blood and removal from the injection site. This avoids large localized concentrations of drug solution which can cause phlebitis or toxicity. Specific problems that can occur due to high local drug concentrations include seizures, cardiac arrhythmias and hypotension. Adult administration rates should not be applied to neonates as the dilutional effects of the systemic circulation following drug administration are vastly different.

The use of the small dosage volumes often encountered in the neonatal intensive care unit can cause difficulty. Often, formulations of a suitable strength to enable precise and easy dosage measurement are not commercially available. The inadvertent administration of the dead space volume if a syringe when flushed can lead to drug toxicity when concentrated drug solutions are used.

Incompatibility between intravenous drugs is important when two or more drugs are mixed in the same line. Careful consideration is equally important whether mixing with a primary infusion fluid or with another drug solution via a 'Y' site connection. Mixing of drug solutions is to be discouraged, although often there is little choice. Incompatibility can be either physical or chemical. Physical incompatibility is the most obvious and results in the formulation of a precipitate or a cloudy solution. Chemical incompatibility is less obvious but results in drug inactivation or even conversion to toxic substances. Pharmacy advice should be sought before attempting to administer drugs together or with an infusion fluid with which compatibility is unknown.

Some drugs are also sensitive to light and can be affected by phototherapy, especially when low infusion rates are used.

Local policies and procedures for intravenous drug use, covering reconstitution, dilution and administration, are essential for safe and effective drug delivery to neonate.

Oral administration

The administration of oral medication is not without complications. The risk of aspiration should be considered, even in the presence of a nasogastric tube. This is particularly important whenever an oral preparation has a particularly high or low pH.

Inadequate flush volumes used to clear tubing following drug administration may result in a proportion of the dose remaining in the tubing. Incompatibilities can also occur with oral dosage forms. The administration of drugs in the presence of enteral feeds can reduce absorption, e.g. phenytoin (Bauer, 1982). The use of hypertonic oral medications may also be associated with the development of necrotizing enterocolitis (White and Harkary, 1982; Atakent *et al.*, 1984).

DRUG FORMULATION

The majority of commercially available drug products are formulated for use in adults, with little consideration given to their potential use in neonates. Many dosage forms are presented in strengths or concentrations that require accurate measurement of small dosage volumes. Appropriate techniques should be used to avoid errors in such measurements, taking into account the dead space of syringe hubs and needles.

The concentrations of drug solutions are important in avoiding pain and phlebitis at the injection site or adverse effects on the gastrointestinal tract. These can be avoided by simple dilution to specified concentrations before administration, and may prolong the patency of an intravenous line or reduce the risk of necrotizing enterocolitis.

The use of certain intravenous preparations orally may overcome some problems, as injections are often formulated without preservatives to minimize irritation at the site of injection. However, this should only be undertaken after pharmaceutical advice has been sought and safety confirmed.

Many drug preparations contain other ingredients as well as the active constituent. These may be preservatives, stabilizers, impurities or even flavourings, and have been associated with adverse effects, including intraventricular haemorrhage, metabolic acidosis, cardiac arrhythmias, seizures and hypersensitivity reactions (American Academy of Paediatrics, 1985). It is important to investigate and assess the constituents of a drug formulation before administration to neonates. Advice can be obtained from pharmacists or drug manufacturers.

REFERENCES

American Academy of Paediatrics Committee on Drugs (1985) Inactive ingredients in pharmaceutical products. *Paediatrics* **76**, 635–43.

Aranda, J.V., Portuguez-Malavasi, A., Collinge, J.M. *et al.* (1982) Epidemiology of adverse drug reactions in the newborn. *Developmental Pharmacology and Therapeutics* **5**, 173–84.

Atakent, Y., Ferrara, A., Bhogal, M. *et al.* (1984) The adverse effects of high oral osmolar mixtures in neonates. *Clinical Paediatrics* **23**, 487–91.

Bauer, L.A. (1982) Interference of oral phenytoin absorption by continuous nasogastric feedings. *Neurology* **32**, 570–2.

Besunder, J.B., Reed, M.D. and Blumer, J.L. (1988) Principles of drug biodisposition in the neonate (Part I). *Clinical Pharmacokinetics* **14**, 189–216.

Bonati, M., Zullini, T.M., Pistotti, V. and Tognoni, G. (1990) Adverse drug reactions in neonatal intensive care units. *Adverse Drug Reactions Acute Poisoning Review* **9**, 103–18.

Harpin, V.A. and Rutter, N. (1983) Barrier properties of the newborn infant's skin. *Journal of Paediatrics* **102**, 419–25.

Hyman, P.E., Feldman, E.J., Ament, M.E. *et al.* (1983) Effect of external feeding on the maintenance of gastric acid secretory function. *Gastroenterology* **84**, 341–5.

Kundsen, F.U. (1977) Plasma diazepam in infants after rectal administration in solution and by suppository. *Acta Paediatrica Scandinavica* **66**, 563–7.

Lyon, A.J. and McIntosh, N. (1985) Rectal aminophylline in the management of apnoea of prematurity. *Archives of Disease in Childhood* **60**, 38–41.

Schulse, K.F., Graff, M., Schimmel, M.S. *et al* (1983) Physiologic oscillations produced by an infusion pump. *Journal of Paediatrics* **103**, 769–8.

Tyrala, E.E., Hillman, L.S., Hillman, R.E. and Dodson, W.E. (1977) Clinical pharmacology of hexachlorophene in newborn infants. *Journal of Paediatrics* **91**, 481–6.

White, K.C. and Harkary, K.L. (1982) Hypertonic formula resulting from added oral medications. *American Journal of Diseases in Children* **136**, 931–3.

17

Ethical issues in the neonatal unit

Gosia Brykczyńska

The field of neonatology is full of paradoxes. The delight and awe of new life are juxtaposed against disease, malformation, pain and premature death. Yet premature babies are born, some alive and some with such a tenuous hold on life that only a mother could dare hope that the child would survive.

It is the aim of neonatology to nurture, treat and heal the premature baby until such time as it can live with its parents without the massive technological, pharmacological and professional support that a modern neonatal intensive care unit can provide. Most prospective parents are not prepared for the eventuality of premature birth and when this does happen, it is usually accompanied by fears of death.

It is against such a background of spiritual and psychological distress that the nurse working in the neonatal unit must function. The nurse may wish that the parent would start to identify with the tiny scrap of humanity that lies before them but the parent, in shock, is immobilized by fear and pain; thus the parent comments: 'This one? No feelings towards it, I'm just numbly sorry for the tiny scrap. . . I need to hold it in my arms, tell it how much we care, tell it how sorry I am that it is not still safely inside me. I am not numb now, I am exploding inside with the need to reach out to this baby. "Touch her" the nurses say. I cannot; its separateness from me is like a screen around it, a barrier that it will not let me cross. My mind cries out to it, baby, we care, don't die' (Cooper and Harpin, 1991).

In analysing the ethical issues inherent in the nature of neonatology, it is imperative to remember that whatever is being discussed and debated, at the centre of the argument will always be a tiny human life. The premature infant is not the cuddly, rounded baby of formula milk advertisements, it is rather a stark reminder that the best place for 'tiny scraps' is the mother's womb, and all other options, however sophisticated, are but distant contenders.

ETHICAL ISSUES IN NEONATOLOGY

The ethical issues raised during the care of these tiny babies fall into several categories. Whereas each child is the product of a unique pair of parents and presents, to some extent, unique medical and psychosocial problems, nonetheless, from a moral perspective, the ethical dilemmas and moral stress that parents and staff experience fall into rather broad general categories.

Thus, there is a group of moral issues which stem from the very nature of the infant's prematurity and call into question the nature of the infant's personhood (Engelhardt, 1977; Tooley, 1983; Cameron, 1991). Moral concerns over the beginnings of life constitute a large category of ethical interest, e.g. When does life start? Can we talk of independent life? Is every infant an autonomous moral agent? Who is in the best moral position to speak on behalf of an infant? (Dunn, 1985; Yu *et al.*, 1986; Iglesias, 1986; Warnock, 1992). Engelhardt (1977) noted: 'Person is an important category to understand because it is through those things, which are persons, that a moral community exists'.

The second large group of concerns deals with problems and the ensuing distress resulting from whether or not to treat (Duff and Campbell, 1973; Trammell, 1975; Lappé, 1981; Kuhse and Singer, 1989). These moral problems address the professional unease surrounding the aggressive treatment of the very immature infant and question the ethicacy surrounding withdrawal of treatment due to advanced disease, malformation, profound physiological immaturity and congenital defects (Fost, 1982; Bailey, 1986; Hack and Fanaroff, 1989; Campbell, 1992; Campbell, Gillett and Jones, 1992).

Recently, a third group of moral problems has arisen concerning the use of fetal material for subsequent research or even therapeutic purposes (Kushner and Belloitti, 1985; IME, 1988; Nelson, 1988; Fry, 1990; Tindall, 1992). The central issue discussed here covers the age-old moral debate of whether or not it is ethically acceptable to use a 'person' as a means to an end. An example may be the use of brain tissue from aborted fetuses for experimental work on cures for neurodegenerative disorders such as Parkinson's disease, or the use of embryonic ovaries for treatment of infertility. The ethicacy of such work is being seriously questioned (Polkinghorne, 1989; Fry, 1990; Lamb, 1992; Singer, 1992; Tindall, 1992).

Lastly, there are those moral issues raised by sociopolitical and economic aspects of the health care system (Campbell, 1992). Neonatal units are suffering from scarcity of finances, adequate equipment, skill mix and research funding. Not enough money or resources are being channelled into perinatal medicine or neonatal nursing, and what is being put aside for neonatology addresses the need for high-powered tertiary intervention once the premature or critically ill infant is born, whereas far more intervention is called for prior to birth, or even prior to conception (Lappé, 1981, Matthews, 1992). Preconceptual care is almost non-existent in the UK, yet perhaps a more appropriate response would be to look at the health of prospective parents, their physical, emotional, psychological and social wellbeing (Lappé, 1981; Van Maanen, 1990). Not all prematurity can be halted but much of the prematurity dealt with in perinatal units is due to stress and unhealthy lifestyles.

These and other ethical issues will be examined, ever mindful of the statement by a bereft mother of a premature infant in a neonatal unit: 'Maybe, in an earlier era, when couples had many children and infant death was a common occurrence, women took the loss of their children in their stride. But I doubt it. Should you try to measure the unthinkable, the death of one's child is off the scale' (Mehren, 1992).

ASPECTS OF PERSONHOOD

In few other branches of nursing is the question of personhood and the nature of the individual so obviously thrust into prominence as in the field of neonatology. Aspects of personhood affect the work of geneticists, embryologists, obstetricians (involved with assisted fertilization programmes) and midwives (involved with prenatal scanning, genetic counselling and the delivery of profoundly handicapped infants). Likewise, neonatal nurses hovering over the fragile life of a child 'born too early' frequently pose the philosophical questions that keep repeating themselves and need to be answered each time anew: What is the nature of this patient-person? Who can be considered an autonomous being? (Lappé, 1981; Tooley, 1983; Goldenring, 1985; Cameron, 1991).

Traditionally, nurses equated an infant's autonomous existence with the capacity to exist independently (Shea, 1985; Dunn, 1985; Singer, 1992). This arbitrary cutoff point to distinguish an autonomous being from a maternal parasitic appendage was so crude and full of inconsistencies that new definitions had to be considered. Gestational age alone, however, is not a sufficient measure of personhood, as Dunn (1985) points out. Any definition based on a physical measurement scale alone runs the risk of logical inconsistency and anomaly. Thus, how does one define personhood according to gestational age-scale of a fetus 10, 20 or 30 weeks old? Is one fetus classified as half a person at 10 weeks, two-thirds a person at 20 weeks and almost a 'whole' person at 30 weeks? Such purely biological definitions of personhood are obviously nonsensical, yet legal definitions of rights to full personhood and human status are still attributed to fetuses and infants on combinations of biophysical measurements alone, usually gestational age and weight.

Until recently, some fetuses at 24 weeks were deemed sufficiently non-persons to be candidates for abortions, whereas premature infants born at 23 weeks were considered sufficient persons for the purpose of expending vast sums of money and health care resources to maintain their tenuous hold on human life. It is not just a question of moral interest that concerns us here, as Kuhse (1985) might claim. For it is a grave burden and responsibility on society to state and uphold a definition of personhood that does logical justice to all fetuses and thereby clarifies the interventionist nature of those concerned with the wellbeing of mother and child (Hack and Fanaroff, 1989; Ackerman, 1992).

If a newborn baby is rejected (for whatever reason) does it make the infant any less of a full person with protective positive rights under law? Do the criteria for rights to treatment and protection depend most significantly on whether or not the child holds value (or interest) to its parents, as Kuhse and Singer (1989) suggest? Obviously, an infant must be seen legally as an autonomous unit of concern, as an individual with its own right to existence, in order for society to be able to intervene on its behalf, to provide nurture, treatment or even a 'dignified ending'. It is a sad commentary on our approach to very preterm infants, especially those stillborn, that in the eyes of the law and society only a 'person' can be formally buried in a civic cemetery and that definitions of 'persons' do not and traditionally have not included all the products of a pregnancy. As Kohner states, there is 'an urgent need for change. Many professionals and many more parents, have expressed their acute distress and concern about hospital disposal practices of babies born dead before the legal age of viability (Kohner, 1992).

The Government's recommendations (Polkinghorne, 1989), that a dead fetus is respected 'in a way analogous to the respect afforded to a human cadaver on the basis of its having been a human person', would suggest that fetuses and fetal material can and should be accorded respect, which surely extends to burial services for the stillborn 22-week-old infant. However, a preterm infant is only accorded that respect in law to the extent that parents and society are concerned for the continued welfare of the child. Philosophical deliberations about the nature of the infant take second place to the question of whether or not this particular child is to be the focus of our concern (Berseth, Kenny and Durand, 1984; Savage *et al.*, 1987). These concerns are not insignificant, however, for the neonatal nurse, who will be nurturing the preterm infant on the very margins of legal viability, questioning possible further intervention for the full-term (but congenitally profoundly damaged infant, e.g. with anencephaly), and unsure about procedures for the somewhat early but viable nosocomially damaged neonate. All these infants are alive, accorded a place in the ranks of society and nurtured with love and affection but, for one infant the status of legal personhood can be very arbitrarily prescribed, whereas for another it is legally binding but unlikely to be ever positively realized. In a cost-conscious health care climate, what will be the consequences of arbitrary definitions of personhood? (Darbyshire, 1989).

TO TREAT OR NOT TO TREAT?

Whether to start treating an infant or not and whether to withdraw treatment or not are questions that the neonatal team must face quite often (Campbell, 1992). The ethos is to treat the critically ill infant, even if there are some lingering doubts as to the long-term consequences and benefits of the intervention (Whyte, 1989; Cameron, 1991). The burden of proof is always to demonstrate that the aggressive medical intervention is fruitless: that the infant is already dying, is about to die, or has a hold on life that is so entirely artificially maintained that there is no rational purpose in prolonging the dying process. Where it can be demonstrated that any medical intervention is excessive, given the expected outcome, the moral issue abates quite substantially. Parents, and society usually in the form of relatives, the multidisciplinary team, clergy and occasionally lawyers, may be briefed, consulted and a decision not to intervene may be taken. In the UK unlike the USA, such instances are rare and practised only in the case of some profoundly multiply handicapped infants with internal abnormalities incompatible with viability. Of interest to note here is the changing notion of profound handicap, such that few today would consider an infant with Down's syndrome as profoundly multiply handicapped, sufficient to withdraw or withhold treatment; but exceptions are still occasionally noted in the press. On the whole, severely handicapped infants are given a chance of a somewhat 'prolonged life', that is, by assisted ventilation or corrective surgery, but if the fundamental abnormalities cannot be corrected or the disorder reversed, the baby may not be expected to live much past its first year of life, if that. These may be called paradigm cases and, in clinical practice, do not represent the greatest problems (Jonsen, 1981).

In typical paradigm cases palliative care can be advocated. Such care is, however, demanding, emotionally draining and largely within the domain of expert nursing. There is nothing routine, second-rate or morally inappropriate, however, in caring for an infant and its family where CARE is the treatment of choice prescribed by the neonatal team (Clarke and Wheeler, 1992). Parents desperately want their child to live, but not usually at any cost. As one mother recalls saying to the doctors during her premature labour: 'Please, no heroics. . . If this baby is not meant to live, let's not force her. I was terrified that she was too small to survive outside my body. I was just frightened that she would live but in an unconscionably compromised fashion. I wanted Emily to feel the joy of life, not merely the burden of it. I wanted her to be that burbling baby on the bunny blanket. I wanted her to be a child in a high chair, a little girl on the beach with a bucket and spade (Mehren, 1992).

Any other position by prospective parents would be surprising. The overt aim may not be perfection but at least some semblance of 'normality'. It is the criteria for normality that tends to guide the decision not to initiate treatment. If the infant's normal baseline state is such that it is incompatible with life, or incompatible even with an assisted attempt at an adapted life, e.g. corrective neonatal surgery for some congenital abnormalities, such as myelomeningocele etc., then there is indeed little point in performing painful procedures and surgery that are not in themselves palliative or life-sustaining but merely life-prolonging (Berseth *et al.*, 1984; Savage *et al.*, 1987). Not initiating treatment can be a difficult decision to take, with obvious far-reaching consequences, especially if the baby's baseline adaptability to life is severely misjudged, as has often been the case in the past. For example, infants with high myelomeningocele were often not treated at birth, leaving nurses and the family in a quandary as to how they should care for them (Zachary, 1968; Lorber, 1971; Bailey, 1986). Some untreated children survived infancy and their medical problems became even more acute than when they were several days old (Drane, 1984).

Not starting surgical or medical treatment tends to hit the headlines far more quickly than withdrawal of treatment, and seems to be more of an emotive issue, presumably because if treatment is initially withheld inappropriately (however inadvertently), the consequences of such an action are far more permanent and devastating, not to mention at times irredeemable. In the former example the infant is seen to be denied a chance of life, whereas the debate to withdraw treatment focuses on evaluating the level of non-response to intervention.

Twenty years ago, Duff and Campbell (1973) opened up the proverbial Pandora's box by starting a public debate concerning withdrawal and non-treatment decisions in the neonatal unit. Yet in the early 1990s Campbell suggests: 'Many units treat all infants, born alive, aggressively, whatever the weight or gestational age but I have not seen any results, to date, to make me feel that routine intensive care is wise, either for the infant or the family who have to live with the consequences. Below 750 g appropriate for gestational age, the risks of major neurological disability increase considerably' (Campbell, 1992).

The main reasons why the neonatal team may suggest withdrawal of treatment is because the infant who may or may not be severely and multiply handicapped, often due to complications from profound prematurity, is not responding to treatment. The most common accusation however is not that treatment was not initiated or withdrawn, but that treatment was too aggressive, to the extent of holding an infant past the natural point of death and therefore provoking even more damage in the process.

CARING OR CURING?

Physicians may be capable of curing only occasionally, but they and the rest of the neonatal team must always be capable of caring. It is difficult, however, to see examples of caring in some of the instances of medical over-zealouness and surgical prowess in handicapped children who are ex-patients of neonatal units.

Fortunately, however, the same technology that contributed to the 'long dying' of some severely handicapped children is now providing equipment that can detect and assess brain haemorrhages almost immediately, thus avoiding long delays in detecting brain damage and inaccurate assessments of the extent of oxygen deprivation, long-term disability and whether aggressive treatment should continue. Undeniably more small infants survive than ever before and, likewise undeniably, more of the survivors have a good quality of life. The problem is how to reduce the number of children who survive neo-natal illness and trauma and subsequently suffer permanent physical, social or even emotional damage. However reluctant neonatal nurses are to join the ranks of consequentialists, it is hard not to concede some professional responsibility for the long-term effects of the work done. Kantian deontological theory may remind the nurse to respect each infant as an end in itself, which would encourage us to query the unquestioning use of infants' organs as potential donor tissue.

More significantly, a Kantian approach to viewing the infant and its parents as an autonomous unit would suggest that the neonatal nurse should query the rightfulness of inflicting unmeasurable pain and suffering in order to achieve some unknown or uncertain benefit. Intended future good does not necessarily justify the infliction of current pain and suffering, and it is an interesting logic that attempts to support such a rationale solely in order to preserve a baby's life. For the severely handicapped or moribund baby, insisting on preserving life at any cost can be as unjust and macabre a proposition as insisting on keeping a comatose elderly relative on a life-support machine. It is not the value of life that is being disputed, rather the level of pain: an unintended painful existence can do enormous harm. Just because we are capable of preserving life does not necessarily mean that we should always do so.

Loving and subsequently caring for an infant does not in any way diminish the physical and social pain which that infant may experience. Whereas it is not the intention of this chapter to promote the quick death of profoundly handicapped or even moribund infants, neither are we advocating that we are morally obligated to sentence an infant to a horrendous, albeit short, existence, just because of the belief that all life is special. People in the health care field are not and never have been morally obliged to maintain life at any cost. Good health care practice demands that the nature of all intentions is carefully assessed (Duff and Campbell, 1973; Jonsen, 1981). Nurses, however, are always obliged to care for all infants to the limits of their capabilities (Van Maanen, 1990). All babies, both those thriving on therapy and those needing assistance with all activities of living and essentially dying, fall under the neonatal nurse's care and require her sensitivity, wisdom and support. Jonsen sombrely comments: 'Once in the nursery, all infants are considered equal' (Jonsen, 1981).

The greatest insults levelled at neonatal nurses occur when misguided physicians and surgeons withdraw from or refuse to treat a terminally ill or non-viable infant and write in the notes that the infant is for 'nursing care only', equating this with less than expert professional loving intervention. To expertly care for a critically ill or moribund neonate takes competence and compassion as well as an enormous commitment in the form of financial investment (Jonsen, 1981; Fost, 1982; Matthews, 1992).

BALANCING THE COST OF NEONATAL CARE

The vast majority of senior neonatal nurses possess at least two and sometimes three registered nursing qualifications, representing, at a conservative estimate, a minimum of 6 years of nursing education, not to mention any number of additional courses, study days and in-house conferences that they might need to attend to maintain clinical competency and credibility. To train a neonatal nurse takes political commitment and moral courage. The underfunding of neonatal nursing courses and lack of secondment represents an 'empirical' departure from the expressed valuing of their work (Van Maanen, 1990). Neonatal nursing is an area of nursing which is unique in its domain and competence is not acquired by osmosis. It is a terrible indictment of our society that infants who could be cared for in neonatal units are not thus provided for because of lack of funding and expertise. It is not chance that promotes the breastfeeding of infants in neonatal units, but research and excellence in care (Pettit, 1992).

It is clear that, within a finite health care budget, some specialities obtain a greater share of the financial pie than others. Thus, if children represent a quarter of the nation's population at least a semblance of proportional funding should reflect this (Matthews, 1992).

Neonatology is classed as high-powered tertiary referral medicine, hospital-based and requiring extremely costly equipment and intervention. Although cost curtailment and cost evaluative audit exercises are conducted in neonatal units, as in all other health care units, some classic cost curtailing measures that have proved effective in other situations, especially those based on medical and biophysical norms, simply do not operate in the neonatal environment. It is almost impossible to predict how long a neonate may stay on a unit, or the possible cost of treatment and cost to the community should the infant be sent home. Increasing the number of neonatal cots and bassinettes is also of questionable value, since the necessary high patient to staff ratio of these units implies the potential for congestion (assuming there would be staff available to deal with the increase in cots), which in turn discourages the family from visiting (Klaus and Kennell, 1970; Hewitt, 1990).

There is an increasing body of knowledge which suggests that very premature infants kept in neonatal intensive care units suffer much worse from emotional and physical problems in later life than children who did not spend time on such units (Yu *et al.*, 1986; Hack and Fanaroff, 1989; Ludman, 1992). Child abuse, delinquent behaviour and, recently, even a suggestion of increased adolescent suicides, have been linked with prolonged stays in neonatal units. One of the insinuated underlying factors has been inadequate or inappropriate maternal or familial bonding with the infant (Salk *et al.*, 1988; Ludman, 1992). Provisions must be made for parents and the family to visit, which requires commitment from staff and financial backing from politicians and hospital management.

The Patient's Charter calls for the inauguration of the 'named nurse' but how many neonatal units can afford such a luxury, which may require the employment of a greater skills mix on the ward? Traditionally, the primary nurse bonds with the family and acts as the family's advocate in the interests of their infant. This approach calls for commitment from the nurse which is reflected in society's esteem and trust. The level of responsibility that is given to the nurse is often great, but the baby belongs to his parents and they need to recognise this. Modern management techniques and principles may not allow such an approach, do not favour staff stability or permanency, and do not adequately reward expertise, given the current salary structure and fixed budgets. If neonatal units are to reflect social justice and equity, far more needs to be done to inject funds, train more nurses and encourage staff stability, and thereby foster expertise and caring.

It is a characteristic of the professional caring which nurses perform that it is something 'lived', not measured on audit reports, so that it is not likely to be noticed by unit managers. Jackie's mother recalls her daughter's first Christmas, spent in the unit: 'We were delighted to see that several of our 'favourite' nurses were on duty. Laura (her nurse), was standing by Jackie. "Come and see, she's got her best dress on for you!" she called. There was Jackie, looking just like a "proper baby" wearing a tiny blue smock for the first time. There was a Christmas card to us from Jackie. I still have it in her photograph album. Father Christmas had brought her a rabbit and that, too, is still around, rather worn and well loved now.' (Cooper and Harpin, 1991). These caring acts can never be quantified but, without them, all the nursing and medical intervention in neonatal units would be sterile, however clinically successful.

CONCLUSION

In looking at the ethical issues pertinent to neonatology and the work of neonatal nurses, it becomes abundantly clear that, although solutions to the problems may be hard to come by, openly discussing the moral dilemmas and causes of moral distress cannot help but clear up misunderstandings (Johnstone, 1988; Drane, 1984; Lyall, 1989). At the core of much ethical distress lies a lack of adequate communication. Either we refuse to hear and see what is being presented to us, or we do not know how to interpret it. In areas where emotions can run high and professional staff can expect to be overworked, fraught and extremely stressed, a staff desensitizing counselling/discussion group is important. This group, if run with the help of a nurse who is aware of ethical issues, could enable the discussion of various issues as they arise (Spinks and Bowering, 1990; Allmark, 1992). The overlap between psychological health and moral integrity is such that it may be difficult to separate out these presenting factors. However, the benefits to staff of being able to voice concerns over moral issues are immeasurable.

Ethical issues occur almost routinely in the expected course of neonatal work. Some of these concerns are predictable and unavoidable given human nature, the norms of society and professional demands. An analysis of problems along with the approach of developing a grounded theory of neonatal nursing and its moral content may serve nurses' interests. Some theorists might say that the benefit of grounded theory is that it can provide a foundation from which various moral frameworks or views can be applied, and against which the true thoughts and actions of nurses can be evaluated. The best way to feel even moderately in control of a situation is to feel that you are responsible for it and can control or predict its outcome. The same holds true in the field of applied ethics. Nurses need not necessarily feel powerless in the face of overwhelming moral problems, but the time to start reversing this trend is not when the press and mass media are camped outside the nursery door. Only by constant and persistent evaluation of moral problems will nurses feel somewhat more in control (Berseth *et al.*, 1984). Such an approach takes moral courage and conviction and may call for occasional manifestations of professional heroism. As Elsea (1985) points out in her advice to paediatric nurses, 'Since few hard and fast rules or easy answers can be applied in ethical decision making, nurses must be prepared to handle ethical dilemmas in a logical way'. Thus, it is precisely because we care about our patients and are ready to care for them, that we can echo the poet and say:

> '. . . here is the deepest secret nobody knows
> (here is the root of the root and the bud of the bud
> and the sky of the sky of a tree called life; which grows
> higher than soul can hope or mind can hide)
> and this is the wonder that's keeping the stars apart
> I carry your heart (I carry it in my heart)'
>
> e.e. cummings 1960

REFERENCES

Ackerman, T.F. (1992) Innovative lifesaving treatments: do children have a moral right to receive them? in *Contemporary Issues in Paediatric Ethics* (ed M.M. Burgess), Edwin Mallen Press, Lewisten, Chapter 3.

Allmark, P. (1992) The ethical enterprise of nursing. *Journal of Advanced Nursing* **17**, 16–20.

Bailey, C.F. (1986) Withholding or withdrawing treatment on handicapped newborns. *Paediatric Nursing* **12** (6), 413–6.

Berseth, C.L., Kenny, J.D. and Durand, R. (1984) Newborn ethical dilemmas: intensive care and intermediate care nursing attitudes. *Critical Care Medicine* **12**(6), 508.

Cameron, N. (1991) The margins of the human race, in *The New Medicine, The Revolution in Technology and Ethics*, Hodder and Stoughton, London, pp. 92–108.

Campbell, A.G.M. (1992) Neonatal intensive care: where and how do we draw the line? in *Philosophy and Health Care* (eds E. Matthews and M. Menlowe), Avebury, Aldershot, pp. 155–75.

Campbell, A., Gillett, G. and Jones, G. (1992) Neonatal and childhood issues, in *Practical Medical Ethics*, OUP, Oxford, pp. 69–80.

Clarke, J.B. and Wheeler, S.J. (1992) A view of the phenomenon of caring in nursing practice. *Journal of Advanced Nursing* **17**, 1283–90.

Cooper, A. and Harpin, V. (1991) (eds) *This is our Child*, OUP, Oxford.

cummings, e.e. (1960) *Selected Poems 1923–1958*, Faber and Faber, London.

Darbyshire, P. (1989) Ethical issues in the care of the profoundly multiply handicapped child, in *Ethics in Paediatric Nursing*, (ed. G.M. Brykczyńska), Chapman and Hall, London pp. 100–18.

Drane, J.F. (1984) The defective child: ethical guidelines for painful dilemmas. *Journal of Obstetrics, Gynaecology and Neonatal Nursing*, **13**(1), 42–8.

Duff, R.S. and Campbell, A.G.M. (1973) Moral and ethical dilemmas in the special care nursery. *New England Journal of Medicine* **289** (7), 890–1.

Dunn, P.M. (1985) Age of foetal viability. *Maternal and Child Health*, **10**(4), 102, 104.

Elsea, S.B. (1985) Ethics in maternal–child nursing. *Maternal and Child Nursing* **10**, 303–4, 308.

Engelhardt, H.T. (1977) Some persons are humans, some humans are persons and the world is what we persons make of it, in *Philosophical Medical Ethics: its Nature and Significance*, (eds. S.F. Spicker and H.T. Engelhardt), D. Reidel Publishing Company, Dordrecht, Holland, pp. 183–94.

Fost, N. (1982) *Putting Hospitals on Notice.* The Hastings Centre Report Aug, pp. 5–8.

Fry, S.T. (1990) Brave new world: removing body parts from infants. *Nursing Outlook* **38**(3), 152.

Goldenring, J.M. (1985) The brain life theory: towards a consistent biological definition of humanness. *Journal of Medical Ethics* **11**, 198–209.

Hack, M. and Fanaroff, A.A. (1989) Outcomes of extremely low birth weight infants between 1982–1988. *New England Journal of Medicine* **321**, 1642–7.

Hewitt, J. (1990) The sibling response to hospitalisation. *Paediatric Nursing* **2**(10), 12–3.

Iglesias, T. (1986) What kind of being is the human embryo? *Ethics and Medicine* **2** (1), 2–7.
IME (1988) Foetal brain tissue transplants in Parkinson's. *IME Bulletin*, **37**, pp. 12–14.
Johnstone, M.J. (1988) Law, professional ethics and the problem of conflict with personal values. *International Journal of Nursing Studies* **25** (2), 147–57.
Jonsen, A. (1981) Justice and the defective newborn, in *Justice and Health Care* (ed E.E. Shelp), D. Reidel Publishing Co., Dordrecht, pp. 95–107.
Klaus, M. and Kennell, J.H. (1970) Mothers separated from their newborn infants. *Paediatric Clinics of North America* **13**, 1015–37.
Kohner, M. (1992) *A Dignified Ending*, SANDS, London.
Kuhse, H. (1985) Interests. *Journal of Medical Ethics* **11**, 146–9.
Kuhse, H. and Singer, P. (1989) The quality/quantity of life distinction and its moral importance for nurses. *International Journal of Nursing Studies* **26** (3), 203–17.
Kushner, T. and Belloitti, R. (1985) Baby Fae, a beastly business. *Journal of Medical Ethics* **11**, 178–83.
Lamb, D. (1992) Organ transplants and anacephalic infants, in *Philosophy and Health Care*, (eds E. Matthews and M. Menlowe), Avebury, Aldershot, pp. 124–34.
Lappé, M. (1981) Justice and prenatal life, in *Justice and Health Care* (ed E. Shelp), D. Reidel Publishing Co., Dordrecht, pp. 83–94.
Lorber, J. (1971) Results of treatment of myelomeningocele. *Developmental Medical Child Neurology* **13**, 279–303.
Ludman, J. (1992) Emotional development after major neonatal surgery. *Paediatric Nursing* **4** (4), 20–2.
Lyall, J. (1989) A human reaction. *Nursing Times* **85**(38), 19.
Matthews, E. (1992) The ethics of rationing, in *Philosophy and Health Care*, (eds E. Matthews and M. Melowe), Avebury, Aldershot, pp. 28–43.
Mehren, E. (1992) Born too soon. *Readers Digest* **140**(841), 149–84.
Nelson, J.L. (1988) Animals, handicapped children and the tragedy of marginal cases. *Journal of Medical Ethics* **14**, 191–3.
Pettit, J. (1992) Establishing successful breast feeding in special care. *Paediatric Nursing* **4**(7), 24–5.
Polkinghorne, J. (1989) *Review of the Guidance on the Research use of Foetuses and Foetal Material*, HMSO, London.
Salk, L., Lipsitt, L.P., Sturner, W.G., *et al.* (1988) Relationship of maternal and perinatal conditions to eventual adolescent suicide. *Lancet* **98**, 624–7.
Savage, T.A., Cullen, D.L., Kirchhoff, K.T. *et al.* (1987) Nurses' response to do not resuscitate orders in the neonatal intensive care unit. *Nursing Research* **36**(6), 307–73.
Shea, M.C. (1985) Ensoulment and IVF embryos. *Journal of Medical Ethics* **13**(2), 95–7.
Singer, P. (1992) Embryo experimentation and the moral status of the embyro, in *Philosophy and Health Care*, (eds E. Matthews and M. Menlowe), Avebury, Aldershot, pp. 81–91.

Spinks, P. and Bowering, P. (1990) Staff support. *Paediatric Nursing* **2**(2), 19–20.

Tindall, C. (1992) Public attitudes and the treatment of neomorts, in *Philosophy and Health Care* (eds E. Matthews and M. Menlowe), Avebury, Aldershot, pp. 135–45.

Tooley, M. (1983) The relevance of the moral status of the fetus; Persons and human beings; The Concept of Person, in *Abortion and Infanticide*, Oxford University Press, Oxford, Chapters 3, 4 and 5, pp. 40–105.

Trammell, R.L. (1975) Saving life and taking life. *Journal of Philosophy* **72**, 131–7.

Van Maanen, M. (1990) Nursing in transition: an analysis of the state of the art in relation to the conditions of practice and society's expectations. *Journal of Advanced Nursing* **15**, 914–24.

Warnock, M. (1992) The good of the child, in *The Uses of Philosophy*, Blackwell, Oxford, Chapter 5.

Whyte, D. (1989) Ethics in neonatal nursing, in *Ethics in Paediatric Nursing* (ed. G.M. Brykczyńska), Chapman and Hall, London, pp. 23–41.

Yu, V.Y.M., Loke, H.L., Bajok, B. *et al.* (1986) Prognosis for infants born at 23–28 weeks' gestation. *British Medical Journal* **293**, 1200–3.

Zachary, R.B. (1968) Ethical and social aspects of treatment of spina bifida. *Lancet* **2**, 274–6.

18

Home oxygenation

Kathy Sleath

A large percentage of preterm babies surviving the neonatal period will generally have been discharged home by the time they reach term. However, most neonatal units will see a small but increasing number of babies with continuing problems who remain in hospital for a prolonged period, and often become labelled as 'geriatric neonates'. These ongoing chronic problems tend to fall into one of the following categories:

- Neurological problems;
- Congenital or acquired gastrointestinal abnormalities needing surgical intervention;
- Bronchopulmonary dysplasia (BPD) or chronic lung disease (CLD).

This chapter will concentrate on the nursing management of the increasing number of babies with chronic lung disease who remain oxygen-dependent for a prolonged period, necessitating discharge home on continuous oxygen therapy and management.

DEFINITIONS

Bronchopulmonary dysplasia (BPD) is described as a chronic pulmonary condition of infants who have experienced respiratory failure. They remain oxygen-dependent for at least 28 days and have associated clinical and radiological findings (Northway, 1967). It is recognized to be a result of barotrauma due to mechanical ventilation and oxygen toxicity following hyaline membrane disease.

Some babies will develop chronic lung disease as a result of other complications, such as recurrent aspiration, patent ductus arteriosus, acute or chronic infections and apnoea of prematurity. They may have been ventilated for a short period only but remain oxygen-dependent at 28 days, and have associated radiological findings of severe hyperinflation alternating with areas of increased density. The term chronic lung disease may be used more widely to include BPD, as it covers the whole spectrum and the management and treatment remains much the same (Southall and Samuels, 1990).

These babies can be very demanding and irritable as they mature and will often stretch a nurse to her limits. Understanding the condition and why the effort required for breathing is such hard work can be of great benefit when planning the care and needs of these babies (and parents), to allow for an optimum environment for growth and development.

PATHOPHYSIOLOGY

These babies consume excessive amounts of energy in their increased effort to breathe. To understand why, each area of the respiratory tract can be considered in relation to the symptoms that the baby suffers.

Small airways

There is dysplasia of the respiratory epithelium and excessive mucus production, which leads to narrowing of the airways. This causes an increased resistance to airflow, thereby increasing the work of breathing.

Alveoli

There are areas of severe hyperinflation alternating with areas of increased density, due to collapse or fibrosis. This causes poor lung compliance with the high intrathoracic pressures needed to expand the lungs, which increases the work of breathing. The emphysematous areas receive excessive amounts of ventilation but are poorly perfused. The increased work of breathing causes overventilation and therefore carbon dioxide retention.

The areas of collapse are inefficient units of ventilation and therefore hypoxaemia is present. To compensate the respiratory rate increases, increasing the work of breathing.

Pulmonary vascular bed

Alveolar hypoxia causes the vascular bed to constrict and the pulmonary artery pressures to increase, which can lead to pulmonary hypertension and right heart failure. This is mainly reversible, but persistent hypoxaemia leads to persistent pulmonary hypertension and irreversible disease (cor pulmonale), and it is this which in the past has led to the significant mortality of these babies. Adequate oxygenation is therefore essential to their survival. Even a mild degree of chronic hypoxaemia can have general effects, such as sleep disturbances and poor growth, as well as the effects which may be associated with acute apnoeic episodes and respiratory infections. This leads to worsening lung damage, heart failure and possibly death (Abman *et al.*, 1985).

The ultimate cure for chronic lung disease is the natural growth and maturation of normal lung tissue which occurs with increasing age and weight gain. It is a long struggle for many babies to achieve this, with many hurdles to surmount during the first year, and it is during this period that a high standard of nursing care and the individual love and care of the family are critical.

MANAGEMENT OF BPD/CLD

Hospitals now run neonatal community services, allowing babies with chronic lung disease to be discharged home, to be cared for by their families. Close monitoring, support and supervision are provided by a team of people who are familiar with preterm lung disease and oxygen therapy, until the baby has ceased to need oxygen and his growth and development are satisfactory. This ensures the minimum risk to the baby and minimal anxiety to the family. These babies remain extremely vulnerable after discharge, although home is undoubtedly the best place for them (Sleath, 1989).

By the time a baby with chronic lung disease reaches the special care nursery, although possibly still fairly small, he will probably be fairly mature. It is usually at this point that the parents will start to feel frustration. Having seen their baby survive the neonatal period, through intensive care, their expectations begin to rise about the probability of taking a healthy baby home. They see other babies of the same age getting better and being discharged or transferred, but their baby's progress seems to have come to a standstill. Parents need a very positive approach with respect to their baby's condition. They need to understand what CLD is, why their baby has it and how it will be managed, including the possibility of taking him home while still on oxygen therapy. Oxygen should not be seen as a barrier to his discharge but as a part of his treatment that will help him recover and grow into a healthy toddler. If this is discussed with the parents they will look forward to discharge like any other parent and, although there will always be a degree of apprehension, this is probably applicable to all parents taking a baby home from a neonatal unit.

Planning nursing care

Babies with CLD can present with minimal symptoms and ongoing problems or have multiple problems. Planning for their care is very much an individual assessment to identify the ongoing symptoms and problems and how to manage them, and also to identify potential problems and avoid them. These can generally be subdivided into:

- breathing
- nutrition and growth
- development and the family.

It is important to remember that the level of care will be gradually reduced as baby and parents are prepared for discharge. One of the hardest things for parents to do is to believe that their baby is safe with less intensive monitoring: they become very dependent on equipment and staff. Parents must be involved with planning and doing as much of their baby's care as possible; this will naturally be determined by their home commitments, particularly when there are siblings to consider.

BREATHING

Oxygen

The main problem for these babies is their inability to maintain adequate oxygenation without additional inspired oxygen. Consequently they need a continuous concentration of inspired oxygen to maintain stable and consistent oxygen saturation.

Once extubated, a baby will be transferred to a headbox with specific concentrations to maintain adequate oxygenation. An older baby needs physical contact and stimulation (Chapter 15) along with encouragement of oral feeding, but removing him from the headbox causes hypoxia, alternating with periods of hyperoxia when face mask oxygen is used during handling. It is also difficult to monitor SaO_2 accurately at these times, because of movement artefacts.

Ideally, once the baby's condition is stable, irrespective of size, nasal oxygen therapy via a single nasal catheter or double nasal cannula depending on unit policy, is the most appropriate way of delivering a consistent flow of oxygen to maintain adequate oxygenation at all times, during sleep, feeding and handling. Both methods have advantages and disadvantages and which is preferable is probably related to the method one is familiar with.

The single catheter, either size 5 or 6 Fr, is inserted via one nostril into the nasopharynx. The distance that this is inserted is determined by measuring the distance from the tip of the nose to the eyebrow in the very small baby, or from ear to nostril in the larger baby. The catheter can then be secured to one cheek and tucked into the baby's clothing at the back to prevent pulling or kinking. This method is generally well tolerated, although some babies may have increased nasal secretions for the first few days, particularly if the catheter is not inserted far enough. It is not easily removed and, during upper respiratory tract infection, can bypass the nasal discharge and still adequately oxygenate the baby.

The double nasal cannula is placed about 1 cm into each nostril and then secured to each cheek. This can sometimes be difficult in very small babies as the prongs tend to slip out easily, but with the older toddler they can be placed in position without any tape. The main concern with this method is that the cannula can easily be lifted out by the more active baby and placed on top of his nose. During upper respiratory tract infections, a higher flow tends to be necessary because of the nasal discharge.

To determine the baby's oxygen flow requirements with either method, continuous SaO_2 monitoring is necessary for at least the first 24 h, with specific attention given to changes in SaO_2 during sleeping, feeding, while awake and when crying or distressed during procedures.

There are a number of low-flow oxygen meters which allow delivery from 1 l/min down to 0.1 l/min, but probably the most useful and widely used is the 100–500 cl/min variety. Humidity measurement can be included in the circuit and is probably useful for small babies in the hospital environment.

Most paediatricians now agree that these babies need SaO_2 to be kept above 90% at all times, but it is not always appreciated how even mild hypoxia can cause pulmonary hypertension, with some babies far more sensitive than others. The only way to identify a baby's response to oxygen and increased SaO_2 is by echocardiogram to measure pulmonary artery pressures. If this facility is not available, it is probably preferable to maintain SaO_2 between 94–97% at all times, to minimize the risk of irreversible pulmonary hypertension and, at the same time, allow for better growth. Most babies, by this time, should be past the risk of retinopathy.

Monitoring

Babies with CLD who remain small and vulnerable and relatively unstable need continuous oxygen monitoring, preferably using non-invasive pulse oximetry (Rome *et al.*, (1984). Once a baby has been established on nasal oxygen therapy and his condition and oxygen requirements have been stable for some days, the necessity for continuous monitoring should be reconsidered. One of the reasons that babies are left on continuous monitoring while in hospital is to help staff care for them safely, knowing that the monitor will detect changes in their condition. At the same time, monitors can create anxiety and a degree of dependency in the parents. It is not unusual to see a mother staring at the monitor rather than looking at her baby. When planning discharge, intermittent monitoring is preferable to give the parents a chance to become familiar with looking at and assessing their baby's breathing pattern and general wellbeing. An apnoea monitor is probably the only one needed continuously at this time.

There will, however, always be an exception. Some babies may be less stable and require variable oxygen concentrations and would probably go home initially with continuous monitoring facilities.

How often a CLD baby's oxygen saturation should be monitored will vary between units, and depends on his clinical stability. For example, intermittent monitoring for three half-hour periods during every 24 h gives a fairly comprehensive overview of how he is coping. Through a sleep, during feeding and after feeding, the SaO_2 and pulse rate are recorded every 2–3 min for each period, ensuring that the signal is good with no movement artefact. This is something a mother can do while she is visiting and this gives her a better insight into accurate monitoring.

An overnight recording of saturations should be done weekly or if there is any increase in oxygen requirements. This gives an overall picture of trends through a prolonged period and identifies any episodes of desaturation during sleep, as these babies are at risk of intermittent sleep hypoxia (Zinman *et al.*, 1992).

Most oximeters have a memory facility to enable one to download 8 h of recording on to a personal computer or a two-channel printer. It is especially useful for older babies, as they have a more regular sleep pattern, enabling accurate monitoring of trends, as quiet and REM sleep states are easily identified.

MEDICATIONS

Some babies may only be receiving vitamins and iron by the time they go home, whereas others may remain on a selection of some or all of the following: diuretic therapy, antireflux therapy, mineral supplements, calorie supplements, bronchodilators and steroid inhaled therapy plus the standard vitamins and iron. The number of drugs that they are on can be overwhelming for the parents, and they must be given the opportunity and time to become familiar with administering them, particularly because of the minute doses involved and also to understand the importance and action of each.

POSITIONING

With the current Department of Health recommendations regarding cot death and the advice to lay babies on their side or supine, parents will be very anxious about what position is safe and right for their baby.

Some babies with CLD, particularly those with severe BPD, may breathe and oxygenate better when nursed prone and tilted at an angle. Prior to discharge they need to be monitored supine and prone to see if there is a significant change in SaO_2 and the issue discussed between staff and the parents. Input from the physiotherapist is useful at this stage as many of these babies adopt a poor position developmentally, because their respiratory effort encourages them to arch their backs and extend their necks to make breathing easier, particularly if they are hypoxic.

GROWTH AND NUTRITION

Growth failure is a significant problem for many babies with chronic lung disease. Growth is essential for the repair and development of lung tissue as well as general development and feeding. Nutrition is a major issue of management (Lucas *et al.*, 1989). Trying to achieve adequate growth can be extremely difficult and frustrating, both for the baby and his carers and requires good nutritional intake and oxygenation. One of the main factors for poor growth is the increased energy expenditure for breathing: studies have shown a 25% increase in energy expenditure, compared with babies without lung disease (Yeh, 1989). Other factors related to growth failure may be chronic hypoxia, poor nutritional intake, gastro-oesophageal reflux, vomiting, emotional stress and deprivation.

An increased oxygen supply may be needed to compensate for the increased respiratory effort and the hard work required to feed; this will make feeding easier to cope with. Hypoxia during feeding can increase the risk of aspiration, respiratory distress, apnoea and bradycardia.

Many babies with CLD or BPD may have their fluid intake restricted to avoid fluid overload and heart failure. Whether restricted or not, a high calorie intake will be necessary to compensate for their high energy expenditure. Low birthweight formulas will provide a high calorie and mineral intake and it may be necessary to continue these formulas after discharge, particularly if the infant is on a fluid-restricted diet or has a poor nutritional intake due to poor feeding. Some babies may need additional calorie supplements as well.

For many babies with CLD breast milk alone will not provide adequate nutrition, and it may be necessary to combine low birth weight milk or other additives with breast milk, or to modify the feeding regimen to ensure a mix of high-calorie bottle feeds as well as the breast feeds. It can be very difficult for a mother to understand why this is necessary, and needs sensitive handling by medical and nursing staff.

Follow-on milk formulas for preterm babies have now been developed as the next step in nutrition, once low birth weight milk is discontinued. These provide additional energy, protein and minerals to allow for catch-up growth to continue.

For the older baby with more severe BPD, early weaning needs to be considered as a means of increasing his energy intake without an increase in fluid intake. This tends to be well received and can make a significant difference to growth as he gets older.

Close liaison and follow-up with a paediatric dietician is essential if the baby is to receive optimal nutritional requirements to promote growth, both in hospital and at home.

FEEDING PROBLEMS

Many of these babies will be poor, disorganized feeders and continue to have oral feeding problems, long after the appropriate postconceptual age for sucking and swallowing coordination has been reached. Most will be feeding orally by discharge, although they may sometimes be still struggling to achieve an adequate intake. These feeding problems will generally be attributed to prolonged ventilation and endotracheal intubation, resulting in hypersensitive palates. For nursing management, the following points should be considered when planning a feeding programme:

- Optimal oxygenation to avoid increased respiratory distress;
- A quiet environment, with minimal distractions to the baby and his feeder;
- A limited number of nurses (with experience of feeding these babies) along with the mother to allow a consistent and regular feeding pattern;
- A clear feeding plan to provide the necessary encouragement and support for sucking and swallowing coordination, taking into account individual preferences for the appropriate teat, temperature of milk, support of the jaw and gentle stimulation to encourage sucking. There may be poor oral muscle tone and poor oral reflexes. Tongue and jaw movements are less controlled, with poor cheek stability and inadequate lip seal.

The mother, with support, is the right person to feed her baby and this helps to develop a relationship and pattern prior to discharge. With many babies, feeding tends to improve once they are at home because of the consistency and the relationship between mother and infant.

The paediatric speech therapist can play an important part in the early management of the sick neonate who has delayed oral feeding, and in assessing oral–motor function. This may be the appropriate person to advise on feeding regimens and oral stimulation, and is often a good source of advice concerning feeding teats and bottles. Management of the disorganized feeder is a subject covered by Vandenberg (1990), and is important reading for neonatal nurses.

Some babies may require nasogastric tube feeding for a prolonged period, and if parents are keen to take their baby home while still tube feeding there is no reason against it, provided that there is adequate support in the community. This baby is generally more mature, with severe BPD, and his mother is by far the best person to get oral feeding established. Tube feeding is far more demanding than oxygen therapy at home, and can leave the mother feeling very frustrated about her baby's inability to feed.

GASTRO-OESOPHAGEAL REFLUX AND VOMITING

Preterm babies have a higher incidence of gastro-oesophageal reflux than term babies (Newell *et al.*, 1989), and for those with chronic lung disease this can be a contributory factor to worsening lung problems (Jolley *et al.*, 1990). If a baby vomits or regurgitates milk frequently, or has intermittent episodes of desaturation or apnoea and bradycardia, reflux needs to be excluded, either by a 24 h pH study or by a barium swallow. If this proves to be positive, treatment can be started. This includes thickening the feeds, giving antacids, e.g. gaviscon, and careful positioning. He needs to be nursed tilted and prone, either supported in his cot or in a reflux chair. This is generally enough to improve the problem. If reflux persists, prokinetic agents such as cisapride have been shown to be effective.

If reflux is not positively identified, there are many other factors which may contribute to excessive vomiting. Diuretics are emetic and can aggravate the situation. Often these babies find it difficult to bring up wind and then vomit when they eventually manage to do so. Excessive coughing can cause a baby to vomit, which can in time develop into a behavioural problem, when they learn that vomiting brings attention. Excessive vomiting can be frustrating and distressing for the parents, particularly after discharge, and it needs early management to minimize the problem whenever possible.

ENVIRONMENT

Mature babies with CLD are easily stressed. Prolonged hospitalization creates insecurity which, added to the stress due to lack of individual love and attention, results in irritable and demanding behaviour. This can lead to hypoxia, which inhibits growth, and this becomes a continuing cycle of events (Figure 18.1)

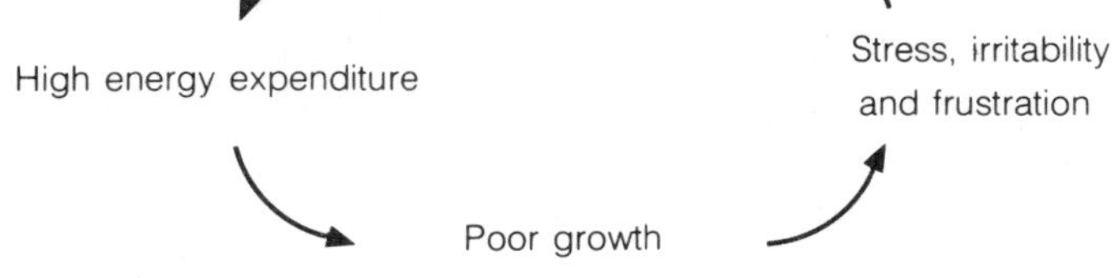

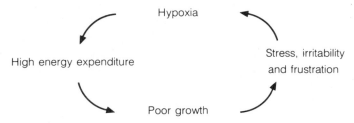

Figure 18.1 Hypoxia cycle.

To provide an optimal environment for growth and therefore recovery, it is necessary to avoid stress and hypoxia, as well as provide a satisfactory nutritional intake; this is not always easy to achieve in hospital, and the ultimate answer to avoid these complications is early discharge home.

DEVELOPMENT

As many as 30% of very low birth weight babies will have moderate to major delay in development because of their prematurity and need for neonatal intensive care. This percentage increases with the smaller baby, with 50% reported for babies less than 800 g (Bernbaum and Hoffman-Williamson, 1986). Babies with added complications, such as BPD, remain even more vulnerable and the developmental delay is not always apparent at the time of discharge.

Even in the nursery it is important that nurses are able to recognize factors that produce stress and the effect that it has on the baby. Care is planned to minimize stress, providing an optimal environment for long-term developmental outcome. Factors such as noise, bright lights, pain and inappropriate and excessive handling can all be reduced by environmental change and planning care (Als *et al.*, 1986). Baby massage is another method which is recognized for its advantage in reducing stress. Chapters 14 and 15 discuss ways to reduce stress and enhance development in the neonatal unit. Teaching parents to understand what causes stress and how to reduce it is an important part of the nurse's role.

Skin-to-skin contact (kangaroo care) between the mother and infant can be a very effective method of reducing stress, resulting in improved oxygenation (Whitelaw *et al.*, 1988; Acolet *et al.*, 1989). The baby is placed naked except for a nappy between his mother's breasts in an upright position. Holding him like this, the mother more naturally talks or sings to her baby and gently strokes his head. Breathing becomes more relaxed as the SaO_2 rises and he becomes very calm and content. It also has a very positive effect on the mother in boosting her confidence in handling her baby, and on the general mother–baby relationship. This is definitely something fathers can do in a similar way.

It may become apparent to the parents, particularly after discharge, that their baby has significant motor delay. He will be compared with their friends' full-term babies whose progress appears to be so much faster. It is important that parents understand, before discharge, that developmental delay is possible because of the prematurity, but the majority will catch up even though it may not be before 2–3 years of age, or even longer for babies with severe BPD and associated poor growth. A full physiotherapy assessment may be helpful to identify any significant problems so that advice can be given to parents on positioning and exercises, which they can do, to allow the baby every opportunity to catch up with his development without forming bad habits.

The parents will need support and encouragement throughout this period if their baby has significant delay. Regular developmental assessments will be done either by the hospital or by the community child development team.

FAMILY

The importance of the parents in caring for their baby cannot be overemphasized, and has been mentioned throughout this book. Families having an infant with CLD may have multiple problems to overcome prior to taking an oxygen-dependent baby home, and will need individually tailored support and advice.

When first approached about taking their baby home on oxygen, most parents will feel extremely anxious about their ability to cope and what effect it will have on their family life. The safety of oxygen in the home and the risks to the baby will be concerns that they immediately voice. The more contact with and care of their baby that the parents have had in the neonatal unit, the more confident they will feel about their baby, understanding his problems and identifying his needs when planning his care.

The mother may have spent a limited amount of time with her baby because of other children or the distance that the family live from the hospital, particularly if there are financial implications. The earlier possibility of home oxygen therapy is discussed with the parents, the easier they will be able to accept it and look forward to the prospect. They have to accept that their baby is not 'normal' and their expectations may have changed slightly, but understanding what CLD or BPD is enables them to accept the problem and allows them to plan and look forward to their baby's discharge.

Some parents may need the opportunity to talk about their feelings and express their anxieties and fears. Often a psychologist, as an independent member of the team, can play an important role during this period. The named nurse/primary nurse or person who is identified to prepare the family for discharge needs to build up a good relationship of trust and communication. Involving many people can cause conflicting advice to be given and, more than anything else, these parents need consistency.

A social worker may be involved, particularly if there are financial or housing problems that make it difficult to take a small, vulnerable baby home. Benefits are available to some families.

Parents may find it helpful to speak to a family who have already taken their baby home on oxygen, or to contact the BPD support group or the Nippers Group.

DISCHARGE PREPARATION AND PLANNING MANAGEMENT AT HOME

With the increasing number of very low birth weight babies who survive but remain oxygen-dependent because of CLD, it is becoming increasingly popular and cost-effective to send them home. To ensure a safe and happy baby without major problems and trauma to the family, there needs to be close supervision and management in the community.

Before a baby is sent home on oxygen, the team available for follow-up needs to be identified. The options currently available are:

- a hospital-based neonatal community nurse whose responsibility is to follow up all preterm babies being discharged, or a combined unit/community nurse who may only follow up babies with ongoing problems;
- paediatric community teams, often with at least one member having neonatal experience and ready to take on the geriatric neonate with ongoing problems;

- discharge into the GP and health visitor's responsibility; this is not uncommon but less frequent nowadays. Major problems may develop because of the lack of experience and understanding of CLD, and therefore these babies will need frequent visits back to the hospital for either day or overnight monitoring and assessment.

There needs to be close liaison between the hospital paediatrician managing the baby and the community team, and some input in the unit prior to discharge, to allow a problem-free transitional period from hospital to home.

Allowing a nurse to make occasional visits when the unit may be quiet does not provide a reliable and supportive service to the family, and may be detrimental to all concerned as some families become very dependent on unit staff. The Royal College of Physicians (1992) gives very clear recommendations as to how oxygen-dependent infants and children should be followed up (and by whom), and guidelines in respect of equipment, monitoring and education and liaison.

CRITERIA FOR DISCHARGE

Once a baby has reached a relatively stable condition with consistent oxygen requirements, and the parents feel ready to take their baby home in the near future, preparation for discharge can begin. Criteria for discharge are as follows:

- The baby is preferably bottle, or breastfeeding (nasogastric tube feeding is considered).
- He is gaining weight.
- Nasal oxygen therapy is well tolerated.
- There are preferably two adults in the home (a single parent will need a local support person who can assist with care and supervision).
- Home conditions are adequate, with a telephone installed.
- No other medical complications.
- Support from the GP and health visitor.

Once a decision is made by the medical/nursing staff and parents, a date is set. This gives the parents time to organize their home life and the hospital time to set up and implement a teaching programme for the parents. The teaching programme includes:

- changing the nasal catheter;
- use of oxygen equipment;
- safety of oxygen in the home;
- resuscitation;
- assessment of breathing
- clinical signs of hypoxia;
- administration of medications;
- environment.

The use of oxygen in the home and the safety factors regarding storing and changing cylinders needs to be discussed. Parents need to understand the risks with smoking and naked flames. In this respect, concentrators are the safer option as there is no need to store a large supply of cylinders, with gas under pressure and, with small children or animals around, there is less risk of damage.

Full resuscitation and the use of an apnoea monitor is explained and practised, with considerable time spent teaching the parents how to assess their baby's normal breathing pattern and how this changes if he is unwell or if the oxygen supply is disconnected. Parents need to see what their baby looks like when severely or mildly hypoxic.

Parents need to understand the risks of respiratory viruses, particularly in the baby's first year, so it is important to stress the need to avoid contact with coughs and colds and crowded environments, such as supermarkets and schools, GP surgeries and baby clinics. This obviously can be very difficult when there are siblings in the family, but it is still important for parents to be aware of the risks. Home visits by the GP or health visitor may have to be arranged.

Prior to discharge, parents are asked to be resident in the unit for at least 24 h and to care for their baby in their own room, away from the unit. This gives them the opportunity to take full responsibility, while support is still close at hand. It also gives them an insight into the baby's needs and demands over a 24 h period, and how these may change their lives.

EQUIPMENT AND LIAISON

Advance planning allows time for the necessary arrangement and preparation of equipment for the oxygen supply, and time for liaison with all concerned with the baby's ongoing management.

There are currently two options available for supplying oxygen in the community, both prescribed by the GP. Oxygen cylinders with a standard bullnose head are supplied and delivered by the local chemist. A system for delivering a low flow (less than 1 l) needs to be supplied by the hospital. For babies on a very low flow of oxygen (less than 100 cl), with the likelihood of coming off oxygen in a relatively short time, cylinders may be the most appropriate method of supply. For babies on long-term therapy, with higher requirements, an oxygen concentrator is the preferred choice of supply. This is a machine which plugs into the domestic electricity supply and takes in ambient air, separates oxygen from nitrogen and other gases and supplies oxygen-enriched gas to the baby, reaching a concentration of 96%. This is also available on prescription and is supplied by companies with contracts to regional health authorities. A low-flow meter needs to be ordered (as an extra item), when arranging for the fitting of a concentrator.

Cylinders can be arranged within a few days but a concentrator may take up to a week to have supplied and fitted in the home. Which method to use needs to be discussed with the GP and parents, and organized in advance.

A portable oxygen system is essential equipment for the family, but not available on the drug tariff, and has to be supplied by the hospital. Who provides the disposable items for these babies depends very much on different health authorities and who is providing the community care. The baby's suitcase is usually packed with at least a month's supply of disposables, and further supplies must always be available.

A discharge summary is completed, with copies made available for the parents, GP and health visitor. Immunizations for these children are recommended and will have been kept up to date. Arrangements for follow-up appointments are made according to local policy, commonly in a month's time.

Parents find the day of discharge full of mixed emotions: it is a day they have waited for but never believed would happen, for a long time. There is excitement mingled with a little apprehension, and it is definitely not a good day to give any more information. Ensure that everything is ready 24 h before and endeavour to make the day as smooth and trouble-free as possible.

An information booklet, which includes all the information and teaching that has taken place, provides a checklist for equipment, and includes a discharge care plan with medications, is useful.

Good communication and liaison between the hospital and the community health team is essential for ongoing management. Babies on diuretics will need frequent urea and electrolyte level tests performed, and these may be done at home; any babies who remain on oral or inhaled steroids will need to have periodic measurement of their blood pressure.

Ideally, a 24 hour on call service should be available to these families. With good support and supervision surprisingly few parents will need to use this service, but it does give that extra sense of security, knowing that someone is always available, particularly in the first few weeks, while they become more familiar and confident in handling the equipment and caring for their baby.

CONTINUING MANAGEMENT

The need to monitor the infant's SaO_2 applies at home just as it did in hospital. While he is still small it is not difficult to monitor through a sleep and feeding cycle, but as he gets older and more active, monitoring can become more of a problem during the day; however, he will be far more stable and consistent with his saturation, and shorter monitoring is sufficient. Babies should be monitored overnight every few weeks, or if there is a change in oxygen requirements or if they are unwell. This is something that parents manage very well and, as babies get older and have a more settled sleep pattern, the information recorded is very accurate.

Complications may occur while at home. Feeding can be a frustrating experience: most infants do better when discharged, but occasionally an infant may slow down and fail to complete feeds. This is especially common if the baby has an upper respiratory tract infection presenting with a 'cold' and a cough. Antibiotics are usually prescribed prophylactically but this depends on the GP. Bronchodilator therapy is usually prescribed at the first sign of a wheeze. This can make a significant improvement. Oxygen flow may be increased a little to ensure good oxygenation. These babies are very vulnerable to episodes of hypoxia when unwell because of increased respiratory effort and sensitive airways. Most hospitals have an open-door policy whereby the infant can be admitted directly to the paediatric ward if necessary.

WEANING FROM OXYGEN

When to reduce oxygen depends very much on the baby's stability. Full monitoring during weaning is crucial, so as not to compromise the infant. Once maintaining saturations above 94%, in minimal oxygen, he will be monitored for a short period in air. If the SaO_2 does not drop below 94%, parents will be advised to disconnect the oxygen for an hour or two each day while he is awake. Over a 2-week period, if saturations remain good, this period off oxygen will be increased until he is off oxygen all day while awake, but he will need to be monitored, in air, during daytime sleeps. If he continues to maintain about 94%, oxygen will be stopped all day, awake and asleep. It is important, at this point, to identify which babies have lower SaO_2 when asleep (Sekar and Duke, 1991). Before stopping oxygen at night, an overnight recording in air will be done and, as previously mentioned, an echocardiogram will be done before a final decision is made.

Babies with severe lung disease can have a significant fall in saturations when asleep, despite having an SaO_2 above 94% in air when awake, and require oxygen overnight. A very small number may still be on oxygen past 2 years of age and these children will continue to need visiting and support, but probably only on a fortnightly or monthly basis.

The baby will continue to be monitored for the first month after stopping oxygen, and a repeat overnight recording will be done before visits are discontinued. The baby can then be handed over to the care of the health visitor.

CONCLUSION

Caring for these babies at home can be hard work for the parents and puts many demands on the family environment and relationships, but it works well provided that the parents are prepared properly before discharge and receive the support that they need once home. Parents are the best people to care for their babies but they are expected to learn, in a short period, what we have been learning over many years. Success depends on good communication and trust during the preparation for discharge; if this is not there, difficulties will arise and parents may end up bitterly regretting the experience, with harmful effects on their relationship with their baby.

With recent changes in the National Health Service, and community care seen as the way forward, there will be more of these babies going home; it is our responsibility to ensure a safe and happy discharge, with appropriate management and care in the community, to enable them to grow and develop happily and safely.

REFERENCES

Abman, S., Wolfe, R., Accurso, F. *et al.* (1985) Pulmonary vascular response to oxygen in infants with severe bronchopulmonary dysplasia. *Pediatrics* **75**(1).

Acolet, D., Sleath, K. and Whitelaw, A. (1989) Oxygenation, heart rate and temperature in VLBW infants during skin-to-skin contact with their mothers. *Acta Paediatrica Scandinavica* **78**, 189–93.

Als, H., Lawhon, G., Brown, E. and Gibb, R. (1986) Individualised behavioural and environmental care for the VLBW preterm infant at high risk for BPD: NICU and developmental outcome. *Pediatrics* **78**(6).

Bernbaum, J. and Hoffman-Williamson, M. (1986) Following the NICU graduate. *Contemporary Pediatrics* **3**, 22–37.

Jolley, S., Halpern, C., Sterling, C. and Feldman, B. (1990) The relationship of respiratory complications from gastroesophageal reflux to prematurity in infants. *Journal of Paediatric Surgery* 25(7), 755–7.

Lucas, A., Morley, R., Cole, T. *et al.* (1989) Early diet in preterm babies and developmental status in infancy. *Archives of Disease in Childhood* **64**(11), 1570–8.

Newell, S., Booth, I.W. and Morgan, M.E.I. (1989) Gastroesophageal reflux in preterm infants. *Archives of Disease in Childhood* **64**, 780–6.

Northway, Rosan, R.C. and Porter, D.Y. (1967) Pulmonary disease following respiratory therapy for hyaline membrane disease. *New England Journal of Medicine* **276**, 357.

Rome, E.S., Stork, E., Carlo, W. and Martin, R. (1984) Limitations of transcutaneous $P\text{O}_2$ and $P\text{CO}_2$monitoring in infants with BPD. *Pediatrics* **74**(2).

Royal College of Physicians (1992) A report of a working group of the Committee on Thoracic Medicine. *Domiciliary Oxygen Therapy for Children*. Royal College of Physicians, London.

Sekar, K. and Duke, J. (1991) Sleep apnoea and hypoxaemia in recently weaned premature infants with and without BPD. *Paediatric Pulmonology* **10**, 112–6.

Sleath, K. (1989) The breath of life. *Nursing Times* **85(44)**.

Southall, D. and Samuels, M. (1990) Bronchopulmonary dysplasia: a new look at management. *Archives of Disease in Childhood* **65**, 1085–95.

Vandenberg, K. (1990) Nippling management of the sick neonate in the ITU; the disorganised feeder. *Neonatal Network* **9**(1), 9–15.

Whitelaw, A., Heisterkemp, G. and Sleath, K. (1988) Skin to skin contact for very low birth weight infants and their mothers. *Archives of Disease in Childhood* **63**, 1377–81.

Yeh, T.F., McClenan, D.A., Ajayi, O.A. and Pildes, R.S. (1989) *Pediatrics* **114**, 448–51.

Zinman, R., Blanchard, P. and Vachon, F. (1992) Oxygen saturations during sleep in patients with bronchopulmonary dysplasia. *Biology of the Neonate* **61**, 69–75.

19

Infant statistics

Marjorie Tew

Neonatal nurses are concerned with those infants who survive birth but need some form of medical care. Most infants do survive birth, as the tremendous growth in the world's population demonstrates, but the proportion of survivors has not always been as high as it is now, nor is it the same in different countries. How widely it is known to vary depends on how accurately infant births and deaths are recorded.

COUNTING BIRTHS AND SURVIVORS IN BRITAIN AND ABROAD

In England, since 1837, it has been a legal obligation to register every death and, since 1874, every live birth, so that calculations of infant mortality rates (IMR) – deaths in the first year per 1000 live births – have been available for over a century. Survival proportions are the complement of death rates: a death rate of 20/1000 births means a survival rate of 980/1000. Registration of stillbirths was not compulsory until 1927; it is probable that, until then, some liveborn babies who died soon after were treated as stillbirths and not registered, so understating both the numerator and the denominator by the same amount, and hence the death rate. In Scotland, a system of registering live births and deaths was introduced in 1855, but stillbirths did not need to be registered until 1939; for Ireland the corresponding dates were 1864 and for Northern Ireland 1961 (Macfarlane and Mugford, 1984a).

Other countries have their own systems of recording births and deaths. These are likely to be most reliable and complete in the richer countries, which can afford the administration costs and where more people are literate. The World Health Organization (WHO) publishes records of these life events from countries which are able to submit the statistics (the African region is poorly represented). Caution is obviously necessary in making international comparisons based on data of variable definition and reliability. In the 1980s, IMRs were generally found to be lowest in the economically developed countries, higher in the former communist countries, and highest in the economically underdeveloped countries; that is, infant death rates are lower where the standards of living and of nutrition are higher, and vice versa. Where the standard of living is higher, the provisions for medical care, including care of the newborn, are also likely to be more liberal.

INFANT MORTALITY RATES IN DIFFERENT PLACES

Within these broad groups there are wide variations in IMRs, as there are also between different regions or districts within any single country, but higher mortality is always strongly associated with greater poverty. The association between low mortality and liberal medical provisions is much weaker, as was shown in a study of the local authority areas of England and Wales in the late 1960s (Ashford, Read and Riley, 1973). Over a long period, Scotland enjoyed superior medical services

Table 19.1 Infant mortality rates per 1000 live births in selected countries

Country	*Year*	*Total*	*Males*	*Females*
Japan	1990	4.6	5.0	4.2
Finland	1989	6.0	6.7	5.4
Netherlands	1989	6.8	7.9	5.9
UK	1990	7.9	8.9	6.8
Australia	1988	–	9.7	7.5
USA	1988	10.0	11.0	8.9
Bulgaria	1988	13.6	15.6	11.5
	1990	14.8	16.8	12.6
China	1989	–	19.0	16.8
Uruguay	1989	–	23.8	18.3
Romania	1986	23.2	26.0	20.2
	1989	25.4	28.2	22.4
Egypt	1987	–	46.5	43.6

– Not printed
Source: World Health Statistics Annual, 1990 and 1991a, Tables 11 and 12

to England but it was economically poorer, and until the late 1970s its IMR was consistently higher. Despite its very high expenditure on medical services, the affluent USA has always had appreciably higher IMRs than less affluent England. Some idea of the range in recent IMRs is given by the sample of countries in Table 19.1, which also shows the typically higher mortality rate of boys.

The absolute number of birth survivors in any country depends, of course, on the actual number of births. If there are many births, a high death rate may still be associated with a relatively large population increase and relatively many infants needing, if not receiving, neonatal nursing. A fluctuating number of live births will obviously create a fluctuating need for neonatal nurses.

MORTALITY RATES AT DIFFERENT TIMES AND DIFFERENT INFANT AGES

IMRs have also varied widely through time. Throughout the 20th century wherever standards of living and of nutrition have kept improving, IMRs have kept falling, but in the former communist countries each of these trends has latterly been reversed, for example in Romania and Bulgaria (Table 19.1). In England and Wales, the IMR per 1000 births, which had been about 150 in the late 19th century, had fallen to 80 by 1920, to 57 by 1940, to 22 by 1960, to 12 by 1980, and to 8 by 1990 (Registrar General 1957, 1973; OPCS DH1 No. 19; OPCS 1990c). Similar downward trends are recorded in other prosperous countries.

Deaths do not occur evenly throughout the first year of life: deaths in the first week far outnumber deaths in the next 3 weeks and, since the early 1960s, deaths on the first day have far outnumbered deaths in the next 6 days for babies of low birth weight. In the first days after birth antenatal and intranatal experiences have the dominant influence on survival, but gradually the baby's environment assumes the greater importance.

Data for England and Wales are available from 1906 for deaths at different infant ages: at 1 day, up to 1 week (early neonatal), from 2 to 4 weeks (late neonatal) and over 4 weeks (postneonatal) (Registrar General 1973; OPCS DH1 No. 19).

These show that, in 1906–1910, 66% of the deaths were postneonatal and 21% early neonatal; by 1931–1935 these percentages were 49% and 36% respectively; by 1961–1965 they were 31% and 60%. Thus, up until that time most of the reduced mortality had taken place at the postneonatal stage. Babies were showing the same reaction to the improving environment as young children, whose death rate was falling fast as they became more resistant to diseases, thanks to more ample and nutritious diets which resulted from better economic conditions and from the decreasing average family size. The impressive decline in the high death rates suffered by these children due to infectious diseases was already well in progress before it was accelerated by the availability of immunizations and antibiotic treatments.

Postneonatal (PNMR) and late neonatal (LNMR) mortality rates fell continuously between 1906 and 1965: the PNMR from 76.9 to 6.0 (a fall of 92%) and the LNMR from 15.7 to 1.7 (a fall of 89%). In contrast, it was not until after 1940 that the early neonatal mortality rate (ENMR) really started to fall. Despite the increased input of resources into maternity care, it was higher in 1937 than it had been in 1921–1925. It eventually fell from 24.5 in 1906 to 11.3 in 1965, a fall of 54%.

After 1965, however, it was the ENMR that showed the greatest decline: by 68% from 11.3 to 3.6 in 1989, while the proportionate fall was less at 35% for the LNMR (from 1.7 to 1.1) and also for the PNMR at 40% (from 6.0 to 3.6). As a result, by 1989, early neonatal deaths made up the same proportion (43%) of the infant death rate as did postneonatal deaths. To some unquantifiable extent, the lesser decline in the LNMR and PNMR probably reflects that some of what might have been early neonatal deaths were being postponed and were taking place at a later infant age, for this was the experience of higher-order births (see below), and an increasing proportion of postneonatal deaths were being attributed to 'certain conditions arising in the neonatal period' (OPCS, 1989). That most did survive the first year is indicated by the continuing fall in the IMR (from 19 in 1965 to 8 in 1990).

EFFECT OF BIRTH WEIGHT ON SURVIVAL

The chance of dying soon is by far the greatest for small babies. These are the ones whose early environment has most likely changed by being given special or intensive care, for which facilities were rapidly extended after 1965. For babies of very low birth weight (VLBW: 1500 g or less), the rate for first-day deaths per 1000 births fell by 56% (from 418 in 1965 to 186 in 1981); it had fallen by only 5% from 441 in 1953 to 418 in 1965. For babies of low birth weight (LBW: 2500 g or less), the rate for first-day deaths also fell by 56% (from 73 in 1965 to 32 in 1981); it had fallen by only 13% from 84 in 1953 to 73 in 1965. This might suggest that the special or intensive neonatal care that most of the smallest and most vulnerable babies were later receiving was saving new lives. The death rate at days 1–6 fell by 42% (from 160 in 1965 to 93 in 1981) for VLBW births and by 53% (from 38 in 1965 to 18 in 1981) for LBW births, but data for the earlier period are not publicly available for comparison (nor are data after 1981) (Macfarlane and Mugford, 1984b). This inference seemed the more plausible since the same sudden change in the survival trend took place in other countries where special and intensive neonatal care was being developed at the same time. Most of the evidence supporting this inference depends on comparing outcomes before and after the introduction of the new treatments. There are dangerous pitfalls in assuming causal relationships from specific observed changes over time; other potentially causal factors may have been changing over the same periods.

For babies weighing over 2500 g, however, the rate of first-day deaths also fell by 57% (from 2.1 in 1965 to 0.9 in 1981, having risen from 1.9 in 1953), while the death rate at days 1–6 fell by 50% (from 2.4 in 1965 to 1.2 in 1981). Most of these heavier babies did not have special or intensive neonatal care, yet their ENMR fell after 1965 proportionately as much as did the ENMR for the low weight babies, and one might have surmised that the beneficent influence causing a lower ENMR might have affected both weight groups similarly. This casts doubt on the inference that it was the introduction of more widely used methods of neonatal care that were the sole or predominant causes of the reduced mortality of the babies who received them, and implies some other cause, at least as potent, contributing to the accelerated decline in mortality at all birth weights after 1965.

WHAT CAUSED THE IMPROVED SURVIVAL OF BABIES?

It had been widely assumed that, because stillbirth and early neonatal mortality rates were decreasing at the same time as the hospitalization and obstetric management of birth were increasing, the latter trends were the cause of the former. No randomized controlled trial had ever been conducted before the increase in hospitalization, to establish the greater safety of hospital births. Such trials are only possible as long as prospective participants are not already biased in favour of one particular policy, a condition that medical propaganda soon ensured could not be met. Evaluation of alternative types of intranatal care therefore had to depend on statistical analyses of actual results, and these consistently showed that such a causal relationship could not exist (Tew, 1986; Campbell and Macfarlane, 1987; Tew, 1990).

By the 1990s this discrediting of the widely assumed causal relationship had at last come to be accepted by impartial judges (Lancet, 1986; House of Commons Health Committee, 1992a), though only with reservations by the Royal College of Obstetricians and Gynaecologists (RCOG) and the Department of Health, and was not accepted at all by many medical practitioners who clung unquestioningly to their indoctrinated beliefs. The births, which obstetric management certainly did make safer, constituted only a small proportion of the total; for the majority, there had to be some other cause of the increased safety.

There is an unquestionable biological link between healthy parents and healthy offspring and much evidence of the continuously improving health status of successive generations of 20th century parents. The mothers who were coming to childbearing age by 1965 were themselves of a generation which had benefited, both as fetuses and as children, from the improved social and nutritional conditions that their mothers had increasingly enjoyed from the late 1930s, and so had developed healthier reproductive systems capable of giving birth to healthier offspring. This generation was, in turn, repeating the experience of preceding generations throughout the century. The cumulative improvement in health status and efficient reproductive systems was beginning to show substantial rewards, and was to go on doing so. There is, therefore, an extremely strong probability that by far the greater part of the decrease in mortality was the result of improved parental health and improved vitality in babies (Tew, 1990).

WHAT CAUSED THE IMPROVED SURVIVAL OF SMALL BABIES?

There is, however, even more reluctance to dispute the equally widely held view that the improved survival rates of small infants (LBW), and particularly of very small infants (VLBW), are due almost entirely to the use of neonatal technology, administered by neonatal nurses and paediatricians. The contribution of improved infant vitality is discounted.

Research had indicated that the most specialized care, using the highest technology, produces better survival results than less specialized care. In Melbourne, Australia, between 1966 and 1969, a controlled trial showed that, for infants weighing 1000–1500 g, better survival rates followed intensive, rather than the routine, neonatal care then given (Kitchen *et al.*, 1979). Other studies have shown better survival rates for the VLBW babies born in or transferred to the larger, most specialized neonatal intensive care units (NICUs) than in smaller NICUs or special care baby units (SCBUs) (Stewart, Reynolds and Lipscombe, 1981; Powell, Pharoah and Cooke 1986; Powell and Pharoah, 1987; Field *et al.*, 1991). This, however, is not necessarily evidence that intensive care is better than any possible alternative.

An English study followed up, at school age, the babies who had been born in a defined area between 1963 and 1971, weighing from 501 to 1500 g and given only careful nursing. It found that 'in terms of survival, handicap and intellectual capacity . . . outcome compared favourably with that of infants born over the same period in areas where intensive methods of perinatal care were used' (Steiner *et al.*, 1980).

Further doubt about the superior life-saving results of neonatal technology was raised by the claims made by paediatricians in Bogota, Colombia, that the survival rate of very tiny infants is as good if they are kept warm between their mothers' breasts, with unrestricted access to their own milk supply. The psychological benefits for mother and child were confirmed by a British paediatrician, but he questioned the statistical reliability of the mortality results claimed (Whitelaw and Sleath, 1985). However, once paediatricians have become convinced that better survival can only be achieved by the use of their sophisticated technological instruments, they consider it unethical to deny the use of these to one subgroup in a randomized controlled trial, so no such trial is ever likely to be carried out to evaluate, without bias, the outcomes of these alternative treatments, one of which would obviously be vastly cheaper, though less scientifically exciting for its professional practitioners, than the other.

Doubts about the life-saving results of neonatal technology are strengthened by the fact that, in the years when a reasonable number of births were allowed to take place outside obstetric hospitals, the specific perinatal mortality rate (PNMR; stillbirths plus EN deaths per 1000 total births, still plus live) was always higher for the births under obstetric management in hospital, by a margin which was far too great to be explained by any plausible predelivery selection of higher-risk cases for hospital. This was the finding in nationwide perinatal surveys carried out in Britain in 1958 and 1970 under the auspices of the RCOG (Butler and Bonham, 1963; Chamberlain *et al.*, 1978). It was also the finding of official data collected by the Chief Medical Officer of England and Wales, published in his annual reports from 1954 to 1964 and, unpublished but made available to the present author, from 1967 to 1973, years which followed the general introduction of special neonatal care facilities (Tew, 1990). The finding was confirmed by Dutch data for 1986, when 43% of all babies were delivered by independent midwives. The data showed that, for babies with gestations of less than 37 weeks (a close proxy for births of low weight), there was a very significantly higher PNMR for babies delivered under the care of obstetricians in hospital, with immediate access to neonatal intensive care, than delivered by midwives either at home or as independent practitioners in hospital (Tew and Damstra-Wijmenga, 1991). These separate findings are brought together in Table 19.2. The data available, admittedly limited, do not even demonstrate significantly better outcomes for the babies of very low birth weight or very short gestation.

Table 19.2 Perinatal mortality rates per 1000 births

A Of low weight (2500 g or less)

		Place of actual delivery	
Source of data	*Year*	*Hospital*	*Home/GP unit*
Perinatal survey	1958(a)	328	161#
British Births Survey	1970(b)	232	79#
Chief Medical Officer			
England & Wales			*Home*
All under 2500 g	1954–58(c)	296	181#
	1959–64(c)	269	162#
Under 1001 g	1967–73(d)	898	868
1001–1500 g	1967–73(d)	621	635
1501–2000 g	1967–73(d)	270	242+
2001–2250 g	1967–73(d)	116	99*
2251–2500 g	1967–73(d)	56	40§

B Of short gestation (36 weeks or less)

Official Dutch Data	*1986(e)*	*Obstetricians hospital*	*Midwives home & hospital*
Under 33 weeks		186	170
33–36 weeks		46	13#

Statistical significance of differences:
* P<0.02
\+ P<0.01
§ P<0.001
\# P<0.0001
P <0.02 was a 98% probability, and P <0.0001 was a 99.99% probability, of the difference being real and not a chance finding.

Sources:
(a) Butler & Bonham (1963), Perinatal Mortality.
(b) Chamberlain *et al*. (1978) British Births 1970, vol. 2.
(c) Chief Medical Officer of the Ministry of Health, Annual Reports for the years 1954–1964.
(d) Chief Medical Officer of the Ministry of Health, unpublished returns.
(e) Centraal Bureu voor de Statistiek (1987) *Monthly Bulletin of Population and Health Statistics* **87**:11 and (unpublished) computer printouts of stillbirths and first-week deaths.

Most of the above statistics appear in Tew (1990) *Safer Childbirth?*

THE INCIDENCE OF LOW BIRTH WEIGHT

Like mortality, low birth weight is strongly associated with poor maternal health, so that the incidence of low birth weight (<2500 g) might have been expected to decrease as general health status improved. This has not happened in England and Wales: low-weight births made up 54.1% of still births and 6.7% of live births in 1959, and 57.6% and 6.5% respectively in 1989. The percentage of live births weighing 2001–2500 g did decrease (from 4.7% to 4.3%) but there was a compensating increase in smaller babies, though some of this apparent increase may have been due to a greater willingness to record as live births, rather than as stillbirths, those feeble premature babies who survived only briefly. The percentage of live births which weighed less than 1500 g increased from 0.77 in 1959 to 0.95 in 1989.

In 1959, of all infant deaths, 43% occurred among the 6.7% of LBW births and 23% among the 0.77% of VLBW births. In 1989, of all infant deaths, 46% occurred among the 6.5% of LBW births and 31% among the 0.95% of VLBW births (Macfarlane and Mugford, 1984b; OPCS, 1989). Thus the contribution made by LBW and VLBW births to the total of infant deaths increased over these 30 years; despite all medical endeavours and claims, their survival rate had not improved as much as that for the heavier babies.

Births of low and very low weight may follow the spontaneous onset of premature labour or the term delivery of babies whose intrauterine growth has been retarded, or preterm labour, obstetrically induced, with the hope of forestalling the adverse outcomes of potentially life-threatening conditions, diagnosed, rightly or wrongly, in the fetus or the mother (see below). How much each of these factors has contributed at different times to the total is not generally known.

Babies who are both of low weight and immature are likely to need more nursing care than those of the same weight but whose vital systems are more developed, as happens in the LBW babies in multiple births and babies small for gestational age, and their relative immaturity is followed by a higher rate of later handicap (Verloove-Vanhorick and Verwey, 1987; House of Commons Health Committee, 1992c). However, data on length of gestation, which can be difficult to determine, are not routinely published in England and many other countries, despite WHO recommendations that they should be.

The causes of spontaneous premature labour are poorly understood, but certain factors are identified with it. It is common in congenitally malformed babies, in multiple pregnancies and after closely spaced pregnancies. Babies of low birth weight are more likely to have mothers who are less than 20 or more than 35 years old, or who have already borne more than three children. Their mothers are more likely to be unsupported, emotionally and socially as well as financially, and they are more likely to suffer stress, to smoke and to drink too much alcohol. These factors are, to some extent, interdependent (Newton and Hunt, 1984). Many studies have found that babies whose mothers have received supportive antenatal care from a midwife are less likely to be born prematurely or of low weight than babies whose mothers receive less personal care in a hospital antenatal clinic, and there is good reason to believe that this outcome depends more on the quality of the stress-relieving, confidence-building care than on the predicted physical risks of the pregnancy (Flint and Poulengeris, 1987; Oakley, Rajan and Grant, 1990; Davies, 1991; Evans, 1991; Durand, 1992).

If, in normal biology, it is the fetus that times its own arrival by initiating the hormonal changes that set in motion the chain of birth processes once it has developed sufficiently to start independent life, spontaneous premature labour may be a signal from the fetus that its uterine environment has become inadequate for its needs. Obstetricians have failed to find reliable emergency therapy for improving the uterine environment in such cases, or for significantly postponing delivery. Alternatively, the initiating hormonal changes may be triggered by some external stimulus, either physical or emotional. Literature is full of stories of spontaneous preterm labour after emotional trauma. In recent decades, nearly all pregnant women have experienced obstetrically directed antenatal care, with its increasing range of screening tests intended to uncover physical indicators of latent potential complications and to promote healthy births. Yet this regimen has failed to prevent the rising proportion of very underweight preterm births to an increasingly healthy childbearing population. One might speculate whether it may indeed be the invasive antenatal interventions themselves, including vaginal and ultrasound examinations, which somtimes act as the trigger for preterm labour, since they can certainly cause more anxiety than they alleviate (Green, 1990; Lorenz *et al.*, 1990).

Fortunately, most of the mothers at above-average risk of giving birth to preterm underweight babies will, in fact, give birth to healthy babies of normal weight and gestation. Most mothers who give birth to twins, triplets or higher-order births are not likely to be so lucky.

MULTIPLE BIRTHS

In an official survey of multiple births in 1980 and 1982–1985 (Botting, Macfarlane and Price, 1990), 49% of the twins, 94% of the triplets and 99% of the higher-order births weighed under 2500 g at birth, with 9%, 28% and 52% respectively weighing less than 1500 g; 9% of twins, 25% of triplets and 48% of the higher-order births did not exceed 32 weeks' gestation. Although the stillbirth rate among all multiple births is over three times as high as among singleton births, the vast majority of them are born alive. Of births in the study, four-fifths of the triplets and nearly all of the higher-order babies received special or intensive care; one-quarter of the triplets and three-fifths of the higher-order babies stayed for 4 or more weeks in the NICU. Neonatal death rates are over seven times as high for all multiple births as for singletons, but for those who survive to the postneonatal stage their relative disadvantage in mortality falls to less than three times (OPCS, 1989).

The limited success of neonatal care in postponing death for higher-order births is illustrated by the 33% decline in their ENMR between 1987 and 1988 (from 81 to 54) but the more than compensating 46% rise in their death rate from 7 days to 1 year (32 to 47) (OPCS, 1989).

The proportion per 1000 pregnancies which resulted in a multiple birth had been declining steadily from 12.7 for twins and 0.12 for all higher orders in 1951–5 to 9.6 and 0.13 respectively in 1976–1980, but the increase in assisted conceptions and in the use of fertility drugs raised these ratios to 11.3 and 0.30 in 1990 (Botting, Macfarlane and Price, 1990; OPCS, 1990a). More of these higher-order babies tend to be more sick and disabled than babies of multiple births who are naturally conceived (House of Commons Health Committee, 1992c). The demands that they make obviously strain the capacity of SCBUs and NICUs, especially if the desirability of tending siblings in the same unit is to be implemented. The extent of the extra strain depends on the number of multiple births occurring, but more particularly on when and where they occur. Though the numbers involved are relatively small and are spread over wide areas, chance may lead to temporary overloading of local facilities.

CONDITIONS NEEDING NEONATAL CARE

Special care is needed not only for underweight immature babies, but also for sick, unstable babies of any weight who have problems that call for continuous monitoring, frequent testing, abnormal administration of nourishment, phototherapy or antibiotic treatment and, most immediately, for those in respiratory distress.

Breathing difficulties of the newborn

A baby's most urgent need is to establish effective breathing and much intensive care is directed at relieving the difficulties of the small minority who fail to do so. Technological advances have made possible a manifold increase since 1970 in the numbers receiving ventilatory support and in their chances of survival. By the late 1980s, just over 1% of live births in the northern region of England were so treated for non-surgical reasons, with about three-quarters of all those ventilated and nearly half of those weighing less than 1000 g at birth surviving until fit for hospital discharge (NRHA, 1989). The cost of care, however, is about twice what it would be for babies of similar gestation who do not have respiratory distress (Mugford, Piercy and Chalmers, 1991), and the ventilated babies are at increased risk of other respiratory disorders in infancy and childhood, since mechanical ventilation impairs healthy lung growth (Skeoch *et al.*, 1987).

Most likely to have immediate breathing difficulties are the very preterm and VLBW babies whose lungs have not had time to develop sufficiently to take over their extrauterine function, but last-minute corticosteroid therapy for mothers in impending preterm labour and surfactant therapy for the neonate have been shown to hasten significant pulmonary development, so that the number of very early deaths is reduced. This, however, causes the number of survivors who need prolonged intensive respiratory assistance to increase (Tyson *et al.*, 1989; Morley, 1991). The medication and subsequent surfactant therapy are very costly, but so far no adverse physical consequences of this particular intervention have been identified, although NICUs cannot provide appropriate social and psychological environments for the long-stay neonate.

The risk of suffering breathing difficulties diminishes greatly as fetal maturity and birth weight increase, but it is aggravated for babies of all weights whose mothers have been given analgesic or anaesthetic medication to relieve pain in labour (Chamberlain *et al.*, 1975). These drugs cross the placenta and have a depressing effect on the fetus's vital instincts to breathe and suck. They are liberally administered under obstetric management in Britain, though not so in the Netherlands, where the Dutch women's self-confident attitude to childbearing avoids the need (Verloove-Vanhorick and Verwey, 1987). Their greater use is particularly associated with the induction and acceleration of labour and operative deliveries.

Operative deliveries and neonatal outcomes

The percentage of births which were induced was 13% in 1964, but doubled to 26% by 1970 and trebled to 39% by 1974; then, at least partly in response to public protests, the increase was halted and, after 1978, reversed to reach 17% by 1984, around which figure it remained to the end of the decade. The strongly upward trend in instrumental deliveries in the 1960s and 1970s was also reversed in the 1980s. The percentage rate for forceps deliveries in England and Wales increased steadily from 8.1% in 1962 to 13.2% in 1977, but then decreased to 10.3% in 1982 and 9.1% in 1985; it was estimated at 9% for England only in 1989–1990. The percentage rate for caesarean sections climbed slowly from 4.7% in 1962 to 5.3% in 1972, and then much faster to 10.1% in 1982. Decisions as to how necessary and advantageous caesarean sections were varied widely between individual surgeons, some favouring a rate of no more than 5%, others a rate upward of 20%. But the American lead was not followed to its extreme; the average rate in England and Wales rose only to 10.5% in 1985 and was estimated at

12% for England only in 1989–1990 (Tew, 1986; House of Commons Health Committee, 1992b).

CAUSE AND EFFECT RELATIONSHIPS

It will be noticed that the substantial increase in inductions and operative deliveries, in the hospitalization of birth, in neonatal intensive and special care facilities on the one hand, and the acceleration in the decline in perinatal mortality on the other, all took place over the same period. Although death rates are acknowledged to be higher in groups where interventions have taken place than in groups where they have not, obstetricians argue that the result would be the opposite if proper allowance were made for the higher predicted risk of the groups with interventions. Caesarean section is the intervention particularly favoured by obstetricians to advance delivery when they judge the risk of preterm birth to be less than that of the diagnosed pathology. As the mortality associated with preterm birth has declined, so obstetricians have felt more justified in cutting short a pregnancy which is diagnosed as pathological.

They had, however, never been able to find data which could prove their point (Tew, 1990) but, never doubting that their theory was right, they were quick to claim that the decline in mortality was caused by the increases in their interventions. Analysis of the trends, however, shows the claim to be invalid: mortality rates went on falling when rates of induction and instrumental deliveries were also falling, while individual studies showed that mortality decreased as much in series where the caesarean section rate did not increase as where it did (Tew, 1986). In a recent study covering 2600 preterm births, the section rate was increased by 61% between 1980 and 1989, while the survival rate increased by 50% but, on statistical analysis, no significant association was found to exist between the two rates; the increased intervention was unlikely to have been the cause of the improved survival (Cooke, 1990).

Special neonatal care was introduced in the 1960s for the increasing number of babies born in poor condition after the obstetric intranatal interventions which were becoming increasingly common. It is probable that some of the contribution that neonatal special and intensive care makes to lower mortality rests in counteracting the excess mortality which would otherwise be caused by obstetric interventions, which may be undertaken as routine procedures rather than in response to unequivocal need in the small minority of circumstances where the risks involved are known, not just hoped, to be justified. At all events, paediatricians believe that, in the modern delivery setting, the human baby cannot survive without their ministrations. The opinion of the British Paediatric Association is that 'All of the babies born in consultant obstetric units require paediatric medical care during the newborn period, (some very urgently and unpredictably at birth in order to resuscitate - even in apparently uneventful pregnancies and labours). Some of the babies require special care and a small proportion of the babies require intensive care' (House of Commons Health Committee, 1992b). On the other hand, apprehension about 'the growing involvement of neonatologists in the care of the healthy newborn' and 'the long term implications of this medicalisation of normal life' is voiced by midwives (House of Commons Health Committee, 1992c).

CONGENITAL MALFORMATIONS

Congenital malformations identifiable at birth have been officially notifiable in England and Wales since 1964. In 1990, in addition to causing many stillbirths, these were notified in respect of 1.3% of liveborn males and 0.9% of liveborn females, with considerable regional variation (OPCS, 1990b). The Department of Health reported that 'a congenital anomaly is present in about 3% of newborn babies. Congenital anomalies are the cause of 25% of deaths in infancy and account for 18% of hospital paediatric admissions' (House of Commons Health Committee, 1991b). Some affected babies require special or intensive neonatal care while their abnormalities are treated, medically or surgically. Efforts to intervene have become ever more ambitious and sometimes iatrogenic complications have been added to the initial defect.

The incidence of congenital malformations is higher among LBW babies, notably those born small for gestational age (Verloove-Vanhorick and Verwey, 1987) but deaths due to this cause make up a higher proportion of the relatively smaller total of infant deaths of babies of normal birth weight. Some malformations, such as cerebral palsy and some heart and kidney defects, are not definitely identifiable until some time – months or even years – later in the child's development, so they are not likely to be prescribed treatment in the neonatal care units. But the risk of cerebral palsy and other defects increases greatly with decreasing birth weight, which is another reason why the VLBW recipients of special neonatal care may go on to need special paediatric care.

The burden that congenital malformations and chromosomal disorders make on neonatal care services is most likely to be reduced by preventative measures which reduce their incidence, in some cases through genetic counselling, in others through the antenatal identification and therapeutic abortion of damaged fetuses, a practice which was made legal in Great Britain by the Abortion Act of 1968. However, therapeutic abortion accounts for less than one-third of the reduced incidence of some malformations, in particular those of the central nervous system, which has fallen in line with the improving nutritional standards of pregnant women and latterly with the vitamin supplementation available to them (MRC, 1991). A parallel decline has taken place in several other countries, the Netherlands, Scandinavia, Canada, Australia, Hungary and also in Eire, where abortion is still illegal (OPCS, 1990b).

Further contribution to lowering the incidence of malformations has been made by the prepregnancy immunization of women against rubella: between 1987 and 1990 the number of notified infections in pregnancy fell from about 200 to 20 (House of Commons Health Committee, 1991a).

SCALE OF PROVISION FOR NEONATAL CARE

Number of cots

How great then is the need for special care for sick babies? In 1959 an official committee (Cranbrook, 1959), advising on the maternity services in England and Wales, recommended an increase in hospital births but, observing a parallel increase in neonatal morbidity, also recommended the setting up of special care baby units. A later committeee in 1971 (Sheldon, 1971) noted that by 1968, 3369 cots in 257 such units were recorded, or about four cots per 1000 live births. As units were set up they were rapidly filled, admitting 12% of babies born in 1970, which prompted the committee to estimate a greater need at six cots per 1000 live births, on the over-optimistic assumption of a future average duration of stay of 15 days. It noted, however, that 90% of these admissions came from the maternity departments in the same hospitals. This might suggest that the need was more likely to be created by hospital treatment, but results showed that, despite more special care, mortality from breathing difficulties was significantly higher for the hospital-born babies (Chamberlain *et al.*, 1975; Tew, 1980). Alternatively, it might suggest that the criteria of need often depended less on the physical condition of the neonate than on the convenient availability of provision, including facilities for intensive care. A review in 1981 of existing evaluative studies found a lack of evidence to justify the use of neonatal intensive care services, and so speculated that 'the supply of neonatal intensive care determines its use rather than the converse' (Sinclair *et al.*, 1981). As the representative of the Neonatal Nurses Association (NNA) testified in 1991, '. . . when you looked critically at the population within the neonatal unit, 40% of those admissions may not necessarily have had to be admitted to a neonatal unit' (House of Commons Health Committee, 1992b). Nevertheless, on whatever criterion and despite improvement in basic maternal health and social conditions, and despite increased antenatal care, the number of babies requiring admission to intensive care units is said, by care providers, to be rising (House of Commons Health Committee, 1992c).

Although there have been changes in the balance of infant morbidity treated, there has not yet been an impartial investigation to quantify the need for different grades of neonatal care and to measure the implicit workload falling on the nurses. Without universally accepted criteria based on research evaluations, provisions vary widely in different areas, partly for historical reasons. The variation may arise also because of different approaches to policy. The technological equipment is expensive to install and maintain, and nurses have to be expensively trained in the skills necessary for its correct usage and interpretation. The number of babies who need the most intensive care is limited. If they were all concentrated in a few regional centres, or even fewer supra-regional centres, these financial costs would be lower; the high nursing skills would be in constant use and fewer nurses would have to be trained and employed in dispersed units. On the other hand, the human and financial costs to the families, separated by long distances, would be very high and some provision for emergency intensive care would have to be maintained at all but the smallest obstetric centres. These arguments obviously conflict and some regional authorities favour one more than the other. A special inquiry by the National Audit Office (NAO) found that, as between the English health districts in 1988, the ratio of special care cots ranged from 1 to 10, and of intensive care cots from less than 1 to 6, per 1000 live births (National Audit Office, 1990).

The British Association of Perinatal Medicine (BAPM), in 1991, defined four levels of care; intensive, high-dependency, special and normal, related to the severity and urgency of babies' morbidity and to the attention required from the specially trained nurses (House of Commons Health Committee, 1992b). In practice these categories cannot always be distinguished from one another. Formerly, many conditions were treated in the SCBU but when, in the 1980s, the disadvantages of separation for both baby and mother came to be realized, neonatal nurses found it manageable to carry out many of the special treatments with the baby in a cot beside his mother in the postnatal ward, where most care is in the normal category. At the same time, more babies were deemed to need intensive care, so that the number of cots in special care units declined by about 12% between 1984 and 1988, while there was a small increase in the actual number of intensive care cots (National Audit Office, 1990), although this fell well short of the requirement of an extra 500 cots then estimated by a working party (made up of professional providers of neonatal care) of the Royal College of Physicians of London (Royal College of Physicians, 1988).

The routine national statistics, however, are unable to distinguish between cots for special and cots for intensive care. The combined total for England fell by 8.2%, from its peak of 4018 in 1976 to 3581 in 1988 (Department of Health, 1988, 1991). This decrease contrasted with the increase in live births, so that the ratio per 1000 live births fell from 7.3 in 1976 to 5.5 in 1988/9. The decline in this ratio was not compensated for by a reduction in the average duration of stay in the cots, for this rose from 8.2 days in 1976 to 8.4 days in 1978, when 16% of all live births were so treated (Macfarlane and Mugford, 1984a) to 11.0 days in 1986 (the last year for which this statistic is currently available). This was probably reflecting the relative increase in the intensive care cots, where babies with longer-lasting problems were being treated, and aggravated the perceived shortage of provision.

Number of nurses

The nursing of sick babies, the constant vigilance, the interpretation of the continuous monitoring and initiation of appropriate action, and the counselling of distressed parents is clearly very stressful. The stress is increased with the more babies that one nurse has to look after at the same time. The Sheldon committee in 1971 recommended staffing ratios of 1–1.5 nurses per special care cot and three nurses per intensive care cot. In 1983 the Maternity Services Advisory Committee and the RCOG jointly noted a shortage of trained neonatal nurses and recommended a minimum ratio of four nurses per intensive care cot. The shortage was confirmed by a Department of Health survey in 1988, and extra funding for training was agreed. Though shortages and the difficulties of retaining trained staff continue to be noted, the Working Group of BAPM and the NNA, in 1991, raised the target ratio to 5.5 nurses per intensive care cot, with 3.5 per high-dependency cot and one per special care cot (House of Commons Health Committee, 1992b).

However, if it is impracticable for authorities to adhere to a rigid categorization of cot by type of care, it is even more impracticable for them to categorize their neonatal nurses in this way, for these will have to be flexibly allocated to meet varying needs as they arise. Consequently, it has proved impossible to collect statistics which make it possible to monitor how satisfactorily staffing targets at each level of care are met, far less to evaluate whether these are the most appropriate for the efficient achievement of their objective. Neonatal nurses cannot be distinguished from other nurses and midwifery staff in the employment information routinely published on a national basis (Department of Health, 1991), but the Department of Health informed the Parliamentary Inquiry that the number (in full-time equivalents) of nursing and midwifery staff employed in neonatal intensive care had increased from 1640 in 1981 to 3210 in 1989, while the number in specialist training had increased from 309 in 1989 to 395 in 1990 (House of Commons Health Committee, 1991a).

If the policy is pursued of discharging infants from neonatal units but continuing their therapy, for example low-flow oxygen, at home, some skilled neonatal nurses will have to be seconded to community nursing staffs.

Reckoning the cost

It is not easy to establish the costs of providing care for sick babies. The task defeated the NAO which, in 1989, sought specific information about the daily costs per baby from all district health authorities in England and Wales and health boards in Scotland. Their rudimentary costing systems were only able to produce estimates which ranged from £45 to £247 for special care and £199 to £777 for intensive care, relating to different sizes of units with different responsibilities (National Audit Office, 1990). To estimate total costs, these figures would have to be linked with data on duration of stay in the different units. An unofficial estimate of the annual cost per cot for the preterm baby has been quoted as £135,000 (House of Commons Health Committee 1992c). Care for sick babies is known to be very expensive, but to find out just how expensive and how the cost compares with other medical treatments, intensive and chronic, must await considerable improvements in cost accounting.

OUTCOMES IN THE LONGER TERM

There has been an impressive investment, in both financial and human terms, in the special and intensive care of sick babies, which most of them survive. There has been much less investment devoted to following up their health and capacities as they grow through childhood and adolescence. Specific studies which have tracked the development up to the age of

4, of babies whose birth weight was less than 1000 g, have found that one in five survivors has a serious motor, sensory or intellectual impairment, and up to half of the others show minor deficits which may depress their future educational attainments (House of Commons Health Committee, 1992c). Survivors with birth weights less than 1500 g are many times more likely to suffer cerebral palsy than those of normal birth weight, and the incidence may be rising. Whether the cause of this is related to factors before birth, their genetic inheritance or early gestational experience or to harmful elements of their neonatal care is not yet known. (Pharoah *et al.*, 1990; House of Commons Health Committee, 1992c; Stanley and Watson, 1992).

It is a sad fact that small, sick babies are more vulnerable to parental abuse and rejection, perhaps as a consequence of early postnatal separation having weakened natural bonds. As was indicated above, premature babies are more likely to come from less stable homes; their poor social environment may end in cancelling the benefits received from special neonatal care.

Recent research has linked adult morbidity with infant disadvantage (Barker, 1990). Some of the graduates of special and intensive care units will inevitably be at greater than average risk of illness throughout their lives. However, despite their traumatic start, most will probably go on to enjoy normal healthy futures.

REFERENCES

Ashford, J., Read, K. and Riley, V. (1973) An analysis of variations in perinatal mortality amongst local authorities in England and Wales. *International Journal of Epidemiology* **2**, 31–46.

Barker, D.J.P. (1990) The fetal and infant origins of adult disease. *British Medical Journal* **301**, 1111.

Botting, B., Macfarlane, A. and Price, F. (1990) (eds) *Three, Four and More*, HMSO, London.

Butler, N.R. and Bonham, D.G. (1963) *Perinatal Mortality*, Churchill Livingstone, Edinburgh.

Campbell, R. and Macfarlane, A. (1987) *Where to be Born? The Debate and the Evidence*, National Perinatal Mortality Unit, Oxford.

Centraal Bureau voor de Statistiek (1987) Birth by obstetric assistance and place of delivery 1986. *Monthly Bulletin of Population and Health Statistics* **11**, 22–31.

Chamberlain, R., Chamberlain, G., Howlett, B. and Claireaux, A. (1975) *British Births 1970 vol. 1 The First Week of Life*, Heinemann, London.

Chamberlain, G., Philipp, E., Howlett, B. and Masters, K. (1978) *British Births 1970 vol. 2, Obstetric Care*, Heinemann, London.

Chief Medical Officer of the Ministry of Health *On the State of the Public Health*, Annual reports for the years 1954 to 1964 Maternal and Child Health, HMSO, London.

Cooke, R. (1990) Trends in preterm survival and incidence of cerebral haemorrhage 1980–9. *Archives of Disease in Childhood* **66**, 403–7.

Cranbrook, Earl of (1959) Chairman, *Report of the Maternity Services Committee, Ministry of Health*, HMSO, London.

Davies, J. (1991) The Newcastle community care project, the project in action, in *Midwives, Research and Childbirth*, Volume II (eds S. Robinson and A. Thomson), Chapman & Hall, London, pp. 104–15.

Department of Health (1988, 1991) *Health and Personal Social Services Statistics*, HMSO, London.

Durand, A.M. (1992) The safety of home birth: the Farm Study. *American Journal of Public Health* **82**(3), 450–2.

Evans, F. (1991) The Newcastle community care project, the evaluation of the project, in *Midwives, Research and Childbirth*, Volume II (eds S. Robinson and A. Thomson), Chapman & Hall, London.

Field, D., Hodges, S., Mason, E. and Burton, P. (1991) Survival and place of treatment after premature delivery. *Archives of Disease in Childhood* **66**, 408–11.

Flint, C. and Poulengeris, P. (1987) *The 'Know Your Midwife' report*, 34 Elm Quay Court, London, SW8 5DE.

Green, J. (1990) Calming or harming? A critical review of the psychological effects of fetal diagnosis on pregnant women. *Galton Institute Occasional Paper*, Second Series No. 2.

House of Commons Health Committee (1991a) Chairman Nicholas Winterton, *Maternity Services; Preconception*, vol II, Minutes of Evidence, HMSO, London, pp. 1–291.

House of Commons Health Committee (1991b) Chairman Nicholas Winterton, *Maternity Services: Preconception*, vol III, Minutes of Evidence, HMSO, London, pp. 293–336.

House of Commons Health Committee (1992a) Chairman Nicholas Winterton, *Maternity Services*, vol I, Report, HMSO, London, pp. v–xciii.

House of Commons Health Committee (1992b) Chairman Nicholas Winterton, *Maternity Services*, vol II, Minutes of Evidence, HMSO, London, pp. 338–650.

House of Commons Health Committee (1992c) Chairman Nicholas

Winterton, *Maternity Services*, vol 3, Minutes of Evidence, HMSO, London, pp. 651–922.

Kitchen, W., Rickards, A., Ryan, M. *et al.* (1979) A longitudinal study of very low birthweight infants. II Results of controlled trial of intensive care and incidence of handicaps. *Developmental Medicine and Child Neurology* **21**, 582–9.

Lancet (1986) Editorial, Home Hospital or Birthroom. *Lancet* **2**, 494–6.

Lorenz, R., Comstack, C., Bottoms, S. and Marx, S. (1990) Randomized prospective trial of ultrasonography and pelvic examination for preterm labour surveillance. *American Journal of Obstetrics and Gynecology* **162**, 1603–10.

Macfarlane, A. and Mugford, M. (1984a) *Birth Counts: Statistics of Pregnancy and Childbirth*, vol 1 (text), HMSO, London.

Macfarlane, A. and Mugford, M. (1984b) *Birth Counts: Statistics of Pregnancy and Childbirth*, vol 2 (tables), HMSO, London.

MRC Vitamin Study Research Group (1991) Prevention of neural tube defects; results of the MRC vitamin study. *Lancet* **338**, 131–7a.

Morley, C. (1991) Surfactant treatment for premature babies – a review of clinical trials. *Archives of Disease in Childhood* **66**, 602–6.

Mugford, M., Piercy, J. and Chalmers, I. (1991) Cost implications of different approaches to the prevention of respiratory distress syndrome. *Archives of Diseases in Childhood* **66**, 767–64.

National Audit Office (1990) *Maternity Services*, HMSO, London.

Newton, R. and Hunt, L. (1984) Psychosocial stress in pregnancy and its relation to low birthweight. *British Medical Journal* **288**, 1191–4.

NRHA (1989) *Collaborative Survey of Perinatal, Late Neonatal and Infant Deaths in the Northern Region*, Newcastle Upon Tyne.

Oakley, A., Rajan, L. and Grant, A. (1990) Social support and pregnancy outcome. *British Journal of Obstetrics and Gynaecology* **97**(2), 155–62.

Office of Population Censuses and Surveys (1989) *DH3 no 23, Mortality Statistics, Perinatal and Infant, Social and Biological Factors, England and Wales*, HMSO, London.

Office of Population Censuses and Surveys (1990a) *FM1 no 19 Birth Statistics, England and Wales*, HMSO, London.

Office of Population Censuses and Surveys (1990b) *MB3 no 6 Congenital Malformation Statistics, England and Wales*, HMSO, London.

Office of Population Censuses and Surveys (1990c) *DH6 no 4 Mortality Statistics, Childhood, England and Wales*, HMSO, London.

Office of Population Censuses and Surveys (1841–1985) *DH1 no 19 Mortality Statistics, England and Wales*, Serial Tables, HMSO, London.

Pharoah, P., Cooke, T., Cooke, R. and Rosenbloom, L. (1990) Birthweight specific trends in cerebral palsy. *Archives of Disease in Childhood* **65**, 602–6.

Powell, T. and Pharoah, P. (1987) Regional neonatal intensive care: bias and benefit. *British Medical Journal* **295**, 690–2.

Powell, T., Pharoah, P. and Cooke, R. (1986) Survival and morbidity in a geographically defined population of low birthweight infants. *Lancet* **1**, 539–43.

Registrar General Statistical Review for England and Wales for the years 1957 and 1973, HMSO, London.

Royal College of Physicians of London (1988) *Medical Care of the Newborn in England and Wales*, Royal College of Physicians of London, London.

Sheldon, W. (1971) Chairman, Report of the Expert Group on Special Care for Babies, *Reports on Public Health and Medical Subjects No 127*, HMSO, London.

Sinclair, J., Torrance, G., Boyle, M. *et al.* (1981) Evaluation of neonatal intensive care programs. *New England Journal of Medicine* **305**, 489–93.

Skeoch, C., Rosenberg, K., Turner, T. *et al.* (1987) Very low birthweight survivors: illness and readmission to hospital in the first 15 months of life. *British Medical Journal* **2**, 579–80.

Stanley, F. and Watson, L. (1992) Trends in perinatal mortality and cerebral palsy in Western Australia 1967 to 1985. *British Medical Journal* **304**, 1658–63.

Steiner, E., Sanders, E., Philips, E. and Maddock, C. (1980) Very low birthweight children at school: comparison of neonatal management methods. *British Medical Journal* **281**, 1237–40.

Stewart, A., Reynolds, E. and Lipscombe, A. (1981) Outcome for infants of very low birthweight: survey of world literature. *Lancet* **1**, 1038–40.

Tew, M. (1980) Facts not assertions of belief. *Health and Social Services Journal* **12**, 1194–7.

Tew, M. (1986) Do obstetric intranatal interventions make birth safer? *British Journal of Obstetrics and Gynaecology* **93**, 659–74.

Tew, M. (1990) *Safer Childbirth? A Critical History of Maternity Care*, Chapman & Hall, London.

Tew, M. and Damstra-Wijmenga, S. (1991) Safest birth attendants: recent Dutch evidence. *Midwifery* **7**, 55–63.

Tyson, J., Silverman, W. and Reisch, J. (1989) Immediate care of the newborn infant, in *Effective Care in Pregnancy and Childbirth*, (eds I. Chalmers, M. Enkin and M. Keirse), Oxford University Press, Oxford, pp. 1293–312.

Verloove-Vanhorick, S. and Verwey, R. (1987) *Project on preterm and small for gestational age infants in the Netherlands 1983*, J.H. Pasmans, B.V., S. Gravenhage.

Whitelaw, A. and Sleath, K. (1985) Myth of the marsupial mother: home care of very low birthweight babies in Bogota, Colombia. *Lancet* **1**, 1206–7.

Appendix A: Normal values

Neonatal electrolyte and urea ranges

Electrolyte mmol/l	*Preterm*	*Neonatal*
Sodium (Na)	130 - 140	130 - 145
Potassium (K)	4.5 - 7.0	4.0 - 6.0
Chloride (Cl)	90 - 115	92 - 110
Calcium (Ca)	1.9 - 2.8	2.0 - 2.9
Phosphate (PO_4)	1.10 - 2.60	1.8 - 3.0
Magnesium (Mg)	0.62 - 1.27	0.7 - 1.15
Creatinine	55 - 150	35 - 48
Urea	1.5 - 6.7	1.6 - 5.2

Blood gas values

Blood		
pH	7.3 - 7.4	
$Pa\text{CO}_2$	4.6 - 6.0	kPa (35–45 mmHg)
$Pa\text{O}_2$	7.3 - 12.0	kPa (55–90 mmHg)
Bicarbonate	18 - 25	μmol/l
Base excess	−7 - −2	mmol/l

Appendix B: Assessment of gestational age

The Dubowitz and Dubowitz method of assessing gestational age involves the scoring of neurological and external criteria within the first 5 days of birth. The total score is read against the graph (Figure B.2) to give a post-birth estimation of gestational age.

SOME NOTES ON TECHNIQUES OF ASSESSMENT OF NEUROLOGIC CRITERIA

POSTURE: Observed with infant quiet and in supine position. Score 0: Arms and legs extended; 1: beginning of flexion of hips and knees, arms extended; 2: stronger flexion of legs, arms extended; 3: arms slightly flexed, legs flexed and abducted; 4: full flexion of arms and legs.

SQUARE WINDOW: The hand is flexed on the forearm between the thumb and index finger of the examiner. Enough pressure is applied to get as full a flexion as possible, and the angle between the hypothenar eminence and the ventral aspect of the forearm is measured and graded according to diagram. (Care is taken not to rotate the infant's wrist while doing this maneuver.)

ANKLE DORSIFLEXION: The foot is dorsiflexed onto the anterior aspect of the leg, with the examiner's thumb on the sole of the foot and other fingers behind the leg. Enough pressure is applied to get as full flexion as possible, and the angle between the dorsum of the foot and the anterior aspect of the leg is measured.

ARM RECOIL: With the infant in the supine position the forearms are first flexed for 5 seconds, then fully extended by pulling on the hands, and then released. The sign is fully positive if the arms return briskly to full flexion (Score 2). If the arms return to incomplete flexion or the response is sluggish it is graded as Score 1. If they remain extended or are only followed by random movements the score is 0.

LEG RECOIL: With the infant supine, the hips and knees are fully flexed for 5 seconds, then extended by traction on the feet, and released. A maximal response is one of full flexion of the hips and knees (Score 2). A partial flexion scores 1, and minimal or no movement scores 0.

POPLITEAL ANGLE: With the infant supine and his pelvis flat on the examining couch, the thigh is held in the knee-chest position by the examiner's left index finger and thumb supporting the knee. The leg is then extended by gentle pressure from the examiner's right index finger behind the ankle and the popliteal angle is measured.

HEEL TO EAR MANEUVER: With the baby supine, draw the baby's foot as near to the head as it will go without forcing it. Observe the distance between the foot and the head as well as the degree of extension at the knee. Grade according to diagram. Note that the knee is left free and may draw down alongside the abdomen.

SCARF SIGN: With the baby supine, take the infant's hand and try to put it around the neck and as far posteriorly as possible around the opposite shoulder. Assist this maneuver by lifting the elbow across the body. See how far the elbow will go across and grade according to illustrations. Score 0: Elbow reaches opposite axillary line; 1: Elbow between midline and opposite axillary line; 2: Elbow reaches midline; 3: Elbow will not reach midline.

HEAD LAG: With the baby lying supine, grasp the hands (or the arms if a very small infant) and pull him slowly towards the sitting position. Observe the position of the head in relation to the trunk and grade accordingly. In a small infant the head may initially be supported by one hand. Score 0: Complete lag; 1: Partial head control; 2: Able to maintain head in line with body; 3: Brings head anterior to body.

VENTRAL SUSPENSION: The infant is suspended in the prone position, with examiner's hand under the infant's chest (one hand in a small infant, two in a large infant). Observe the degree of extension of the back and the amount of flexion of the arms and legs. Also note the relation of the head to the trunk. Grade according to diagrams.

If score differs on the two sides, take the mean.

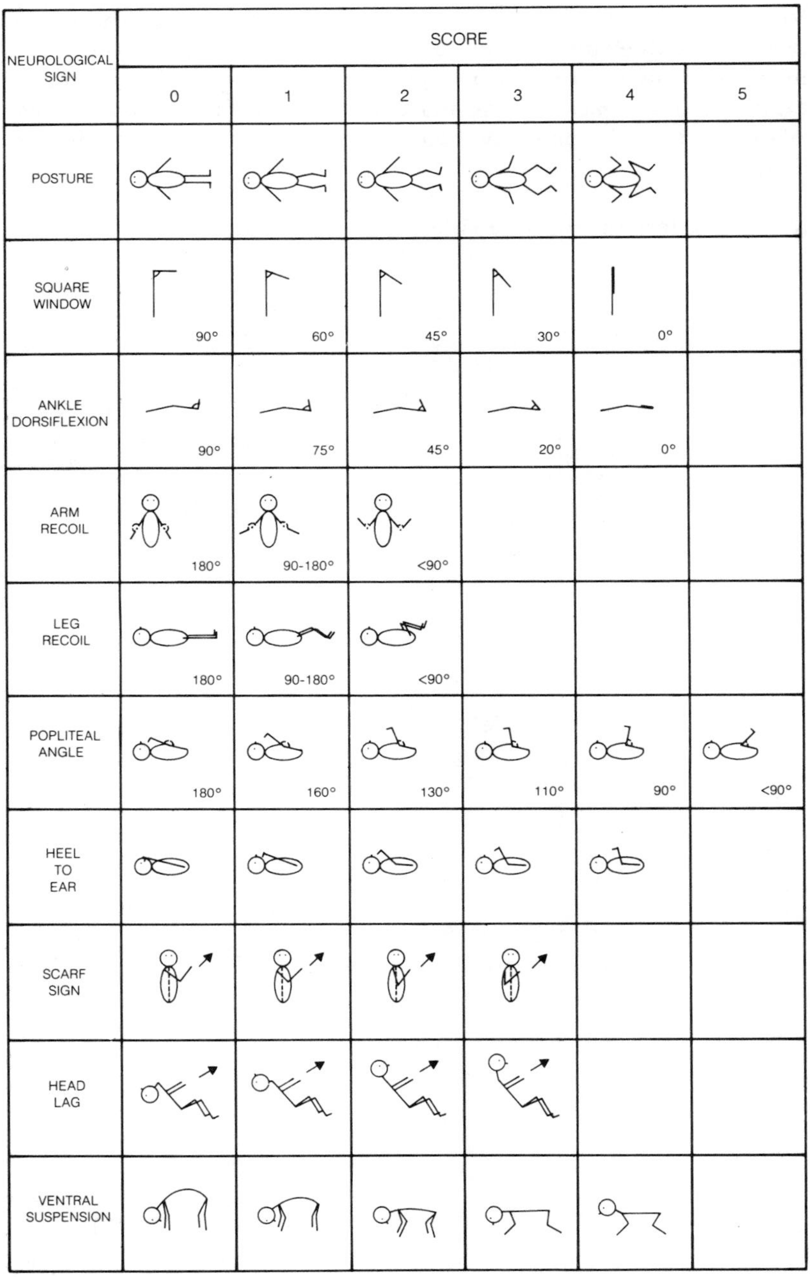

NEUROLOGICAL SIGN
SCORE
0
1
2
3
4
5
POSTURE
SQUARE WINDOW
90°
60°
45°
30°
0°
ANKLE DORSIFLEXION
90°
75°
45°
20°
0°
ARM RECOIL
180°
90-180°
<90°
LEG RECOIL
180°
90-180°
<90°
POPLITEAL ANGLE
180°
160°
130°
110°
90°
<90°
HEEL TO EAR
SCARF SIGN
HEAD LAG
VENTRAL SUSPENSION

Figure B.1 Scoring system for neurological criteria.

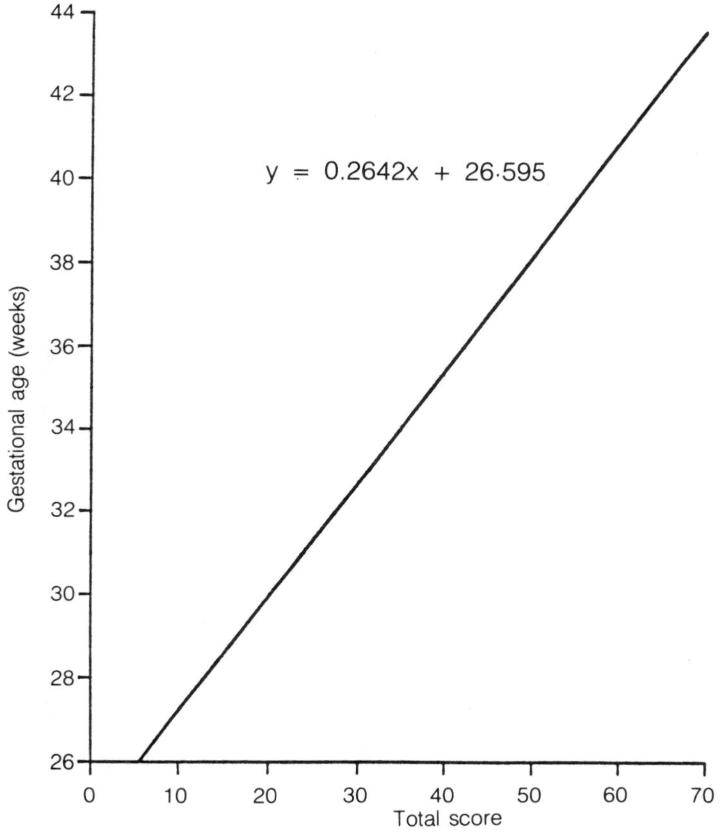

Figure B.2 Graph for reading gestational age from total score. Reproduced by kind permission of the authors and *Journal of Pediatrics*. Dubowitz, L.M.S., Dubowitz, V. and Goldberg, C. (1970) Clinical assessment of gestational age in the newborn infant. *Journal of Pediatrics* **77**(1), 1–10.

Table B.1 Scoring system for external criteria

External sign	Score* 0	1	2	3	4
Edema	Obvious edema of hands and feet; pitting over tibia	No obvious edema of hands and feet; pitting over tibia	No edema		
Skin texture	Very thin, gelatinous	Thin and smooth	Smooth; medium thickness. Rash or superficial peeling	Slight thickening. Superficial cracking and peeling especially of hands and feet	Thick and parchment-like; superficial or deep cracking
Skin color	Dark red	Uniformly pink	Pale pink; variable over body	Pale; only pink over ears, lips, palms, or soles	
Skin opacity trunk)	Numerous veins and venules clearly seen, especially over abdomen	Veins and tributaries seen	A few large vessels clearly seen over abdomen	A few large vessels seen indistinctly over abdomen	No blood vessels seen
Lanugo (over back)	No lanugo	Abundant; long and thick over whole back	Hair thinning especially over lower back	Small amount of lanugo and bald areas	At least ½ of back devoid of lanugo
Plantar creases	No skin creases	Faint red marks over anterior half of sole	Definite red marks over > anterior ½; indentations over < anterior ⅓	Indentations over > anterior ⅓	Definite deep indentations over >anterior ⅓

Nipple formation	Nipple barely visible; no areola	Nipple well defined; areola smooth and flat, diameter < 0.75 cm.	Areola stippled, edge not raised diameter < 0.75 cm.	Areola stippled, edge raised, diameter > 0.75 cm.
Breast size	No breast tissue palpable	Breast tissue on one or both sides, < 0.5 cm. diameter	Breast tissue both sides; one or both 0.5–1.0 cm	Breast tissue both sides; one or both > 1 cm.
Ear form	Pinna flat and shapeless, little or no incurving of edge	Incurving of part of edge of pinna	Partial incurving whole of upper pinna	Well-defined incurving whole of upper pinna
Ear firmness	Pinna soft, easily folded, no recoil	Pinna soft, easily folded, slow recoil	Cartilage to edge of pinna, but soft in places, ready recoil	Pinna firm, cartilage to edge; instant recoil
Genitals Male	Neither testis in scrotum	At least one testis high in scrotum	At least one testis right down	
Female (with hips ½ abducted)	Labia majora widely separated, labia minora protruding	Labia majora almost cover labia minora	Labia major completely cover labia minora	

Adapted from Farr and associates, Develop. Med. Child Neurol. 8:507, 1966.
*If score differs on two sides, take the mean.

Index

Page numbers appearing in **bold** refer to figures and page numbers appearing in *italic* refer to tables.